THE SPECIALIST CHICK SEXER

R. D. MARTIN

Forewords by
John Kerin
and
Hitoshi Miyata

Bernal Publishing
Melbourne

“to my predecessors, former colleagues
and our successors”

Forewords

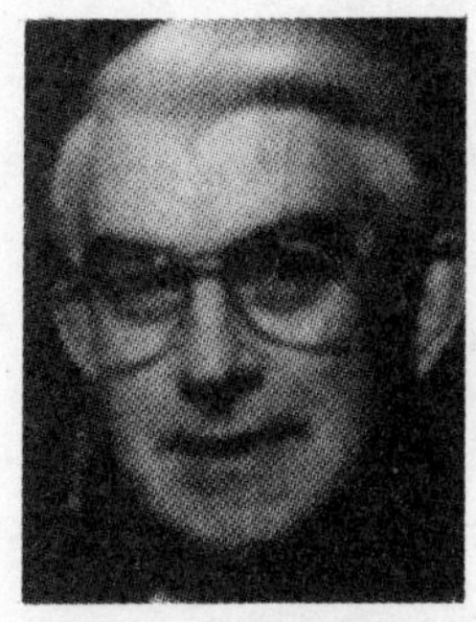

Until we can successfully breed only female chickens there will be a need for chicken sexers particularly in the egg-laying industry. This unique book tells not only of the history and science (or is it art?) of chicken sexing but also about the people who have played such a vital part in our poultry industries.

I grew up on a poultry farm and was there for the first thirty-three years of my life. Although I had vague ideas about being a veterinarian, one of the early possible career paths that caught my attention was chicken sexing. Allegedly, they were highly paid, they would never be replaced by machine and they were in a growing industry. But nothing much developed by way of pursuing the interest so I eventually became an economist and then a politician—it was all downhill from those halcyon, contemplative days on the poultry farm!

Just as once every bird was vaccinated by hand in the vent for laryngotracheitis and then a "mass produced" way was found, I was staggered in later life to learn that chicken sexing was carried out by looking at the bird's feathers after a few days old—vent sexing had been all but replaced by feather and colour sexing—so I was told.

However, I now learn that there is every possibility of the traditionally skilled sexers coming back into their own and that numbers may increase well above their nadir in the mid 1970s, due to the fact that the newer system does not perform as well.

When one thinks of skill, one thinks of Japan but today vent sexers are being taught in both the United Kingdom and Japan. Japan and Australia are the only countries which do not employ overseas chick sexers—we have about 25 at present.

The Japanese have now devised a method of holding two chicks in their hand and this technique allows up to 1700 chicks per hour to be sexed—an increase of up to 100%! And the oldest chick sexer in Japan is a 73-year-old woman who in 1993 still sexed 100 chickens in 6.45 minutes with 100 per cent accuracy!

This fascinating book will not have a large readership but nevertheless is essential in recording where we've been, where we are at and where we are going in the realm of chicken sexing.

I'm not sorry I didn't become a chicken sexer but considering some of the people I had to deal with when I was active in politics it may have been more rewarding to regard the back ends of chickens than the minds of some of my protagonists. Perhaps, one day the country and the city will see eye to eye and all people will get immense pleasure and interest from this valuable work?

John Kerin
Chairman, Australian Meat and Live-stock Corporation
March, 1994

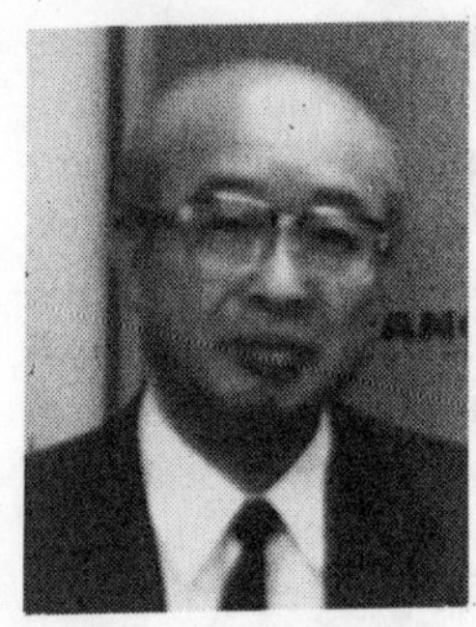

The theory of vent or cloacal chick sexing was discovered by three Japanese veterinary scientists in 1924 on the basis of their long studies, and was successfully brought into practical use by several pioneering poultrymen in Japan through their painstaking efforts in the 1920s through the early 1930s.

Before this theory was made known, poultry farmers had to rear all the chickens hatched, wasting feed and labour on the cockerels for 30 days or so before their sex could be discerned by outer appearance. If the chickens are sex-determined after hatching, only the pullets for layers may be reared, thereby bringing about far more profits to the poultry industry. The practical use of vent chick sexing was, therefore, long-awaited.

Accordingly, when the theory of vent sexing was made public, poultrymen welcomed the news with great expectations, and devoted themselves so that their dreams might come true.

In 1929, an organisation aiming at marketing guaranteed sexed chickens, as well as training and qualifying chick sexers, was established in the Aichi Prefecture, in Central Japan, which was then the centre of the Japanese poultry industry.

In this way, the technique of vent sexing became the specialty of the Japanese, and with the improvement of the technique of Japanese chick sexers, and the increasing number of them year after year, the time was ripe for the propagation of this technique to the world.

In 1934, as the first Japanese expert chick sexers, Mr Hikosaburo Yogo visited New South Wales and Mr Hideo Kataoka visited Victoria respectively, to teach sexing commercially. They exhibited miraculous skills to Australian poultry people. Unfortunately, the outbreak of World War II interrupted the exchange of Japanese experts with the Australian poultry industry in 1940, with Mr Kataoka and Mr Shiraishi leaving Australia as the last experts to visit.

After the war, the opportunity to resume the interchange with Australian poultry industry came in 1947. A chick-sexing course was held in Kobe City at the request of the Australian and New Zealand soldiers then stationed there as Allied Occupation Forces in Japan. This class was taught by such experts as Mataichi Sakai, Nobuyoshi Tanaka and Koji Kato, who had visited Australia in the 1930s, and it was a great success.

Since the late 1950s, more Japanese expert chick sexers have been sent overseas by our association than in the pre-war days, mainly to Europe and the United States. At one time, the number of experts sent abroad exceeded 150. To our great regret, none of our experts have had the chance to work in Australia after the war. However, we are proud to say that experts such as Mr Yogo and Mr Kataoka, who introduced this technique to Australia in the 1930s, played an important role in the development of the Australian poultry industry.

It is more than 70 years or so since this vent chick-sexing technique was originated and developed in Japan. For a while dependence was placed on the so-called sex-linkage—applied autosexing, such as feather sexing and colour sexing, owing to a temporary shortage of vent sexers throughout the world. However, vent-sexed chickens have shown much better performance in egg productivity, cost-effectiveness, and so on. We are optimistic about the future of commercial vent chick sexers throughout the world.

We look forward to the completion of *The Specialist Chick Sexer* by Mr Robert D. Martin, a grand-pupil of Mr Hideo Kataoka, the first Japanese expert to cross the Pacific to Australia in the 1930s, and we hope for the better development of the poultry industries of both countries, Australia and Japan.

Tokyo, Japan, 15 June 1994
Hitoshi Miyata
Executive Director
Zen-Nippon Chick Sexing Association

Contents

PART II

List of illustrations

PART II

Acknowledgements

A special thanks to the following people who have freely given their time, access to their records, correspondence and photos.

Bill Stanhope, former Principal Poultry Officer, Victorian Agriculture Department, Ass Editor *Australasian Poultry* Melbourne.
Frank and Mavis Evans, of Dundas, Sydney.
Arthur and Aileen Pamment, Kenthurst, Sydney.
Ray Parkin, Wisemans Ferry, New South Wales.
Hartley Hall, Frankston, Victoria.
Dr Hu Hisiang-Pih, Chinese Academy of Agriculture Science, Kijias, Beijing, China.
Zen-Nippon Chick Sexing Association, Tokyo.
Koji Kato, Nagoya, Japan.
John Hammond, Baxter, Victoria.
Max Akam, Frankston, Victoria.
Doreen De Carteret, Mornington, Victoria.
Onko Wallbrink, Ringwood, Victoria.
Norm Bell, Altona Hatchery, Forrestfield, Western Australia.
Jong Ho Yoo, Korea Chick Sexer Services Association, Seoul, Korea.
Kel Staples, Greenacres, South Australia.
Charlie Bode, Eltham, Victoria.
Gordon Lowe, Elizabeth, South Australia.
Ron Mason, Eaglehawk, Victoria.
Krystyna Eva Gawecka, Pornan, Poland.
Cliff McDowell, Epping, New South Wales.
Hisao Iwaya, Sendai, Japan.
Ian Bestwick, Kent, UK.
Watt Publishing, (Poultry Group) Mt Morris, Illinois, USA.
Takashi Hobo of Hobo Sexing, Waregem, Belgium.
Dr S. Hart, Bonn, Germany.
David Nitta, 'Amchick', Philadelphia, USA.
Hector McLeod, Scotland.
Rob & Lyn McDonald, Upper Yarra Emu Farm, Launching Place, Victoria.

For interpretation:
Keiko Kuwasaki, North Balwyn, Victoria.
Mayumi and Yoshimi Yamazaki and their daughter, Yumi Goto, Sendai, Japan.
Takamitsu Hashimoto, Tokyo.

Other acknowledgements are listed in the main text. There were many bits and pieces from my own records and scrap books collected since I was in my teens. The source of much of this information has not been recorded, as I was even less scrupulous at keeping records then than I am now.

A special thanks to Marlene Martin for enduring a year of 'chick-sexing talk', proofreading and putting up with an impatient husband, and finally, to my son, Matthew, for introducing me to the mysteries of the PC computer.

Terminology used in the text

Breed—a group of fowl breeding true to type, carriage and characteristics distinctive of the breed name they take.

Broiler—a young table bird of either sex usually not more than ten weeks of age.

Brooder—equipment used to produce heat during the first weeks of a chick's life.

Cages—a system of housing fowl. Birds are confined in wire cages either singly or in multiples.

Chicks—usually refers to a fowl from day-old until removed from brooder.

Chick Sorter—a person who separates the sexes of day-old chicks by either the feather or colour method.

Cloaca—the common external opening for the digestive, urinary and reproductive tract.

Cockerel—a male bird aged from a day-old to the end of its first breeding season.

Colour sexing—the method of sexing chicks by their colour.

Crossbred—a chicken produced by crossing two or more different breeds or varieties.

Cull—the removal from the flock of an unprofitable or unsuitable bird.

DNA—(deoxyribonucleic acid) an organic compound found in chromosomes as a double spiral and controlling and transmitting genetic characters. Plays a central role in protein transmission of hereditary characteristics from parents to offspring.

Embryo—a young organism in the early stages of development, as before hatching from the egg.

Eminence—the actual appendage or sex organ, sometimes referred to as the process, phallus, or genital eminence. In this study it means the male and sometimes female degenerate genital eminence between the lateral folds of a chick.

Excreta—waste matter from the intestines.

Feather sexing—the method of sexing the chicks by examining the wing feathers.

Folds—the protective layer of skin covering the eminence, lying inside the rim of the cloaca.

Genetic engineering—alteration of the structure of the chromosomes in living organisms to produce effects beneficial to farmers in agriculture and so on.

Geneticist—a person who studies or specialises in genetics.

Green chicken—is one that has very recently hatched from the incubator and contains considerable moisture content. For a chick sexer a green chicken is very soft and very fragile to work with. In less than three or four hours the chick 'dries out' and is much easier to handle.

Grand Parent Stock—GPS parents of Parent Stock (PS), can usually only be sexed by specialist chick sexers.

Hatchability—number of chicks produced from all eggs set in the incubator.

Hen—a female fowl after the first adult moult.

Hyperdermia—the act of pressing the cloaca.

Incubator—a machine used for the artificial hatching of eggs.

"Machine" method—a misnomer, as it is in no way a machine, but it is a term that has been generally used in the poultry industry since this method was introduced. The optical way of sexing day-old chicks.

"Machine"—an optical instrument for sexing day-old chicks.

Parent Stock—PS purebred stock used for producing offspring which can usually be sexed by feather or colour sexing. Parent stock can usually only be sexed by specialist chick sexers.

Prefectures—regional districts in Japan.

Primary Stock—PS same as parent stock.

Pullorum—a disease of poultry. (*Salmonella typhi-murium*)

Pelvic bones—thin terminal portion of the hip bones that form part of the pelvis.

Poults—young turkeys.

Primaries—the long stiff flight feathers at the outer tip of the wing.

Pullet—a female bird from day-old to the end of her first laying season.

Purebred—a chicken produced from parents of the same breed.

Rim—the outer edge of the cloaca.

Secondaries—the large wing feathers adjacent to the body.

Sexer—a person who divides chicks into male and female groups at day-old by either the cloaca method or the "machine" method. A specialist chick sexer.

Sexing—the act of dividing birds into male and female groups.

Specialist Chick Sexer—a person who sexes chicks or turkeys by the cloaca/vent or "machine" method commercially.

Vent method—usually referred to as the cloaca (1) method or sometimes, in Australia, the hand method; the method of sexing chicks and turkeys by examining the cloaca.

Vent—the external opening from the cloaca. Sometimes in this study the term cloaca is used for this area. The common name for the cloaca or anus where the sex organs are contained.

Preface

Why write this book?

The men and women interviewed and written about in this book have sexed millions of day-old chickens, many have been commercial chick sexers for over forty years, and all have something to contribute to those who will follow after them.

Maybe just one comment they make could trigger in the student a clue, a spark, that is relevant to a particular student's thinking for success.

Maybe a student needs to think better of himself, or herself, to have a dream and be able to turn that dream into a practical application for success.

R.D.M.

Introduction

From 1929 to the early 1940s was a period of economic depression throughout the world, yet it was during this decade that the poultry industry experienced two events which had a profound influence on the industry's future growth and stability.

The two events were the development of the electric forced-draught egg incubator in the early 1930s and the development and introduction by the Japanese of day-old chick sexing.

The larger forced-draught incubators revolutionised the production of day-old chickens: not only in the quality of the chickens but also in hatching percentages of eggs set. Up to the development of these forced-draught incubators hatching results of around 50 per cent of all eggs set were considered satisfactory. With forced-draught incubators these figures gradually improved till 90 per cent of all eggs set were achieved. The latest mammoth steel cabinet incubators sometimes achieve higher percentages than this. These improvements in hatching results and later being able to separate the sexes as soon as they were hatched enabled the egg-producing industry to expand and to greatly reduce costs.

The benefits to the egg industry of being able to distinguish the sex of day-old chickens were better utilisation of shedding, and reducing feed costs for replacement egg-laying stock. The unwanted day-old cockerels could be disposed of after sexing, a saving in brooder space and valuable feed, both big savings in costs.

The farmer no longer had to rear and feed unsexed chickens until he or she could pick out the cockerels at five to seven weeks and then either sell them, usually below costs, or rear them until they were at a marketable age and weight, which took up to three times as long as it now takes today's meat chickens. Most times the farmer would lose money on these sales as the markets were flooded with these unwanted by-products of the egg industry.

With the developments in sex-linked genetic stock with its resulting easy separation of the sexes as they are unloaded from the incubators by hatchery-trained staff, the specialist chick sexer is now needed only by the hatcheries and breeders who produce parent stock or for sexing turkeys.

This is a far cry from the 1930s, 1940s and 1950s when many hatcherymen built their business reputations partly on the accuracy and reliability of their chick sexer.

There is, however, in some countries a move away from the egg replacement stock which has been genetically bred for easy separation of the sexes at day-old. How far this trend will develop depends on any economic gains from the change back to vent-sexed replacement stock.

As we will see in Part II of this study, the future of the specialist chick sexer looks brighter than the casual observer might at first assume.

In the history of the 60-plus years of the specialist chick sexer there have been several threats to the commercial chick sexer as an occupation.

Earlier, there were threats of being able to treat eggs so that only females would hatch. Feather and autosexing breeds have always been available. Then in the 1950s the Japanese introduced the "Chick-tester", an instrument which enabled a skilled operator to sex chickens with 100 per cent accuracy after only a few months' practice.

This new and easier to learn 100 per cent method prospered mainly where there was a shortage of skilled vent sexers.

The Japanese stopped teaching this method in 1966, and no-one manufactures any of these so called "machines" now.

The vent sexers were more than able to hold their own with these "machine sexers" both in accuracy, speed and in many cases, injury to the chick. There are still very skilled commercial users of this method who can sex at the rate of 1200 plus an hour with accuracy comparable with the best vent sexers. They work side by side with their vent colleagues and there is no doubt that they will be commercial chick sexers until they decide to retire.

But, as Australia's most experienced and accurate "machine" sexer said when I went to interview him for this study, "The 'machine' is finished!"

The biggest change that has brought about some reduction in the number of specialist chick sexers throughout the world has of course been the growth of feather and colour sexing of day-old chicks.

This change has been made possible by the concentration of the breeding and hatchery industry around the world under the control of few large breeding companies. As far back as 1988 it was said that 75 per cent of the western world's egg-laying replacement breeding stock was in the hands of five companies.

Because of their size, they are able to employ highly skilled geneticists and other technical staff to undertake research and development work.

These developments have reduced the need for specialist chick sexers to sex replacement layer stock, and in some cases broiler breeders, but the specialist chick sexer is still an essential part of the poultry industry and there does not appear any likelihood of this changing.

In 1994 there are still chick-sexing schools being held in Japan, Korea and England, as well as students being taught by individual chick sexers in Australia, as the need arises.

When I floated the idea of writing a "history of chick sexing" to some of my former Education Ministry colleagues, their reactions were . . . "A history of what!"

Thirty years ago, when I was a commercial chick sexer, when a stranger asked me what I did for a living they responded with: 'The Japanese had something to do with that, didn't they?"

It seems the greater the technology the narrower the field of knowledge.

It is little wonder that Bill Stanhope, the former Principal Poultry Officer of the Victorian Ministry of Agriculture, stopped advertising the Ministry's chick-sexing examinations in the 1980s because of the embarrassment caused through media attention.

Most of the men and women who learnt chick sexing from the visiting Japanese experts between 1934 and 1940 were in their teens or early twenties.

They were the first generation of commercial chicken sexers. It was from one of these 'first-generation' chicken sexers, Charlie Bode, of Melbourne, that I learnt the technique. I was fifteen years old when I attended Charlie Bode's Saturday-afternoon classes at Research and eight weeks later sat for my first government chick-sexing examination. After some innocent expectations, disappointments and luck I became a second-generation chick sexer. It was a vocation I worked at, and enjoyed, for twenty years.

On retirement to my farm I taught an equally naive but enthusiastic twenty-one-year old, John Hammond, the techniques of chick sexing and gave him most of my clients. John Hammond then joined a third generation of commercial chick sexers.

In Part I we will see why being able to tell the difference between male and female day-old chickens is so important to the egg industry.

When the broiler-meat industry started to grow in the 1950s, being able to sex day-old chickens was also important to the poultry-meat industry. The pullets grow more uniformly if separated from the cockerels at the time of hatching and reared separately until they mature ready for marketing. This practice of rearing the sexes separately is not followed in all broiler-industry countries.

In doing research for this sixty-year study of chick sexing, I first tried to contact the first generation of Australian chick sexers living in Victoria, all of whom I had known or met. Of the original ten, only two,

Hartley Hall, and Charlie Bode, my teacher, are still available.

Hartley Hall, a friend and colleague of over forty years, was holidaying in Queensland so I had to start on my connections from the second generation of chick sexers. Not too many of this group of fourteen were traceable either. Some of them had worked through most of the period I have designated the third generation as well as their own second-generation period. The most remarkable of these in Victoria, in my view, was Max Akam.

Max sexed chickens commercially until he was sixty-three and he more than held his own with the new 100 per cent accuracy of the third-generation "machine" chick sexers.

As I got further into my research I learnt that there were other chicken sexers with equally impressive records, particularly in New South Wales. One of the first generation in NSW has sexed chicks until he was 71.

Later, I also learnt that there was a 73-year-old Japanese woman, Yoshino Tanaka, chick sexer still sexing one to two days a week and in America there are many chick sexers still working in their 60s and 70s.

If this study tends to have more detail of the Australian experience it is only because I was able to collect more documentation, had more direct oral information, and of course had my own involvement in Australia's chick-sexing fraternity for twenty years. Also, in the case of Victoria, Bill Stanhope had saved the Agriculture Department's early documentation covering the 1934–1956 period.

I also had to rely heavily on my Australian colleagues and their diaries, some of their old copies of Australian/Victorian poultry journals and the Victorian State Library.

I have had a great deal of help and encouragement from members of the chick-sexing fraternity in Japan, England, Belgium and America and also some correspondence from several organisations in Europe.

I am greatly indebted to Hitoshi Miyata, Koji Kato, Yomio Mano and Takamitsu Hashimoto of the Zen-Nippon Chick Sexing Association for their hospitality and help with my research. They gave me ready access to their records in Tokyo and at their school in Nagoya. Also a special thanks to Koji Kato for permission to use four photos from his book, *World of Chick Sexer* 1991.

I hope that in this study I have done them all justice and given some idea of their achievements over the past sixty years of chick sexing.

Australian chick sexers in particular were in a unique position, being in the Southern Hemisphere. They had the spring, the chick-hatching season, at a time when the Japanese chick sexers were not sexing in their own country and so were able to come to Australia to sex chickens and to teach Australians the skills.

Likewise Australian chick sexers were free to travel to the Northern

Hemisphere spring to sex chicken in Europe's main hatching season, which many did from 1937 until the mid-1950s.

The individual historical studies in Part I are about their achievement and their contributions to the poultry industry in Australia and overseas.

Even with such a small group there were many family tragedies, many business successes after their chick-sexing careers had finished and even some comedy. One even became an Olympic and world champion sculler.

Among the comedy two events come to mind: not comedy to the participants at the time, I am sure, but viewed from the distance of time, they have the ingredients of a first-class comedy.

A Victorian first-generation chick sexer who operated in a country area serving a series of small farms also ran a mixed-farm business between chick-hatching seasons. This gentleman ran his farm with the help of his wife and two other women. He advertised in rural papers for his female staff of live-in farm workers.

Some stayed for only brief periods but eventually he seems to have settled down with two. These two were so satisfied with their position that they were removed from the payroll and "promoted" to the status of wives.

When one of the unchurched wives showed she was fertile and wanted her child to be born in wedlock, my enterprising fellow chick sexer worked out a plan.

He dressed one of his farm wives as a man and had her "married' to the other farm wife. The "wedding" was performed by a member of the clergy at Frankston, a Melbourne beachside suburb. He got away with it.

Eventually trouble started when one of the wives wrote home to her mother and related the story.

The authorities did not appreciate my former colleague's loving endeavours at keeping harmony among his 'wives'.

He was released from prison after serving a two-year sentence.

He had difficulty while in prison. The authorities did not get his two artificial legs serviced regularly enough and when he was released he had difficulty walking for several months.

He did not return to chick sexing.

When this entrepreneur went to prison I inherited his chick-sexing business, which kept me working long hours each weekend.

My predecessor had spread his work over four days during the week and had more time to fraternise with his clients and their families. I was always in a hurry and hardly ever went up to the homes of the farmers to chat.

As a result they all thought well of my predecessor but were less enchanted by his young replacement. My chick-sexing ability was never taken into their assessment when comparing us. For my part I was glad to get the work as I had been a commercial chick sexer for only three years and was still working up a name for myself.

Even earlier than this incident I obtained another good client through the philandering of another colleague. On this occasion my predecessor usually finished sexing his client's chickens between 11 p.m. and 1 a.m.

The farmer always helped the chick sexer by counting what had been sexed and putting another box of unsexed chickens in front of him. This was the usual arrangement in Australia between the farmer and the chick sexer.

Often at this place the farmer would go off to bed at about 10:30 and the chick sexer would work the last couple of hours by himself.

On one occasion the farmer could not sleep and got up. He noticed out of the window that the chick sexer had left. "That's good."

After making a cup of tea he noticed that his fifteen-year-old daughter was not in her bed. "That's not so good."

He called the police and together they started searching.

Eventually they found the chick sexer and the daughter snuggled up together. No harm had been done. The daughter was lucky. My fellow chicken sexer was also lucky the police were there to protect him from the wrath of the farmer.

You may think that all my clients were obtained as a result of the misdemeanours of my fellow chick sexers, but this is not so. Almost without exception chick sexers worked hard for long hours and kept their minds on the soft bits of down in front of them.

For first- and second-generation chick sexers, that is from 1934 till about the early 1960s, the work was seasonal, lasting for about sixteen weeks. For many it was a seventeen-hour day and always a seven-day week.

The financial reward was good, but you had to work long hours, be reliable and be accurate. This did not give much time for anything else.

With the growth of the broiler industry in the 1960s, third-generation chick sexers had work almost all the year around, until feather sexing started to relieve them of their importance and only the well-established and, in some cases, lucky ones survived as full-time chick sexers.

Of the 140 candidates who have passed the various government chick sexing examinations in Australia, 24 have been women. Of these 24, eight were "machine" chick sexers from the third generation. Not all candidates who obtained a government certificate became commercial chick sexers. Likewise, there were a few chick sexers who sexed commercially in some areas who did not have a government certificate, no doubt there were some women sexers among these also.

In Queensland Dorothy McCulloch was one of the key people responsible for the training of generations of Queensland chick sexers from 1936 onwards. Miss McCulloch learnt from the visiting Japanese expert, Mr Kiyoski Ozowa, in 1934. By 1935 Dorothy McCulloch had become one of Australia's most proficient commercial chick sexers.

In New South Wales there were women chick sexers from 1935 onwards. There were at least four husband-and-wife chick-sexing partnerships in NSW.

In the 1930s in Victoria at least three women learnt from the Japanese.

Women chick sexers in Australia came to the fore commercially in the third generation, with the advent of "machine" sexing. They were very fast and very accurate.

Most worked commercially for ten years, until feather sexing pushed them out of the industry.

In 1994, out of the 20 commercial chick sexers still practising in Australia only two are women.

In Australia most women have tended to work at it part-time or in partnership with their husbands or partners, some of whom they later married.

With the growth of the poultry industry since the 1950s, large private and public companies entering the industry, the disappearance of most small family farms, and the introduction of strains that could be feather sexed, the decline of the individual commercial chick sexer was almost complete.

Individual chick sexers became less well known, except among their peers. The 'stars' of the past were gone.

Commercial chick sexers started working in teams of up to eight, arriving at a hatchery to work their way through a batch of 50 000 chickens in a day. Sometimes they might be required the followed week(s), other times not for several weeks.

In Australia in the 1990s, chick sexers fly interstate regularly to work.

While most chick sexers today are less known than their predecessors, they are, as a group, much faster and more consistently accurate, which in the end is what counts.

In order to write this sixty-year history in an objective way and step outside a subject I have spent half of my working life in, I have written in the third person throughout Part I, even when I am writing about myself.

When I have written about a particular chicken sexer's speed or accuracy I used documented evidence such as examination results, letters, or witnesses, mostly their clients. In some cases I have worked with a particular chick sexer and we have checked each other's work.

At many large egg farms all the chickens are reared and checking on accuracy is not difficult as accurate records are usually kept. Except for a brief period during the war and a couple of years after, no-one in Australia was engaged as a chick sexer on a large scale without passing a government examination and building a good reputation for accuracy and reliability over many years. There have been exceptions, but it is a general rule.

At no time during this study did I depend on the glowing memories of the participants for evidence of speed, accuracy or the number of chickens handled in a day or year.

In Part II I have written in the first person as I am very much involved by way of researching statistics, correspondence, visits, interviews and some practical update. It seemed to be the best way of presenting the evidence and opinions of others as well as my own.

In looking at future prospects, any historian or researcher can base predictions only on what is happening now and on looking at the experience from the past.

This book will not teach you how to sex day-old chicks. It is not a skill learnt from a book.

Teaching is a task for an experienced commercial chick sexer able to sex chicks with almost a 100 per cent accuracy.

For an advanced student or a practising commercial chick sexer a reading, or a re-reading, of this study could help a 95 to 97 percenter advance to a 98 or 100 percenter.

Most of the individual histories relate to Australian chick sexers, but their experiences and observations are not so very different to chick sexers world wide.

With close reading of their comments and observations as well as some of the Japanese masters, the reader will notice a common theme, with those who have mastered the skills which go towards making a top commercial chick sexer.

There are no hidden secrets. There is, however, practice, practice and practice, together with perseverance—together with an understanding of the biology behind the method of being able to distinguish quickly and accurately the differences between the degenerate eminences of the male and female day-old chick.

R.D.M.

PART I

(A history)

The beginning . . . Japan, North America, Australia

The Japan Chick Sexing Association 1934–1940

England 1935–1940

Canada, England, France, Belgium and Australia 1935–1936

United States 1935–1940

The difficulties

Japanese chick sexers in Australia 1934–1940

Australia: Individual histories

The golden age of chick sexing

The third generation 1966–1994

The teachers

DR KIYOSHI MASUI

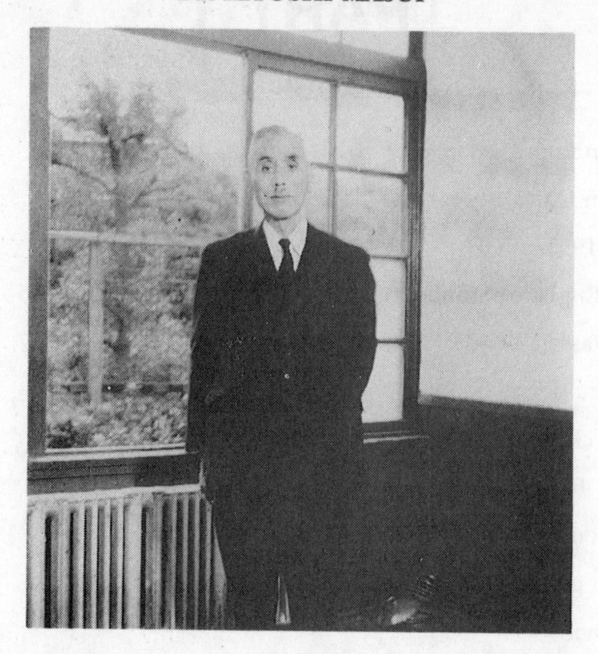

Dr Kiyoshi Masui in conjunction with Professor Juro Hashimoto developed the commercial sexing of day-old chicks by examination of the cloaca.

Dr Masui produced his legendary paper on determining the sex of day-old chicks in 1927 at the World's Poultry Congress in Ottawa, Canada.

He was always active in the commercial chick sexing profession. In 1948, he ran the chick-sexing school at Kobe for Australian and New Zealand Servicemen. He was born in 1888 and died on 6 August 1981.

(Photograph taken by Jack Whyte when he was a student of Dr Masui at Kobe 1948.)

The beginning

Two Japanese visitors are walking through a crowded market in the Shantung district of China when they notice a stallholder surrounded by a group of giggling children. The children are watching the old stallholder examine the vents of some newly hatched chickens.

It does not take the two foreigners long to work out that the seller of eggs and day-old chickens is picking out some male chicks for one customer and some female chicks for another.

The two knew enough about birds to know that male chickens must have some kind of tiny penis or genital eminence tucked away inside the edge of the vent. Seeing the vendor of chickens examining these newly hatched chicks in the sunlight in that crowded place excited the two visitors.

Back home, poultrymen had had to wait until other sexual characteristics developed in their chickens before they could distinguish male from female: cockerels from pullets. This development often took up to ten weeks, and with some breeds of poultry even longer.

In some light breeds, which are bred mainly for egg production, such as white leghorns, the cockerels could be picked out at about four weeks.

As the two travellers leave for Japan, a skill that had been known in the Orient for a long time was about to begin a journey which would take it to a Japanese University, three scientists, two Japanese poultry farmers and by 1934 would spread to the poultry industries of three continents.

In one of these continents there is a small boy asleep in his bed.

The seven-day clock strikes. The magpies are warbling. There is the excitement of a new day.

The boy hears his grandfather in the kitchen. He smells toast, then there is silence.

Seven-thirty. He hears his grandmother's quiet movement in the kitchen. There is a gentle chirping of newly hatched chickens. Instantly the boy is out there, dipping his hands in the hatful of soft black, white-tipped, marvels of nature.

As the wide-eyed boy sits beside the warm stove nursing the hatful of chickens he listens to his grandmother relate how she had read somewhere about a gadget that had a weight attached to a string, and if you held it over an egg or a chicken it would swing one way or another depending on which sex the egg or chicken was.

His grandmother was not too convinced in this belief, but she did experiment with her wedding ring attached to a thread of cotton over some of the chickens from the hat, without any conclusive evidence.

Another method of determining a chicken's sex, which she had more faith in, was the belief that rounded-end eggs produce pullets and pointed-end eggs produced cockerels.

It was half a century later before the boy was to read the sources of his grandmother's beliefs, also worldwide beliefs, along with many other gadgets which were supposed to tell you the sexes of newly hatched chickens.

Little wonder then that the two Japanese travellers were met with scepticism when they returned from China with news of their observations.

Nevertheless after some laboratory studies at Tokyo University in 1925 by three Japanese scientists, Dr Kiyoski Masui, Dr Juro Hashimoto and Dr Ohno, the possibility of telling the sex of day-old chicks became a reality.

By 1927 Drs Masui and Hashimoto were able to present a paper at the World's Poultry Congress in Ottawa on "The Rudimentary Copulatory Organ of the Male Domestic Fowl with Reference to the Differentiation of the Sexes of Chicks".

But there was still the need to bridge the gap between the anatomical studies from the laboratory of the Tokyo University and the practical commercial application.

The labours of two Japanese farmers, Mr Kojima and Mr Sakakiyama, helped bridge the gap between the laboratory and the poultrymen on the farms in Japan.

In March 1925 Mr Kojima, a poultry farmer from Nagoya, read in the local newspaper an article titled "The Sexing of Baby Chicks by their Genital Eminence".

He tried what he had read on some newly hatched chicks.

First, he studied the position of the genital eminence in adult birds and then worked his way down to day-old chicks.

He used chicks that were 60 days old, then 30 days, then he examined younger and younger chicks until he was able to successfully examine day-old chicks.

By this method he was able to teach himself the technique of being able to find the genital eminence in day-old chicks.

All professional chick sexers are indebted to the energy and perseverance of this poultryman from Nagoya, who came from very poor circumstances.

By 1933 Doctors Masui and Hashimoto were able to write and publish in English their book, *Sexing Baby Chickens.* Dr Masui, Professor of Veterinary Anatomy at Tokyo University, later became vice-president of the Japan Chick Sexing Association, a semi-government body whose members played a major role in the development of chick sexing as a skill which could be used commercially for the benefit of the poultry industry throughout the world.

In their book (English translation 1933 Journal Printing Co Ltd Vancouver pp. 48, 49) Mr Tokuzo Yamaguch, then editor of the *Japan Poultry Journal,* and later executive secretary of the Japan Chick Sexing Association, writes of Mr Kojima: "The reader should not forget to thank him for his great effort in actually working out a practical method. The poverty of this investigator was so great that it was with the greatest difficulty that he met ordinary living expenses on his little home farm. The man never considered it possible, in fact, to leave home for any cause.

"The situation became even more complicated as he applied himself to work which involved additional expense.

"Before [Mr] Kojima could find the position of the genital eminence in a day-old chick, he found that he would have to consult with Dr Masui, one of the co-discoverers who lived in Tokyo. That meant travelling from Nagoya to Tokyo, and [Mr] Kojima was so poor that he was unable to afford the expense of staying at any of the hotels in Tokyo. Therefore he used to take a night train, in which he got free lodging as he travelled.

"Then he would work all day long at Dr Masui's laboratory in Tokyo and go home from Tokyo by a night train.

"His financial position would not permit him to purchase any meals in Tokyo, so he used to take his lunch to the city with him. The hard work facing this man in sexing chicks in those days is well illustrated by the fact that he could find no more than 20 male genital eminences in 100 chicks that he examined. Still undaunted, he applied himself more earnestly to his work. In his concentration he was actually forgetful of sleep and other comforts. It has been stated that he studied the anatomy of five to six thousand chicks in his investigation. It is difficult to imagine to what extent this man sacrificed himself and actually suffered dire want as he never relinquished his study in the pursuit of his great purpose.

"In August, 1928, more than three years after he began his practical studies and trials [Mr] Kojima found himself sufficiently skilled to be able to sex chicks with great certainty. Verily, it was a splendid reward for such enthusiasm and perseverance. The most interesting thing in connection with his findings is perhaps the fact that the genital eminence is found in some female chicks. This was not reported by either Drs Masui or Hashimoto in their paper. Accordingly he extended his studies to the genital eminences of females.

"These female eminences as discovered by [Mr] Kojima were studied and classified later by Dr Masui by his scientific method. While [Mr] Kojima was doing the work, Yuzo Sakakiyama (later Councillor of the Japan Chick Sexing Association) was wondering if there were any copulatory organs in chicks which correspond with organs of ducks. In 1925, he read the report by Masui and Hashimoto *The Japan Zootechnic Report* and did a great deal of work on its application in a practical way. That he was an earnest student may be appreciated from the fact that he studied it for six months and used more than 3000 chicks in his work. These two men, Kojima and Sakakiyama, are the pioneers of the practice of chick sexing in Japan. The former was very skilful and practised most with chicks which had not been fed, while the latter worked with chicks which had been fed.

"Since many hatcheries began to sell sexed chicks, however, the sexing is applied mostly to the chicks which have not been fed. Under the present conditions the sexing is done by a professional expert or experts before the chicks are shipped or fed."

In Masui and Hashimoto's book they show how the Japanese egg industry made great advances from 1927 onwards. Their brief outlines help to explain why being able to sex chicks at a day old was so important economically to the Japanese poultry industry.

In 1925 the Japanese Government set up five poultry-breeding establishments in the main poultry centres in Japan.

These poultry-breeding centres were used to supply Japanese poultry breeders with breeding stock bred from the best breeding strains from Canada and America, plus some from Europe.

Japanese students and officials had for several years made tours of inspection of some of the most advanced poultry districts in America.

They learnt the latest methods of commercial egg production and the economics of production.

In America and Europe they inspected and purchased highly productive stock used as foundation stock all over Japan.

This brought about a tremendous growth in the poultry industry in Japan. From 1927 the average egg production grew from 107.2 to 122.8 eggs, with individual records at government breeder farms of 342, 344, 348 and 352 eggs for individual birds in twelve months.[1] These great improvements took place during a worldwide depression. This great expansion of the Japanese poultry industry brought about an enormous

---

1 A report from *The Imperial Zootechnical Experiment Station* by M. Kamio, 1928.

surplus of unwanted (and unsaleable at economical prices) white leghorn cockerels.

This wasteful feature of having to raise surplus cockerels in a country where grain was dearer than in most other poultry-industry nations was the economic background against which Drs Masui and Hashimoto, and later others, set out to find a way of discovering a way to tell the sex of day-old chicks.

For many years it has been generally acknowledged that a way of being able to determine either the sex of the embryo in the hatching egg or the day-old chick was highly desirable in the interests of economic efficiency of production. This rapid growth in the Japanese egg industry made this development even more pressing for Japan than most other egg-producing nations of the world.

As in America, Europe and, to a lesser degree in Australia, Japan's poultry industry had become a diversified business.

There were breeders of high-producing strains, breeder hatcheries and commercial hatcheries catering for small egg farmers, as well as the growing number of specialised egg and poultry farms.

Hatching in large force-draught incubators had made remarkable progress.

Large specialised egg farms had sprung up in every part of Japan. There was also a growth in hatcheries.

The City of Nagoya was the centre of this growing chick hatchery industry.

By 1936 there were hatcheries in the Nagoya district with sales of over one million chicks each year. There were more than 120 commercial hatcheries, which together produced total sales of approximately thirty million chicks in a year.[2]

In a census taken in 1935 the poultry population of Japan was shown to be approximately fifty-two million birds, most of which were for table-egg production.

As we have seen earlier, this growth in the poultry population, of mostly white leghorn stock, caused a serious problem with its surplus of white leghorn cockerels. A way had to be found to eliminate this wasteful by-product.

Similar conditions existed in many other countries, where egg production had become established on an intensive commercial scale.

Until the technique of being able to identify the sexes of day-old chicks had been mastered, all chicks had to be raised for several weeks, until the males could be removed and disposed of. This involved additional expenses in feeding, housing, equipment capital, and labour.

---

2 *Sexing Baby Chicks and Work of The Japan Chick Sexing Association* 1936 published by The Japan Chick Sexing Ass., Nagoya, Japan.

Against this background, it can be seen how important the work of the Japanese scientists and the two practical Japanese poultrymen were, not only to the poultry industry of Japan, but to the poultry industries of the rest of the world.

During the years 1927 to 1931 other research and experimentation had been done outside Japan.

However, except in the case of ducklings, they had not had any success.

Research by Dr Henneppe of the Netherlands had shown that the sexing of day-old ducklings by means of the presence or absence of the male copulatory organ is simple, rapid and accurate method of determining the sex.

The method proved to be 100 per cent accurate with ducklings at one- to four-days old.

These results were confirmed in results announced at The National Poultry Institute at Harper Adam's College, England.

However, it was found in the case of day-old chicks: "there was a difference in the physiological structure and appearance of the male and female vent, and that this difference was more easily discernible as sexual maturity approaches, and is quite apparent by six weeks in lightweight cockerels. Sexing young chicks is not sufficiently accurate to be [of] economic importance to the industry because it allows too great a pullet error, it takes too long, and is a difficult and complicated method to learn."[3]

Other investigations outside Japan followed: Dr Lewis W. Taylor and Ms E. MacDonald of the Division of Poultry Husbandry, University of California, found "the differences in the copulative organs of chicks they studied and classified confirmed the findings of Dr Masui's method of sex determination.

"However, the difficulty in applying the method—the cloacal method—needs a deft hand, good eyesight and long practice to obtain a reasonable degree of accuracy. This was considered a disadvantage."[4]

Another American researcher, Alex L. Romanoff of Cornell University stated: "Yamaguch (1928) reported in *Reliable Poultry Journal* in an article, 'New Way to Distinguish Sex of Baby Chicks' and Masui (1932) described a method, which is supposed to give very satisfactory results and which is commonly used in Japan ... We have tried to use this method but presumably it must still remain dependent on Japanese skilfulness."[5]

---

3 "Sex Determination at Hatching" by Helen M. Molyneux. N.D.P., in the *Feathered World*, Jan 1930.

4 "Sexing Day Old Chicks" by Lewis W. Taylor, *Nulaid News*, California, July 1933.

5 "Morphological Study of the Differentiation of sex in Chicks" by Alex L. Romanoff in *Poultry Science*, Sept. 1933.

While all these findings are being announced, back in Japan, following the work of Kojima and Sakakiyama in making the sexing of day-old chicks a practical proposition, there was a three-year period of learning and practice before chick sexing became firmly established in Japan.

During this period many people in Japan set up chick-sexing training schools, and some hatcheries began selling chicks with a guaranteed percentage of males or females.

There were many doubtful chick-sexing experts and agents appearing in Japan. Many were responsible for the sale of chicks of doubtful sex, many not always of the accuracy claimed for them.

These practices brought about the establishment on 15 May 1930 of The Japan Chick Sexing Propagate Association.

This organisation was brought about through the efforts of Mr Hiroji Takahashi, then president of the *Japan Poultry Journal*.

The association's aims were to protect poultrymen from dishonest practices, to conduct the teaching of experts in chick sexing, and to hold examinations and publish the results.

The association soon had 120 first-class experts qualified and they cultivated a new profession of chick sexing throughout the hatcheries of Japan.

CANADA AND THE UNITED STATES

March 1933

In March 1933 the Japan Chick Sexing Propagate Association sent Tokuzo Yamaguch, editor of the *Japan Poultry Journal* and a director of the association, and chick-sexing expert Hikosaburo Yogo to Canada and the United States to introduce chick sexing.

Arrangements were made with the University of British Columbia, at which Mr Yamaguch had been a student.

In a series of lectures and laboratory demonstrations at colleges and experimental stations in British Columbia, Washington, Oregon and California, the history of chick sexing and the technique were explained and clearly demonstrated by the Japanese.

Before this visit in 1933, there had been a few unattached Japanese, some Chinese and some other operators who did some commercial chick sexing randomly at a few locations in America. They did not sex great numbers of chicks and the results reported were not impressive.

The main reason for the lack of performance of these independent operators seemed to be that they undertook the task of chick sexing without any qualifications or backing from any organisation, either in Japan or China.

This pre-1933 experience of independent operators had generated a certain amount of doubt and mistrust among poultrymen, in America

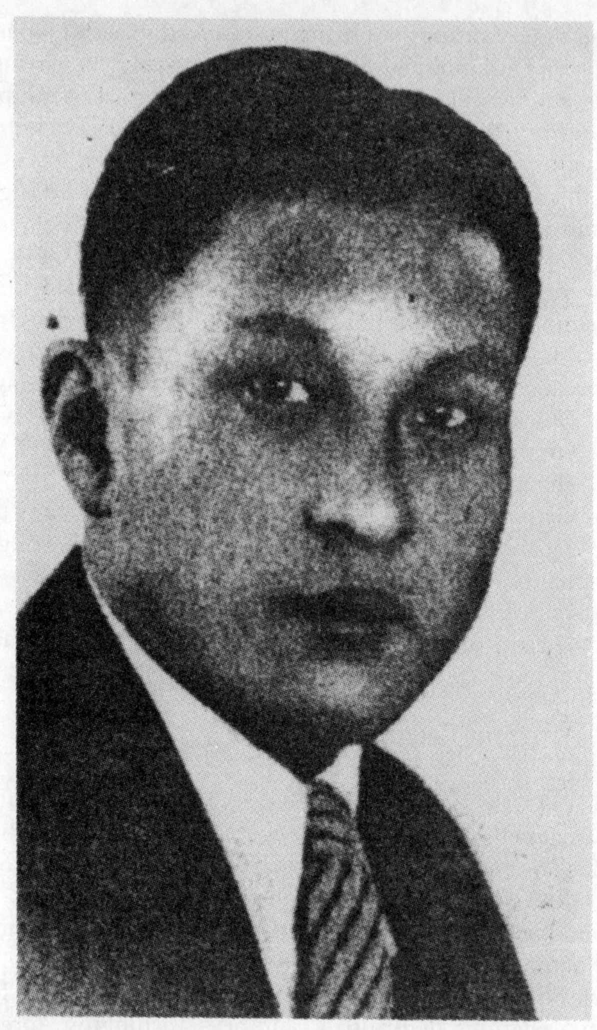

Hikosaburo Yogo, an early Japanese expert who introduced chick sexing to Canada and America in 1933, Australia (Sydney) 1934 and England 1935.

and elsewhere. This experience, together with the findings of research on the sexing of day-old chicks, conducted outside Japan, as shown above, only added to the scepticism of the poultry industry in America.

During the 1933 series of lectures and demonstrations organised by the Japan Chick Sexing Propagate Association, Mr Hikosaburo Yogo first demonstrated on batches of 50 to 100 chicks. After sexing them, the chicks were dissected to check on accuracy. The work of Mr Yogo was found to be 96 to 100 per cent accurate.

In all the demonstrations given at the University of British Columbia and later at several hatcheries and poultry farms, Mr Yogo's errors were never found to be more than 4 per cent.

The Strawberry Hill district, an intensive and thriving poultry district in the 1930s, was close to the university, and became the first district in America to practise chick sexing on a large scale. Some 15 000 day-old chicks were sexed in the district in the spring of 1933 by Mr Yogo.

Below is a record of his performance in 1933 as recorded in Masui and Hashimoto's book *Sexing Baby Chicks*:

Commercial tests in British Columbia 1933

No. of chicks sexed in commercial hatchery	23 400
Time required for the work	4 days
No. of chicks called pullets in one lot	11 800
No. of cockerels found among the pullets	39
Percentage of error	0.32%
No. of pullets left	11 761
Percentage of accuracy	99.68%
No. of chicks called cockerels in 1st lot	10 800
No. of chicks called cockerels in 2nd lot	2000
Pullets found among cockerels @ 5 weeks 1st lot	146
Pullets found among cockerels @ 5 weeks 2nd lot	42
Percentage of errors, 1st lot	1.24%
Percentage of errors, 2nd lot	2.10%
Percentage of accuracy, 1st lot	98.76%
Percentage of accuracy, 2nd lot	97.8%

The above results were recorded at the Bolivar Hatcheries, where 23 400 chicks were sexed in four days by Mr Yogo.

Other tests on accuracy were carried out by the Washington Cooperative Hatchery at Bellington. A check on 500 cockerels resulted in one pullet being found.

Another successful demonstration was given by Mr Yogo at the International Baby Chick Convention at Grand Rapids, Michigan on August 8. In this demonstration, there were over 1000 Canadian and American poultry farmers. Mr Yogo was able to sex 200 chicks in 13 minutes 27 seconds with a 100 per cent accuracy.[6]

During the spring hatching season of 1933 some 15 000 chicks were sexed by Mr Yogo in the Strawberry Hill district. They were sexed in commercial lots for various poultry farmers at the Chick Sexing Farm of Colin Brothers of the newly formed Chick Sexing Association of America, who in 1933 held the copyright of Masui's and Hashimoto's book *Sexing Baby Chicks* quoted from earlier.

So successful was this first sponsored overseas visit by the Japanese expert, Mr Yogo, that the Japan Chick Sexing Propagate Association was asked to send their expert to many other poultry industry nations of the world. By this time, however, many other small associations were established in Japan and tried to imitate the work of the Japan Chick Sexing Propagate Association.

This caused great concern in Japan and it was soon realised that if the chick-sexing business was to have any future it was necessary to establish one well-organised association, rather than the many small organisations with interest in only in the business end.

This was particularly important now that Japanese experts were being sought by overseas countries.

After much discussion in many meetings, these small organisations amalgamated and established a new association.

On 28 October 1933 the new association came into being. It was named the Japan Chick Sexing Association, later to be called the Zen-Nippon Chick Sexing Association.

This association has made a great contribution to the profession of chick sexing, not only in Japan but to most of the poultry industry nations of the world.

6 As reported in the *Victorian Poultry Journal* June 1, 1934 in an article by Prof E. A. Lloyd, Professor of Poultry Husbandry, Faculty of Agriculture, University of British Columbia, Vancouver, B.C.

The Japan Chick Sexing Association

ITS WORK AND EARLY HISTORY OVERSEAS 1934–1940

The first change the new association made was to establish a higher standard of qualification for their chick-sexing candidates. They changed the requirement for a first-class certificate to 95 per cent accuracy, from 92 per cent. The first-class candidate now had to sex 200 chicks within 30 minutes. Previously it had been 100 chicks in 20 minutes.

In October 1934 the association established a new training school in Nagoya. The students at this school were taught throughout the year, unlike later schools in other countries, where chick-sexing classes were conducted mainly during the spring hatching season.[1]

In the Nagoya School students were graded into three classes: primary, junior and senior. A student must pass through each class by qualifying at an examination at each level. All examinations were carried out on white leghorn chicks.

For students to get from primary to junior they were required to sex 100 white leghorn chicks in 20 minutes with an accuracy of 86 per cent or more. They were then classed as third-class experts.

For students to move from junior to senior they were required to sex 100 white leghorn chicks in 20 minutes with an accuracy of 90 per cent or more. They were then classed as second-class experts.

To graduate, a student was required to sex 200 white leghorn chicks in 30 minutes with an accuracy of at least 95 per cent or more. They were then classed as first-class experts. (In 1994 a first-class expert must be able to obtain at least 98 per cent accuracy.)

For those who were unable to attend the school in Nagoya for the examination, the association held examinations in various prefects of Japan.

As well as these examinations, the association conducted at its school

1 In New South Wales, Australia, during the 1930s and 40s, classes were usually held during January, February and March, because Australian instructors were available only during this time of the year.

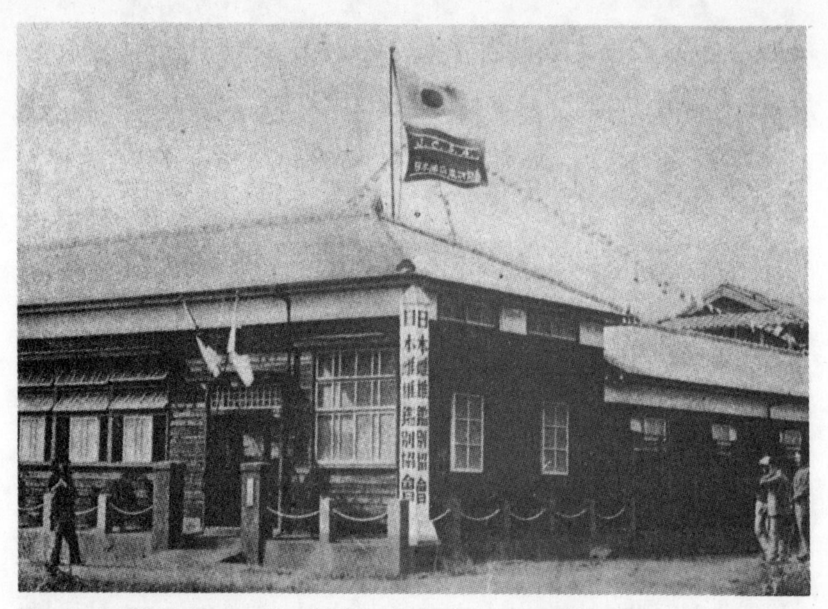

The Japan Chick Sexing Association where the chick sexing system is propagated worldwide. 1934

(Photo and caption courtesy Zen-Nippon Chick Sexing Association, Tokyo.)

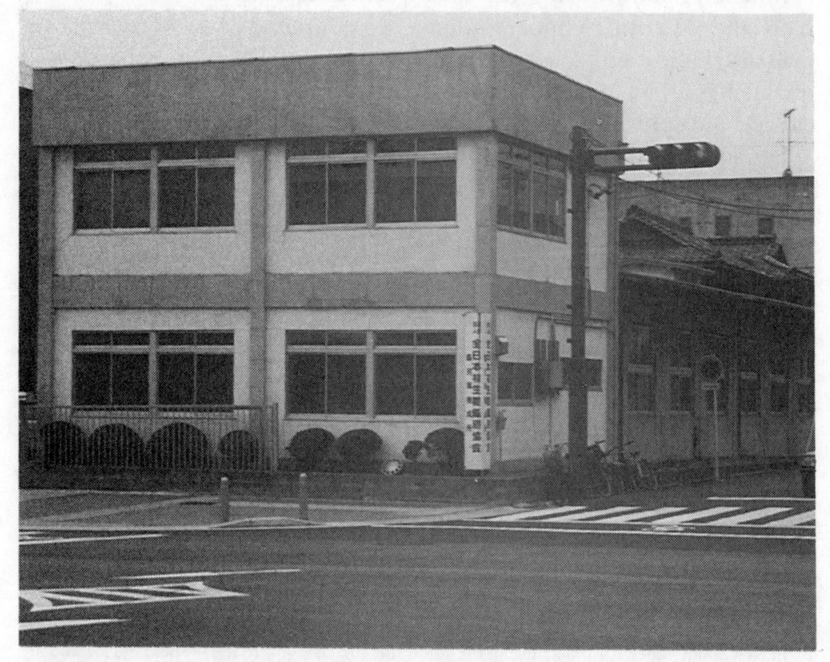

The Zen-Nippon Chick Sexing School at Nagoya, 1994. The only official and permanent chick-sexing school in the world.

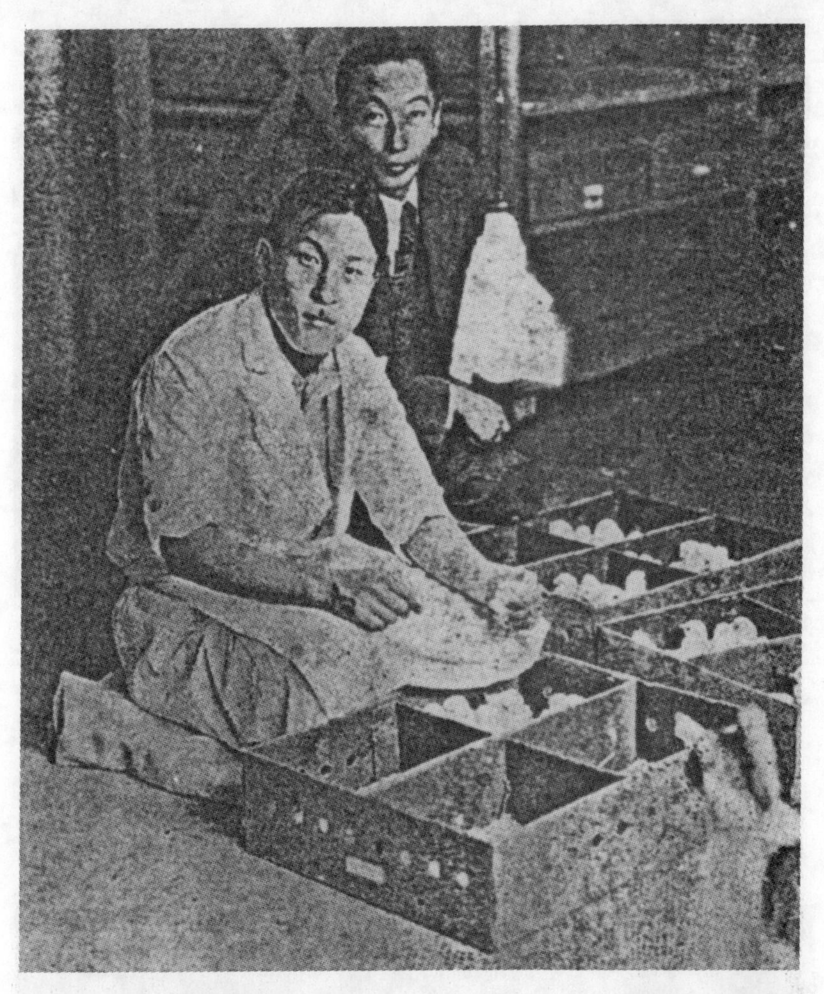

Hikosaburo Yogo sexing chicks in 1929. One of Japan's first chick sexers, he introduced the art of chick sexing to America in 1933 and with Hideo Kataoka to Australia in 1934. In 1935 he went to England to hold classes and sex chicks commercially.

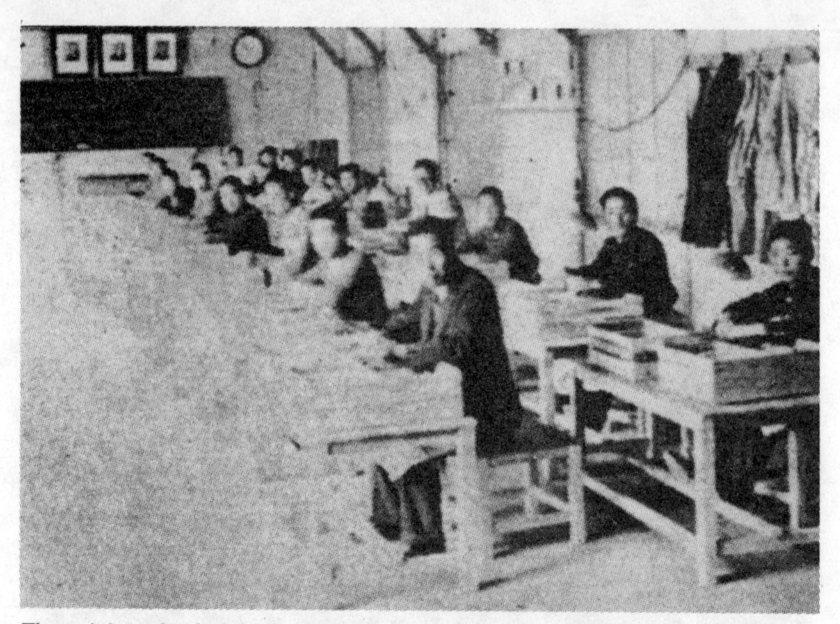

The training school of the Japan Chick Sexing Association, Nagoya, Japan, 1934

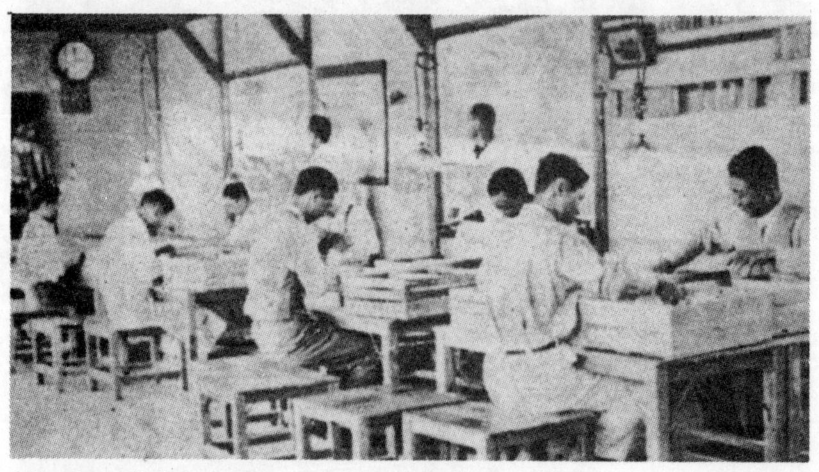

Scene from Chick Sexing Contest in Japan at the J.C.S.A. 1934.
(Both photos: courtesy Zen-Nippon C.S.A.)

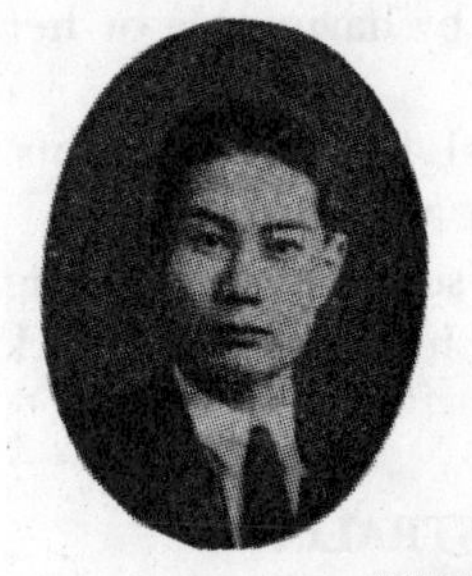

Mr Nobuyoshi Tanaka

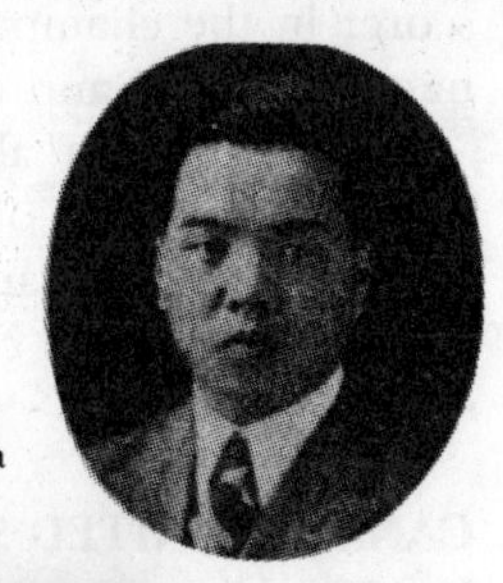

Mr Hideo Kataoka

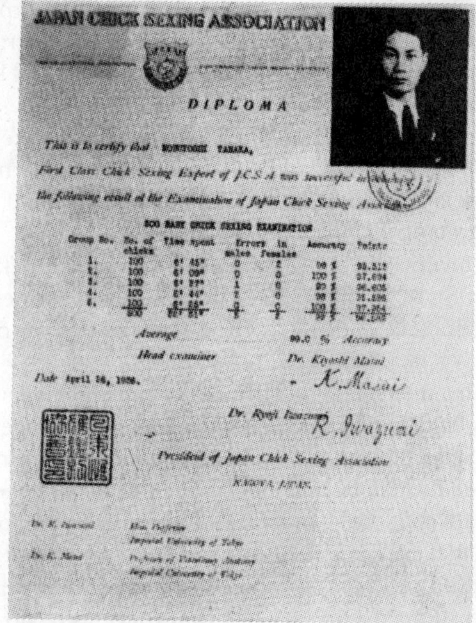

JAPAN CHICK SEXING ASSOCIATION

DIPLOMA

This is to certify that NOBUYOSHI TANAKA,

First Class Chick Sexing Expert of J.C.S.A. was successful in obtaining the following result at the Examination of Japan Chick Sexing Association

500 BABY CHICK SEXING EXAMINATION

Group No.	No. of chicks	Time spent	Errors in males	Errors in females	Accuracy	Points
1.	100	6' 45"	0	2	98 %	[illegible]
2.	100	6' 09"	0	0	100 %	[illegible]
3.	100	[illegible]	1	0	99 %	[illegible]
4.	100	[illegible]	2	0	98 %	[illegible]
5.	100	[illegible]	0	0	100 %	[illegible]
	[illegible]	[illegible]	[illegible]	[illegible]	[illegible]	[illegible]

Average 99.0 % *Accuracy*

Head examiner *Dr. Kiyoshi Masui*

Date April 26, 1936.

Dr. Ryuji Iwazumi

President of Japan Chick Sexing Association

NAGOYA, JAPAN.

Dr. K. Iwazumi [illegible]
Imperial University of Tokyo

Dr. K. Masui *Professor of Veterinary Anatomy*
Imperial University of Tokyo

1936

The above Certificate is issued from the Japan Chick Sexing Association to the First-class Expert who is officially sent to Foreign Country.

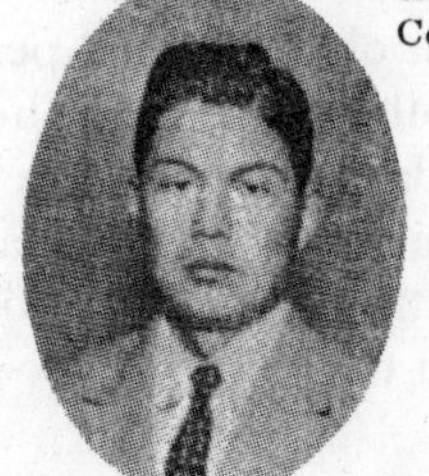

Mr Tomeichi Furuhashi

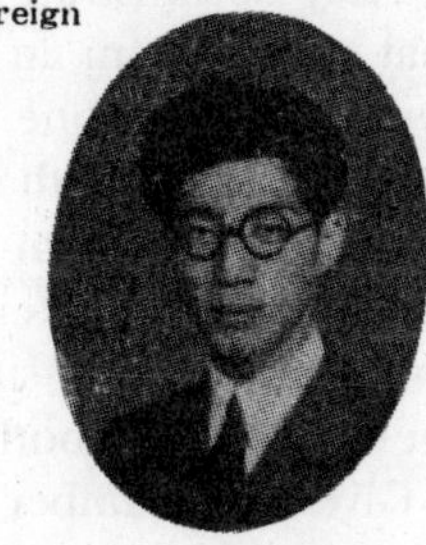

Mr Koji Kato

in Nagoya two chick-sexing contests and one championship series each year, to raise the professional standing of their experts. The highest scorer in the championship series was honoured by having his or her name recorded and was given a trophy.

The association also published regular official reports of events, results of tests and other news from the school in Nagoya.

The most important role of the association was sending chick-sexing experts to overseas countries to work and to teach the skills of chick sexing.

CANADA, UNITED STATES, FRANCE AND AUSTRALIA

In 1934 the Japan Chick Sexing Association sent five experts to Canada and the United States, one to France, and two to Australia. There was a third chick sexer who went to Brisbane, Australia, in 1934. However, he went privately, not endorsed by the association.

It is interesting to note that the Japanese chick sexer who went to Brisbane in 1934 did not follow the accuracy requirements of the newly formed chick-sexing association in Japan, but adopted a 90 per cent accuracy requirement.

When the Queensland Government introduced chick-sexing examinations in that State in the 1930s it followed this 90 per cent requirement for a second-class certificate and the test was on only 100 chicks in 20 minutes.

There was also a first-class certificate requiring 95 per cent accuracy on 200 chicks in 30 minutes, but no other encouragement to chick sexers in that State to improve their accuracy further. Complaints from hatcherymen in the 1950s and 60s about the accuracy of chick-sexing in that State forced the Government to follow the other States of Australia, and make 97 per cent or more a requirement for a first-class certificate, and 93 per cent for a second-class certificate.

These observations do not suggest that there were no accurate chick sexers in Queensland, where one of Australia's top women chick sexers was among the first students to learn in 1934.

They do illustrate the point which the Japanese had already learnt: that tuition from an expert who is capable of often obtaining 100 per cent accuracy is one of the essentials for teaching others the skills. The other essential is that there has to be a high standard of accuracy set for a student to aim for, and to achieve, before beginning commercial chick sexing or attempting to teach others. Over time, there have of course been many successful exceptions to this, but this rule has stood the test of time, both in Japan and Australia.

Given the number of highly skilled chick sexers it has produced over the years since 1934 New South Wales has always dominated chick sexing in Australia. It is also the only State in the Commonwealth which

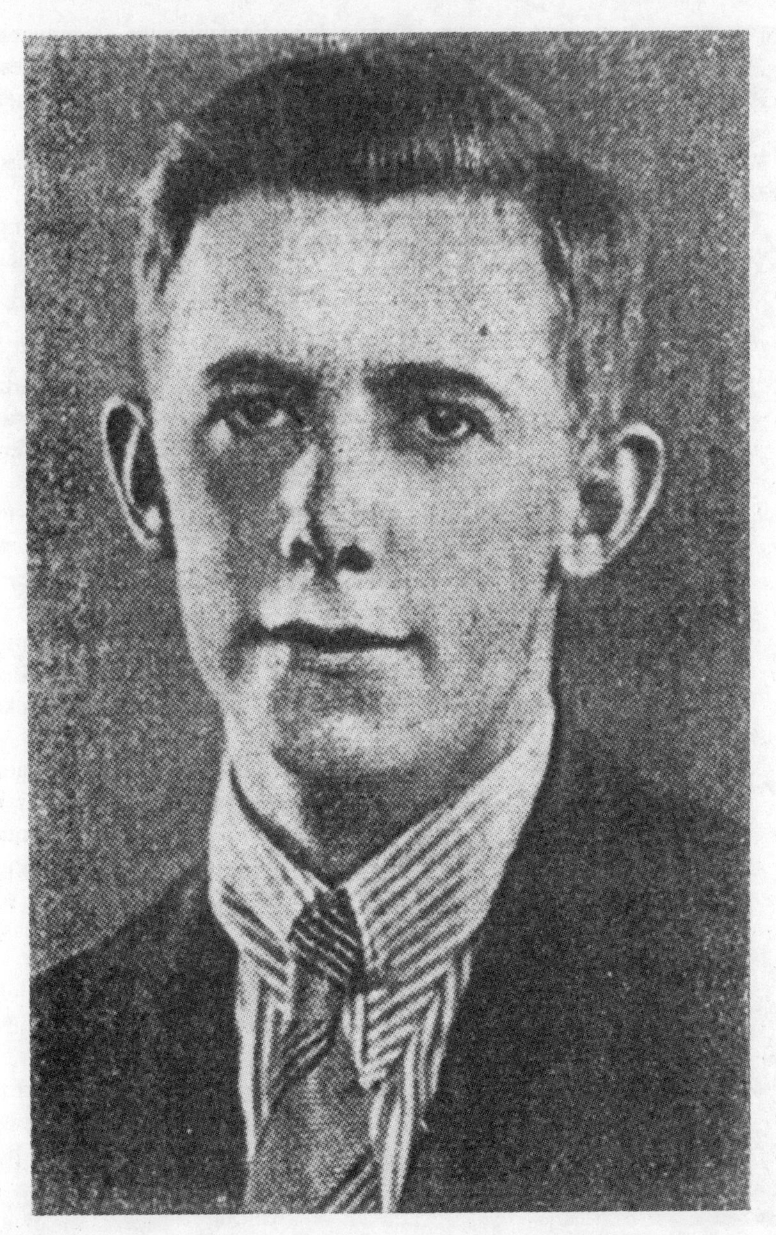

Frank Evans, of New South Wales, the dean of Australian chicken sexers. Frank Evans has taught more successful chick sexers than anyone else in Australia. He was also the first outside Japan to sex chicks at the rate of 1000 chicks an hour with a 99.9 per cent accuracy at an official examination in 1937. It was 14 years before anyone in Australia equalled his accuracy at an examination. No-one has equalled his speed.

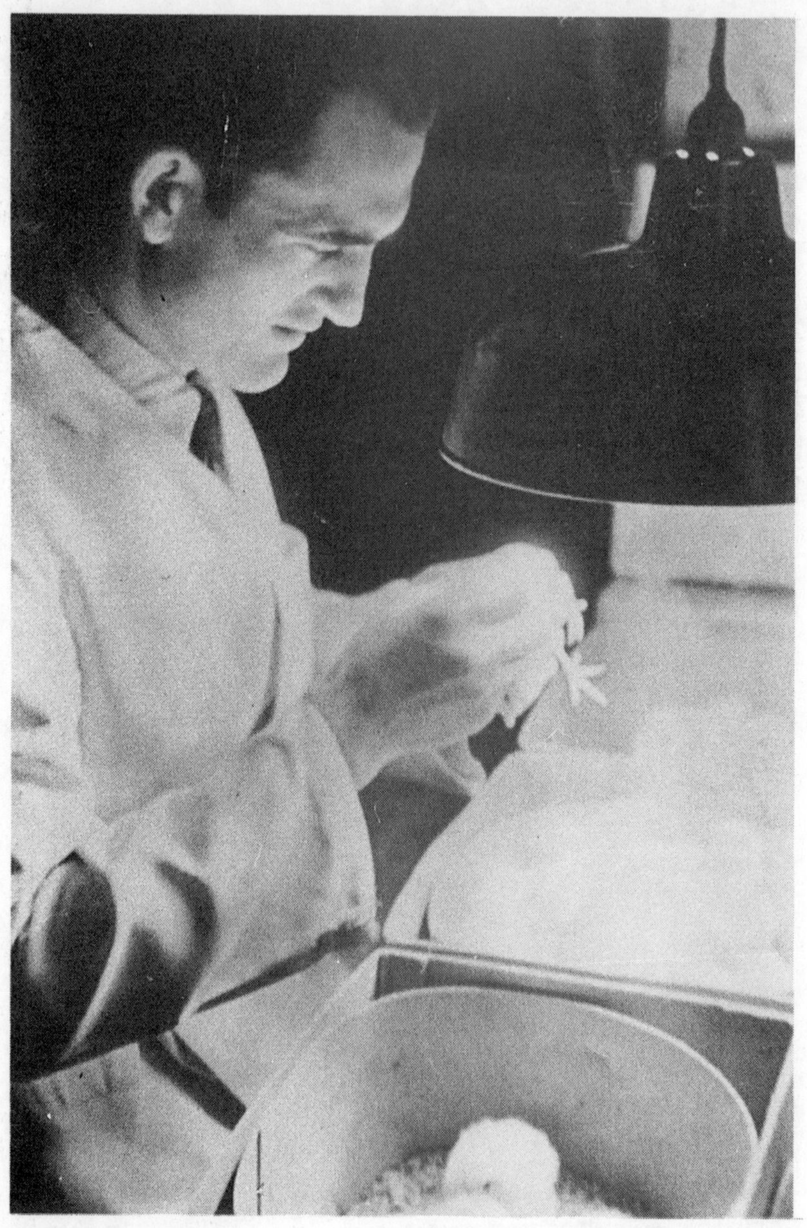

Australia's first commercial chick sexer (October 1934), Hartley Hall, of Melbourne, sexing chickens in 1948 for Australia's largest poultry farm, Carter Brothers, of Werribee.

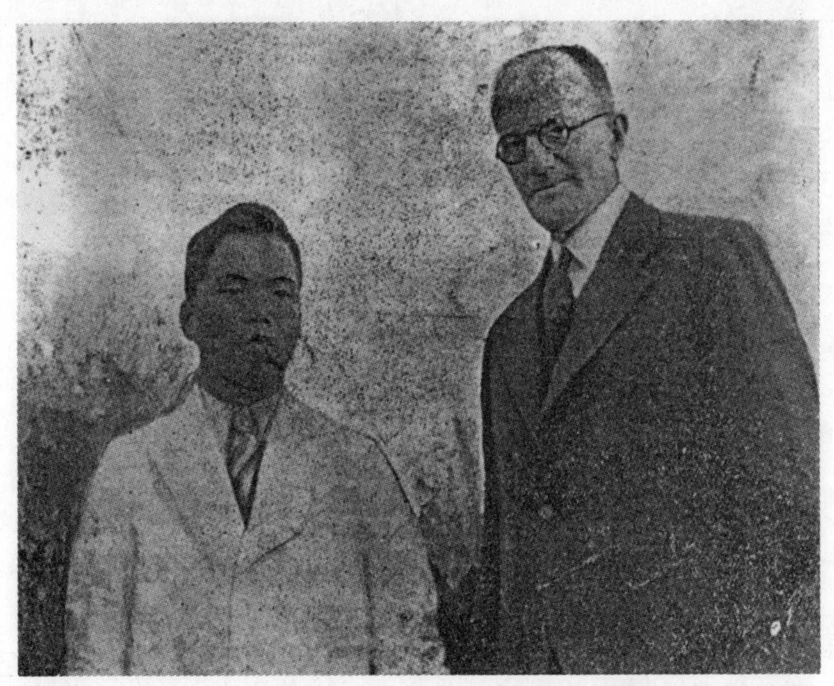

Hideo Kataoka and George Mann at Hall's hatchery, Melbourne 1934

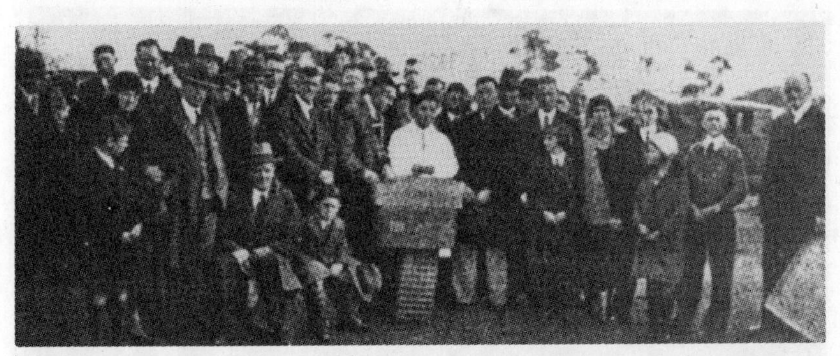

1934: Hideo Kataoka's first demonstration of chick sexing to Victorian poultry farmers and hatcherymen at Seth Hall's hatchery at Heidelberg, Melbourne. In the photo are teenagers and future chick sexers: Harry Pettigrove, Hartley Hall, Keith McLister, Doreen Lloyd and, extreme right in long pants, the youthful Charlie Bode. To the right of Bode is the man who brought the experts to Australia, George Mann.

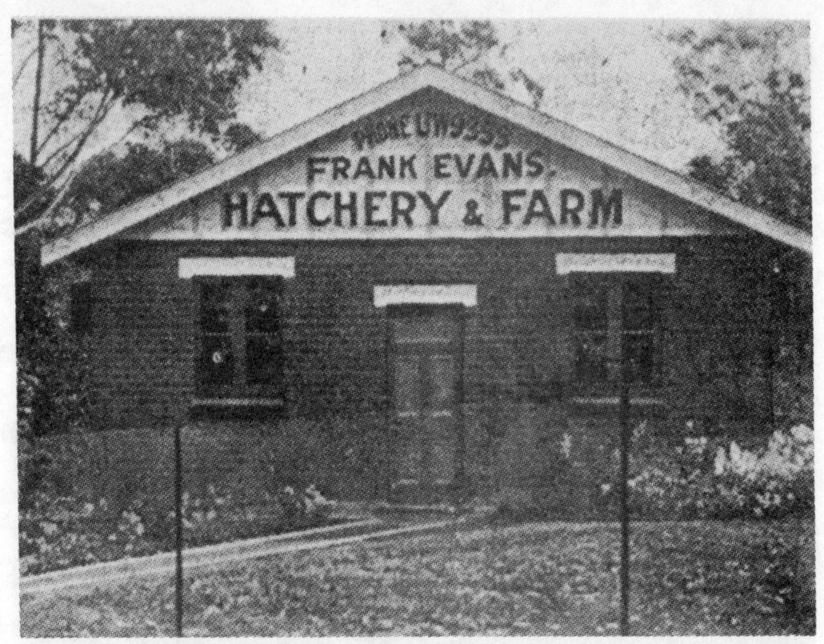

Frank Evans' father's hatchery at Dundas, Sydney, where Frank Evans held his chick-sexing classes in 1935.

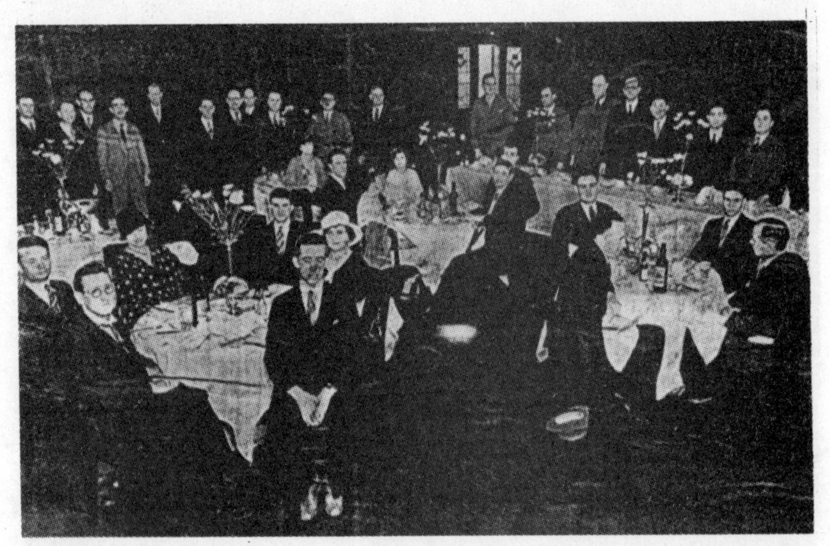

A Sydney farewell to the Japanese chick sexers in 1934. In the picture are the four visiting chick sexers, some of their students and the Australian businessmen who sponsored this first visit.

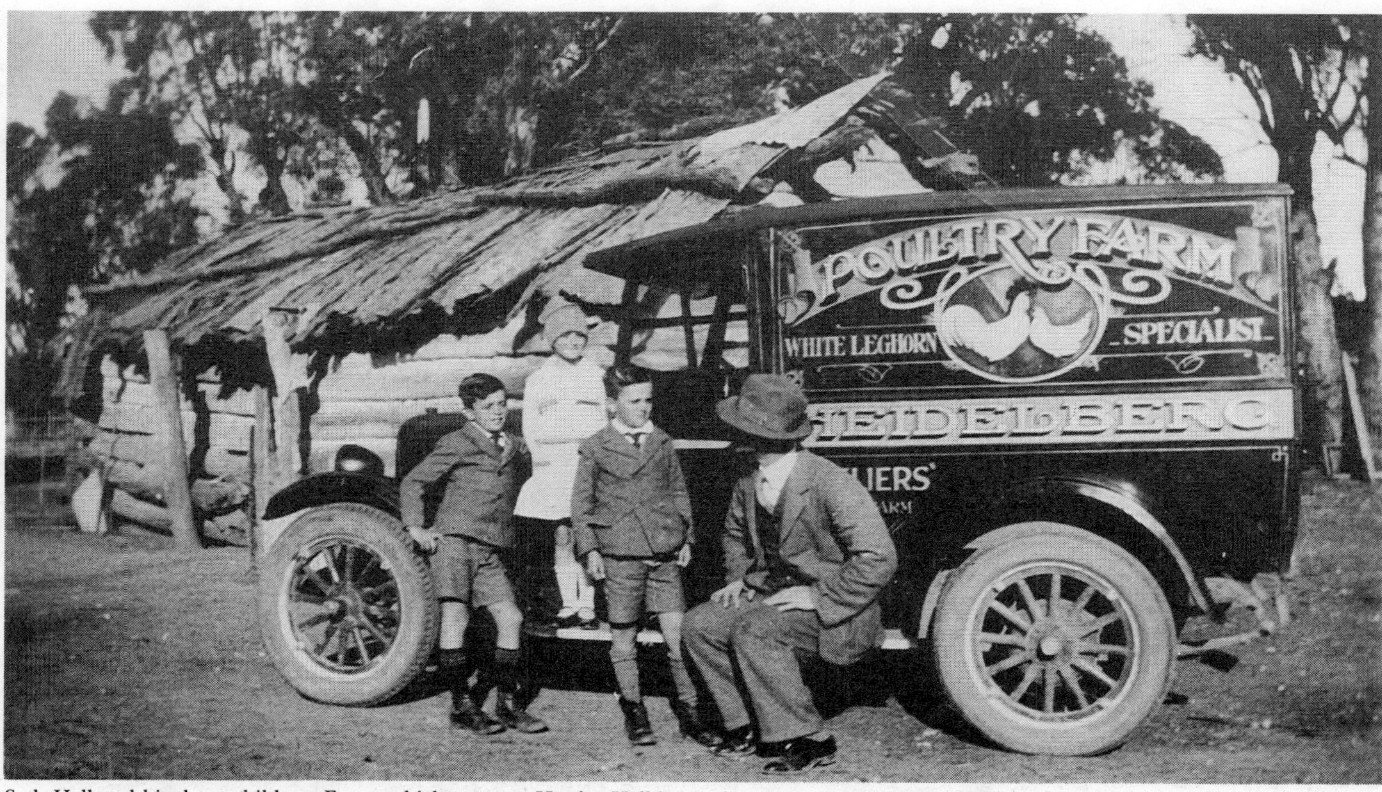

Seth Hall and his three children. Future chicken sexer, Hartley Hall is standing next to his father. c.1926.

has never been short of chick sexers and for many years (up to the mid-50s) supplied chick sexers to Europe.

This was mainly so because it had three outstanding teachers: in 1934 Mr Yogo; in 1935 Japan's champion sexer for speed and accuracy, Mr Tomeichi Furuhashi and the third 100 percenter, one of Mr Yogo's students from his 1934 class, Mr Frank Evans. By 1935 Frank Evans was one of Australia's top commercial chick sexers, and became unarguably Australia's most successful teacher of chick sexing. He had more students with special-class certificates (98 per cent or higher) than any other teacher in Australia.

Frank Evans was the first person outside Japan to sex 300 white leghorn chicks at an official examination in 19½ minutes with a 99.9 per cent accuracy, that is, one error in 300 chicks.

Australia was one of the first countries outside Japan which had annual Government chick-sexing examinations, and a chick-sexing organisation to teach the skills to others and set a code of ethics and rules for its members.

CANADA, ENGLAND, FRANCE, BELGIUM AND AUSTRALIA 1935–1936

Again in 1935, the Japan Chick Sexing Association sent experts overseas, five to Canada, five to England (for the first time), one to France, two to Belgium and five to Australia. There had been Japanese chick sexers in England in 1934 but they worked there in a private capacity and had not been endorsed by any chick-sexing organisation.

In 1936 the Japanese association sent six experts to Canada, two to England, one to France, four to Belgium and four to Australia. From 1934 to 1936 the association had sent 43 experts overseas to work and, in most cases, to teach. See list below:

Year	*Names of countries*	*Names of experts*	*Total No. of experts*
1934	Canada and the United States	H. Yogo	
		K. Kubota	
		T. Yamamoto	
		K. Kondo	
		R. Aihara	5
	France	Shinji Saito .... (Villers-en-Vexin)	1
	Australia	H. Yogo .... (N.S.W.)	
		H. Kataoka .... (Victoria)	2

Year	Names of countries	Names of experts	Total No. of experts
1935	Canada	H. Yogo .... (British Columbia)	
		Shiro Tanaka ...... (British Columbia)	
		Y. Masuda .... (Alberta)	
		Y. Hoshi .... (Manitoba)	
		Saichi Suzuki ....(Quebec)	5
	England	Hiroji Tamaoki .... (Felstead, Essex)	
		Nobuyoshi Tanaka . . (Andover, Hants.)	
		Tomeichi'Furuhashi ... (Lincolnshire)	
		Yoshiharu Sugiura .....(Leicestershire)	
		Hiroshi Takahashi .....(Leicestershire)	5
	France	Shinji Saito .... (Villers-en-Vexin)	1
	Belgium	Junichi Hobo ...... (Caster-Anseghem)	
		Ihei Suzuki ....(Caster-Anseghem)	2
	Australia	Mataichi Sakai .... (N.S.W.)	
		Koji Kato .... (N.S.W.)	
		Saichi Hasegawa ....(Victoria)	
		H. Kataoka ....(Victoria)	
		G. Fukushima ....(Victoria)	5
1936	Canada	H. Yogo .... (British Columbia)	
		Hideo Sato .... (British Columbia)	
		Shogo Uryu .... (Alberta)	
		Minoru Suzuki .... (Manitoba)	
		Yoshiharu Sugiura .... (Manitoba)	
		Shozo Yamamoto ....(Quebec)	6
	England	Isamu Ikeda ....(Essex)	
		Kunio Takahashi .... (Hants.)	2
	France	Shinji Saito .... (Villers-en-Vexin)	1
	Belgium	Junichi Hobo ...... (Caster-Anseghem)	
		Kiyomi Horii .... (Caster-Anseghem)	
		Shigeru Tsuruta ... (Caster-Anseghem)	
		Isamu Ninomiya .. (Caster-Anseghem)	4
	Australia	Koji Kato .... (Queensland)	
		Tomeichi Furuhashi .... (N.S.W.)	
		Nobuyoshi Tanaka ....(Victoria)	
		H. Kataoka ....(Victoria)	4

Summary

Year	No. of Experts
1934	8
1935	18
1936	17
Total	43

(List courtesy: Zen-Nippon Chick Sexing Association)

UNITED STATES 1935–1940

The Japan Chick Sexing Association taught many of the chick sexers who later went to America to live and work.

The founder of the American Chick Sexing Association, Mr S. John Nitta, went to Japan in the early 1930s and learnt the skill from the Japanese. Upon his return he established in 1937 the American Chick Sexing School, the first and probably the only commercial and licensed chick-sexing school in America.

The American Chick Sexing Association (Amchick) has, over the years, supplied chick sexers to South America and Europe as well as to all the States of America. By the 1970s and 1990s it could justifiably claim that it is America's oldest and largest chick-sexing service. The association is now run by Mr David K. Nitta, the son of the founder.

There are, and have been other chick-sexing and poultry-sexing services in America over the past 60 years, such as: Mid-West Sexing Service, International Chick Sexers Association, Pacific Chick Sexing Association, and the United Chick Sexing Association, as well as hundreds of smaller groups and independent operators.

The American Chick Sexing Association has tended to work in a close relationship with the Japan Chick Sexing Association. By the mid 1950s the American Chick Sexing Association had over 300 chick sexers working in America, Canada, Mexico and Europe. It was by far the largest, most extensive chick-sexing service in America.

During World War II there were many Japanese-American chick sexers who served in the special Marine division of the US Forces made up of Japanese-Americans who served in Europe.

Australia: New South Wales ... Victoria ... Queensland 1934

In selecting experts to send overseas, the Japan Chick Sexing Association chose those with high chick-sexing skills, of good character and a high standard of professionalism. They also had to have a sound knowledge of the theory of chick sexing and of poultry husbandry in general.

In the course of research and interviews for this study, it was found that the association's choice of overseas experts was very successful.

They were all highly skilled and remembered wherever they went as gentlemen (if this term can be used; sadly it is going out of use) and men of very high professional standard. I found no record of any women experts who went overseas in the 1930s and 40s, even though there were 20 women experts in Japan in the 1930s.

Before an expert was sent overseas he had to qualify for a Japan Chick Sexing Association diploma. To qualify a candidate had to be tested on 500 white leghorn chicks. After each 100 chicks, the time was recorded; then the next 100 were sexed. Again the time taken was recorded.

When the 500 chicks had been sexed, they were dissected and the accuracy recorded. Points were allocated by a formula based on speed and accuracy, with points deducted for any injury or chicks killed during the examination.

Chick sexing has always been regarded as a profession in Japan. This is one of the main reasons Japanese commercial chick sexers are so accurate and have a professional approach to their work. This professionalism and skill was demonstrated by the first Japanese experts to visit Canada and America in 1933 and Australia a year later.

The first Japanese chick sexing experts to come to Australia visited Sydney, Brisbane and Melbourne in 1934.

They were met with some scepticism in Australia, but after the first chickens they sexed were killed and examined by a veterinary surgeon and found to be 100 per cent accurate, chick sexing was readily accepted in Australia by most poultry farmers and hatcherymen.

The Japanese expert who came to Brisbane in 1934 to conduct the first chick-sexing class was Mr Kiyoshi Ozawa, who, as we have seen, was not sponsored by the Japanese association. Among his first students were Mr Oscar Johnson and Miss Dorothy McCulloch. In 1935 they continued their lessons under the tuition of Mr Suzuki, who came to Brisbane that year. Within five years of Mr Ozawa's visit to Brisbane chick sexers became key people in the State's chicken hatcheries.

The first Japanese expert to arrive in Sydney in 1934 was Mr Hikosaburo Yogo. He had just come from the successful season in Canada and America reported above. He was also a director of the Japan Chick Sexing Association. His family owned one of the largest hatcheries in Japan.

At the school conducted by the Japan Chick Sexing Association, Mr Yogo said, students were given two weeks' theory and then practised on the young birds. Anatomy was the secret of the science and 90 per cent or better was necessary for the first-class certificate in Japan.

Mr Yogo arrived in Sydney aboard the SS Aorangi on Friday 15 June 1934. He began commercial chick sexing on Saturday 16 June. All were amazed at the speed with which the work was done.

While 5000 chicks a day was considered a good day's work, Mr Yogo had, while in Canada, sexed 10 000 chicks in one day. The total number of chicks sexed in Canada and the adjoining State of Washington, USA, by the five Japanese experts there in 1934 was two million chicks. Their commercial accuracy was 96 to 98 per cent.

Mr Yogo was brought to Australia by Mr George Mann, of Mann and Gamble Pty Ltd, as was the Japanese expert who went to Victoria, Mr Hideo Kataoka.

During his first week in Sydney Mr Yogo averaged 2000 chicks a day. The numbers steadily increased to 5000 chicks a day. He eventually had more work than he could accept in the time available. His time had been allocated to a particular group of hatcheries at set times each week.

Mr Yogo also gave a series of public demonstrations. The first, for the Department of Agriculture, NSW, was attended by the Under Secretary of Agriculture, the Chief of the Stock Department and government poultry experts. One hundred chicks were sexed in four minutes thirty seconds. Twenty-five of the chicks sexed as cockerels were then killed, as well as eight of the pullets. All were found to have been sexed correctly.

Another demonstration was held at the Parramatta Town Hall on 30 June 1934, arranged by the Parramatta Poultry Club. Again, a hundred chicks were sexed in four minutes thirty seconds. There were fifty-seven pullets and forty-three cockerels. All the cockerels and 12 of the pullets were then killed, examined and found to have been sexed correctly.

A further demonstration was held for the veterinary students at the Sydney University, one hundred again being sexed. All the cockerels and a number of pullets were killed and checked. Again all had been sexed correctly.

While Mr Yogo's services were, by necessity, restricted to the number of hatcheries he could properly serve, there was no restriction on the chick-sexing classes. They were open to all.[1]

Classes were held on Saturday afternoons at George Mann and Son's Hatchery at Dundas. There were twenty-seven students at the beginning of the course, twenty finished. The classes were made up of the sons and daughters of hatcherymen, as well as the younger partners from several hatcheries.

The two most successful students from this initial class were Mr Frank Evans, of Dundas, who obtained 98 per cent accuracy at the end of the course examination, as well as gaining 100 per cent accuracy at many of the tests held in class. The other very successful student from this first chick-sexing class was Mr A. A. (Bert) Tegel, who gained 93 per cent accuracy. Later they combined to conduct classes at the Parramatta School of Arts for several years. Eventually Frank Evans became the State's sole instructor for many years, with outstanding results.

By 1935 Sydney had two chick-sexing classes, one run by the visiting Japanese expert, Mr Tomeichi Furuhashi, who held the world record for speed and accuracy. He was assisted by a student from Mr Yogo's class of the previous year, Miss Mavis Heath, who later married the Australian expert conducting the other class in Sydney in 1935, Mr Frank Evans.

Mr Evans' class was held at his father's hatchery in Leamington Street, Dundas. Frank Evans was to become one of the top commercial chick sexers in the State, as well as the most successful teacher of the art of chick sexing in Australia. He also had successful students from New Zealand, South Australia, Western Australia and Victoria, as well as in Belgium in the late 1940s.

Chick sexing in NSW was well on the way to being firmly established by 1935–36, a lead which it seems to have held throughout the sixty years of chick sexing.

In 1936 NSW chick sexers introduced the art to South Australia. Japanese chick sexers did not visit Adelaide, Perth or Tasmania because, in the 1930s, the poultry industry in those states had not developed sufficiently to make their going there worthwhile.

Victoria was the first State to send chick sexers to Europe (1937–38). No-one from Victoria went overseas after the war.

One of the Victorians who went to England in 1937–38 was Eric Marchant, who learnt the skill in Sydney and was brought to Melbourne by Clark, King and Co and stayed on in Victoria to become one of the

---

1 Reported in the *Victorian Poultry Journal* July 2 1934.

State's most colourful and accurate commercial chick sexers.

Fred Wrigley, another very successful commercial chick sexer in Victoria, and later chairman of the Victorian Egg Board, also had come from Sydney.

The first Japanese chick-sexing expert to visit Melbourne in 1934 to sex commercially and teach was Mr Hideo Kataoka. In 1935 he was joined by Mr Chimiyamura Kagawa and Mr Genbe Fukushima. They were backed in Melbourne by a consortium of six, made up of incubator and poultry supply manufacturers, hatcherymen and poultry farmers.

Chick-sexing classes were held in Melbourne in this year, and then every year until 1940.

Hartley Hall, the son of a hatcheryman at Heidelberg, was one of Hideo Kataoka's first students in 1934 and went on to become a successful commercial chick sexer and was one of the first four Australian sexers to go to England in 1937. Hartley Hall was the first commercial chick sexer in Victoria. He was a top commercial chick sexer in Victoria for two decades, until he retired to other business interests, yet he never sat for any chick-sexing examinations. According to research, he was the only successful student to do this.

Mr Kataoka came to Melbourne every year for six years. It was a condition of their permit to work in Australia that all Japanese experts must teach Australians the art of chick sexing, a task most did with skill. In 1935 Mr Kataoka contracted to sex chicks exclusively for Carter Brothers, of Werribee, and hold classes at their farm on Saturday afternoons.

It is interesting that no other country imposed this condition of teaching on Japanese experts contracted to sex chickens, but most experts from the Japanese association did teach overseas.

This condition of teaching was no doubt a big plus for prospective Australian chick sexers and no doubt one of the reasons why Australia was able to supply chick sexers to Belgium, Denmark, France, Ireland and England for a decade from the mid-1940s.

The person responsible for introducing chick sexing to three of the Eastern States of Australia was George Mann, of Mann and Gamble Pty Ltd of Sydney, manufacturers of Petersime Incubators. An important role in Victoria was also played by J. R. Hall of The Farm and Pastoral Supplies of Melbourne.

One of the Japanese experts to come to Victoria in 1935 was Mr Saichi Hasegawa, former chief instructor of the Japan Chick Sexing Association's school in Nagoya, Japan. He was also in charge of the classes in Victoria.

In 1936 Mr Nobuyoshi Tanaka, then managing director of the Japan Chick Sexing Association, visited Melbourne.

In 1937 and 1938, as well as Mr Hideo Kataoka, who worked exclusively for Carter Brothers of Werribee, Mr Shogo Uryu was engaged by Mr McFarlane of La Pollastre Mammoth Hatchery, Pascoe Vale South, but did not work only for him.

Mr McFarlane, a major hatcheryman, employed at one time or another all of the Japanese chick sexers who came to Victoria from 1934 till 1938, and kept records of their work. Victorian Agriculture Ministry papers of 1939 showed he had this to say about their accuracy:

> 1934: The first year of sexing introduced Hideo Kataoka. During his visit he sexed about 5000 for me as a trial or experiment. [There is no record of his accuracy at McFarlane's. However Carter Brothers engaged Hideo Kataoka for six seasons and they are recorded as saying that Kataoka made from one error in 300 to one error in 900 chicks.]
>
> 1935: Genbe Fukushima, Koji Kato and Haich [Saichi] Hasegawa sexed about 80 000 chicks. The results would average 98 per cent, but I think Hasegawa was below par.
>
> 1936: My third year of sexing I had 99 000 sexed by Nobuyoshi Tanaka and his sexing was the best I have ever had, as he did not average one mistake to the 1000.
>
> 1937: I indented Shogo Uryu and he sexed about 98 000 for me besides sexing about 122 000 for other neighbouring hatcheries. His accuracy was about 99.8 per cent or about one mistake in 500. I reared 12 000 pullets in my yards for 16 cockerels this season.
>
> 1938: I again indented Shogo Uryu and this season he sexed 122 000 for me beside 198 000 for eight other hatcheries. Shogo Uryu also conducted a class twice weekly and gave tuition to ten different students but none could obtain 85 per cent.

The same papers showed that in a letter to the Department of the Interior, Canberra, dated 1 November 1935, reporting on the four Japanese sexing experts they had brought to Australia that year, Messrs Mann and Hall had commented: "Their behaviour and general character has been excellent, their proficiency as chick-sexing experts beyond question, and the important phase of their work—that of training young Australians in the art of chick sexing—has been particularly well carried out."

Even allowing for the vested interests of the writers of the above letters and their, at times, patronising comments about the behaviour of these professional men, it can be seen that these Japanese experts were true professionals in every sense of the word. I have spoken to

Australian men and women who worked with these early experts who introduced the art to North America and Australia. All spoke well of their gentlemanly conduct and true professionalism, a tradition most of their Australian successors have tended to follow.

England (1934) 1935–1940

Before the Japan Chick Sexing Association sent their five chick sexers to England in 1935 there had been two independent Japanese chick sexers who went to England in 1934, Mr Nishitami and Mr Yto. According to the accounts written about their performance in the *Victorian Poultry Journal* September 1934, "they were very satisfactory".

Mr Yto worked at Mr Evans' Kilworth Hatchery and Mr Nishitami worked in Yorkshire.

There was some comment that these early independent Japanese were reluctant to pass on their skills. Teaching did not really start in England until the arrival of the Japan Chick Sexing Association's experts in 1935.

In 1935 there was also a chick-sexing class at the Midlands Agriculture College. This class was run by Mr Owen S. Forsyth, who had attended the demonstrations and classes given by Mr Yogo at the University of British Columbia in 1934. Mr Forsyth's brother, Ralf Forsyth, was an assistant professor at the University of British Columbia.

In 1934 two chick-sexing demonstrations were held in Kent. These demonstrations were arranged by Mr W. C. Blacklocks, of Beach House, Lydd, Kent and Mr W. D. Evans, of Kilworth Hatchery. Their aim was to set up chick-sexing depots in England the following year.

Mr Evans had Mr Yto give lessons to 15 people at his hatchery, but none were able to achieve sufficient accuracy or speed to make it commercially worthwhile. At the time, Mr Evans was convinced "that not one Englishman in 10 000 could hope for success".

Mr Evans told a meeting at Sevenoaks what a big advantage it was rearing replacement pullets separately: "no overcrowding in the brooders, best rearing season in my 14 years' experience".

Mr Evans went on to explain that if poultry farmers in Kent were sufficiently interested in sexing to be able to guarantee to supply him with 6000 chicks a week for this purpose, he would arrange for a Japanese expert to come over, and he would open a depot at either Sevenoaks, Tonbridge or Maidstone. The charge would be tuppence a chick sexed, and although a weekly total of 6000 chicks was not sufficient to cover the cost of the service—at least double this amount was required—he was prepared to take this risk.

He would reserve a certain amount of the expert's time each day for the smaller farmer who had only, perhaps, 100 chicks to be sexed, and it was his eventual intention to open a chain of chick-sexing stations or depots all over England.

Mr Yto then gave a demonstration. He was very fast and 100 per cent accurate. The audience was impressed by Mr Yto's speed and accuracy and "astonished by the ruthless rapidity with which he ripped open a chick for postmortem examination. It was done in a flick of his thumb nail. The chicks in this demonstration were Light Sussex breed.[1]

The National Poultry Council (London) originally considered forming a chick-sexing board which would license and control British chick sexers. The aim was to be able to replace the Japanese chick sexers with British chick sexers.

In 1934 the 12 Japanese chick sexers who came to England independently had been paid £50 000 according to the National Poultry Council. It was estimated that in the 1935 hatching season they would earn £100 000.

The council also claimed that the 1934 Japanese experts would not teach their skills to the English poultrymen.

The Japanese experts were paid a penny ha'penny a chick, with a contract guaranteeing them a minimum of 5000 chicks a week during the season.

There were fewer than a dozen English chick sexers by 1935.[2] Teaching did not really start in England until the arrival of the five Japanese experts sent by the Japan Chick Sexing Association in 1935. The five experts were Mr Hiroji Tamaoki (worked in Felstead, Essex), Mr Nobuyoshi Tanaka (worked in Andover, Hants.), Mr Tomeichi Furuhashi (worked in Lincolnshire), Mr Hiroshi Takahashi (worked in Leicestershire), Mr Yoshiharu Sugiura (worked in Leicestershire).[3]

They demonstrated their skills, taught and did commercial chick sexing.

NATIONAL POULTRY COUNCIL CERTIFICATES

The first official chick-sexing tests organised by the National Poultry Council took place on 31 December 1935. The test consisted of sexing 200 chicks in 30 minutes with an accuracy of 92 per cent in order to gain a certificate, or of sexing 250 chicks in the same time, but with an accuracy of 95 per cent, to gain a certificate with honours. Of the five

1 *Feathered World* June 1934
2 *The Adelaide Chronicle* 7 Nov. 1935.
3 *Sexing Baby Chicks and Work of The Japan Sexing Association*, Nagoya 1936.

candidates who presented themselves for examination, two gained certificates with honours.

This first official examination was held within two years of the first Japanese experts' arrival in England.

By 1936 there were restrictions placed on the number of Japanese chick sexers allowed to work in England. In 1937 four chick sexers from Victoria, Australia, travelled to England to do a season's chick sexing. World War II prevented them from returning the following season.

At the outbreak of hostilities there were twenty Japanese chick sexers working in England. On their release in 1945 they again started teaching chick sexing in England.

France 1934   Belgium 1935

The Japanese association sent Mr Shinji Saito to work in Villers-en-Vexin, France, in 1934 and each season until the outbreak of World War II.

In 1935 the Japanese association sent Mr Junichi Hobo to work in Caster-Anseghem, Belgium. By 1936 Belgium had four Japanese experts working there. They were Mr Kiyomi Horii, Mr Shigera Tsuruta, Mr Isamu Ninomiya and Mr Junichi Hobo again. They all worked from Caster-Anseghem. At the outbreak of war they were interned and later sent back to Japan. At least one, Mr Hobo, returned to Belgium on a permanent basis after the war.

The difficulties

In Japan members of the Japan Chick Sexing Association of Nagoya originally were granted licences for three levels of ability in the art.

To gain entrance to the third level, the candidate had to be able to sex 100 white leghorn chickens in 30 minutes with an accuracy of 80 per cent.

To gain a second-class certificate the candidate must be able to sex 100 white leghorn chickens in half an hour with an accuracy of 86 per cent or more.

In order to qualify for a first-class certificate, a chick sexer must have a second-class certificate and be able to sex 100 white leghorn chickens in 30 minutes with an accuracy of 92 per cent.

Many of the first American, European and Australian chick sexers who entered commercial chick sexing were no more accurate than these very early candidates for membership to the Japan Chick Sexing Association.

Even as late as the 1940s many offering their services as commercial chick sexers were not able to sex above 90 per cent accuracy.

As more chick sexers qualified and some of these early sexers' accuracy improved, the overall commercial accuracy improved. From about 1950 onwards any operator who could not achieve an accuracy of at least 95 per cent would not have been able to find employment year after year.

The documentation covering the Japanese chick sexers who came to Australia to sex commercially in the 1930s and 40s shows that they were capable of almost 100 per cent accuracy, a long way from the original requirements for a candidate applying to join their chick-sexing association in Japan.

In 1936 Mr Nobuyoshi Tanaka, managing director of the Japan Chick Sexing Association, and one of the two Japanese experts sexing commercially and teaching in Melbourne, stated at a press interview with the Melbourne *Argus* (9 October, 1936) that: "... in Japan there were about 200 special-class experts, and probably 800 holding the first class certificate. Practically all chickens in Japan were white leghorns. There were a few Rhode Island Reds and some of a similar Japanese breed—Nagoya."

By 1936 the Japan Chick Sexing Association required its candidates for a first-class certificate to be able to sex 200 chicks with a 95 per cent accuracy or more.

In 1994 the Zen-Nippon Chick Sexing Association has 385 (vent) expert chick sexers having certificates with 99 per cent or higher accuracy, tested on 500 chicks. For a second-class certificate the candidate has to average 96 per cent or better on 300 chicks. In 1994 there are 30 people in this class, but they are classed as non-qualified chick sexers.

There are 22 women expert chick sexers in Japan, which is 5.7 per cent of all chick sexers in Japan.

The Zen-Nippon executives make the point, as does Mr Ian Bestwick of Chick Sexing Specialists (Great Britain), "sexers must be 99 per cent accurate all day long to get by these days as breeding stock is exported all around the world".

Carter Brothers of Werribee, who employed Mr Hideo Kataoka full-time to sex their chickens from 1935 to 1940, state that he made only one mistake in each batch of 900 chickens.

Each of their thirty brooder rooms held 900 chickens, hence the 900 figure check. Carters had an all white leghorn flock, not always the easiest chickens to sex. They were also very methodical in counting and checking the number of chickens and any errors as they transferred each batch of 900 from the brooders to the layer sheds.

Many of the Australian chick sexers who learnt from these highly skilled Japanese experts were also very accurate, as were many of the next generation, who learnt the art from their fellow countrymen and women.

Yet as the following pages will show, many of the commercial chick sexers in Australia and overseas had lapses in their accuracy which the early Japanese experts seldom had.

Before explaining the biology behind the vent method (cloacal-vent method) of sexing chickens, and why it is so difficult to learn and so few become highly skilled in the art, it is also necessary to be aware that:

1) only the top Japanese experts were selected by the Japan Chick Sexing Association to go overseas. Japan had many expert chick sexers to choose from.

   For example in the 1950s Japan had 200 experts with special-class certificates, which now required an accuracy of 98 per cent or more and a far greater speed than the original Japanese standards. There were also 600 experts who held first-class certificates, who had to be able to sex chicks with a 95 per cent accuracy or more and with the same speed as the special-class holders.

Australia in 1950 had approximately twenty sexers with the 98 per cent accuracy or more special certificates and thirty-nine with first-class certificates, which required an accuracy of at least 95 per cent.

2) because of a shortage of commercial chick sexers many Australians were able to become commercial chick sexers before they had been properly trained or had enough experience recognising the processes of cockerels before working with unsexed chickens. The Japanese state that it is necessary for a student to work through at least 250 000 cockerels before they are ready to examine and readily identify the many different types of female and male processes. Very few Australian students would have had access to such large numbers of day-old cockerels, particularly in the days before the industry grew, and therefore had had to learn as they worked as commercial chick sexers.

   This situation seems to have applied less in New South Wales than in other States. There never seems to have been any real shortage of chick sexers in NSW. To prosper commercially in that State an operator needed to be near the 98 per cent mark, or higher.

At least two Victorian chick sexers, Hartley Hall and Bob Martin, readily admit that they were, by circumstances, initiated into sexing large numbers of chickens before they had reached sufficient accuracy. Both became accurate commercial chick sexers.

But many who start before reaching a standard of at least 95 per cent accuracy never obtain the high commercial accuracy of the Japanese or their Australian colleagues.

To fully understand why high accuracy takes so much study and practice we need to look at the biological knowledge on which cloacal chick sexing is based. Without this understanding it is impossible to reach a high degree of accuracy. Also, it helps explain why the skill is so difficult to master.

Just before a chicken is due to hatch some parts of the embryo's growth slow up and do not resume normal growth again until about three days after it is hatched.

It is believed this growth is temporarily diverted to the chicken's muscles in order for it to be able to break out of the egg shell. There could be other reasons, but what is important to the chick sexer is the fact that growth of the process, or genital eminence, is slowed up just before hatching.

The process or genital eminence is especially important in determining the sex of day-old chickens.

The genital eminence, or more correctly named the process as it does not serve as a genital organ, appears at about the sixth day of incubation.

Its size and shape remain the same for both sexes until about the twelfth day of the chicken's embryonic development. Then folds develop which make it easy to locate and identify both the process and these lateral folds.

A difference in the processes of the male and the female begins to appear on the fourteenth day of incubation, and increases until it is quite distinct at the time of hatching, and for some two or three days afterwards.

Studies have shown that during this period of embryonic life the process of the male continues to develop, while in the female it diminishes. Some females will have no process or very small ones by the time they are hatched. The student chick sexer's difficulties start when he or she has to learn to separate the 15 per cent of females with processes from the male processes.

It has been shown that there are about 134 different variations of processes. The chick sexer's task is to be able to rapidly distinguish these contracted female processes from the male processes. About 85 per cent of females do not have a process, or it is so small that it can be easily distinguished. Once the student has learnt the technique of folding back the chicken's vent, he or she should be able to sex with at least 80 per cent accuracy. Greater accuracy then comes with being able to instantly recognise the male processes and open the vent in such a way that the female process is not made to look bigger than it actually is. With practice and trial and error it is possible to separate these processes with great accuracy and speed, even though they do at first look the same.

Some breeds are easier to distinguish than others which is one of the reasons why a less experienced chick sexer can be praised at one farm and found unsatisfactory at another.

White leghorn chickens are often more difficult to distinguish than other breeds, a point several Japanese experts in Australia had to point out to their disappointed students.

After chick sexing became more established in the industry, some poultry breeders started breeding from the mistakes they found in their pullets. After doing this for several years, these farms would become a chick sexer's nightmare, because they were breeding from cockerels which in most cases had been difficult to sex at day old.

This difficulty in learning to distinguish the various processes was the reason the optical method of chick sexing was so readily taken up by new students when it was introduced in the 1950s.

After only a few weeks' practice it was possible to be able to sort the sexes with 100 per cent accuracy. With this so called "machine" method the operator was able to view the testicle of the male chick or the ovary of the female chick. It was a fairly clear-cut decision, but it still required a skill but with less concentration than the cloacal method.

Even with this improved method, many commercial chick sexers managed in time not to always be 100 per cent accurate.

This is one of the reasons why the skilled vent sexers were more than able to hold their own with the much easier to learn "machine" method, and eventually made this method obsolete.

What characteristics does a prospective chick sexer need?

Other attributes are needed. Keen eyesight, and the obvious physical capacity to be able to stand working under a strong light for long hours. Many said that small hands were necessary, but experience has proved them wrong. The hands do need to be soft and pliable, and the fingers nimble. Besides physical attributes, a commercial chick sexer needs to have certain mental attributes.

A book on sexing day-old chickens written in 1935 by Charles S. Gibbs, a research professor of veterinary science at Massachusetts State College, Amherst, *A Guide to Sexing Chicks* states what he believes a prospective chick sexer's inherent mental attitude should be: "He should be kind in disposition, gentle in manner, with a natural liking for chickens, and withal a keen interest in the application of biologic science to the welfare of the poultry industry."

Many of the commercial chick sexers have these "inherent mental attitudes" but not all. Some do not see anything in front of them other than the vents which they are examining. When sexers started working in teams of six or more, some were better at politicking with the management than concentrating on the job in front of them.

For a chick sexer to continuously achieve a high standard of accuracy, which is what commercial chick sexing is all about, he or she also needs egotism, something Professor Gibbs in those early days would not have been aware of.

Whether it is open or more subtle, almost all successful commercial chick sexers are boastful of their accuracy, speed and of their gentleness. Most boasts include all three, plus the number of chickens they sexed in a day.

All chick sexers want to be 100 per cent accurate. They are always working towards that goal. When they achieve it, they work to hold it. Speed is also essential to a commercial chick sexer.

Without this strong, overweening pride in their accuracy and speed, a chick sexer would never be able to achieve and hold the high commercial accuracy which, in the 1990s, is essential.

It has been said that some "old timers" will boast that they have sexed so many chickens they could sex chickens with their eyes closed. This situation of course never arises, unless 50 per cent accuracy is all they are aiming for.

However there is some basis to this claim, in as much as a commercial chick sexer handles the chickens at the rate of 800 to 1700 or more an hour and would not be able to dwell on the variously shaped "processes" (both male and female) that all texts on chick sexing discuss at length.

To be a successful commercial chick sexer a great deal of intuitive ability is necessary. There is no time for conscious reasoning. This is one of the reasons why it is essential to practise on thousands of cockerels before beginning on unsexed chicks.

In the course of research for this book and listening to conversations between "old time" (vent) chick sexers, one still sexing commercially at 66, said that "Some of the cockerels have nothing there, but I know they are cockerels."

This is intuition at work.

He was not conscious of anything that showed it was a cockerel, yet he knew it was. I suggest that his subconscious was aware of something about the "process" or "lateral folds" which told him it was a cockerel.

The size and shape of the processes are relative, and there is no way of judging them except intuitively.

A commercial chick sexer must be constantly on the lookout for rare types and to discover ways and means of differentiating them from those he or she has already learnt.

To be 100 per cent accurate is a continuous learning procedure, particularly with the industry's genetic breeding practices, which for feather- and colour-sexing aims are working on the sexual genes, which can also affect what the chick sexer is examining to determine the chick's sex. According to Frank Evans, Australia's most experienced chick sexer, modern genetic breeding has made sex determination more difficult. Yet today's chick sexers are faster, as a group, than their predecessors and, in most cases, more consistently accurate.

A prospective student of chick sexing by the vent method may be a little disheartened by the many types of processes and the little or no apparent differences between some male and female processes, but after a lot of practice it is much simpler than it first seems.

When commenting on his outstanding results in the 1937 government chick-sexing examination, when he sexed at the rate of 1000 chicks an hour with only one mistake in 300 chicks (at that time the first person outside Japan to achieve this) one of New South Wales former top commercial chick sexers said, "I was like an athlete, I was at my peak, I had sexed over a million chickens. I just went ahead, it either had a process—a cockerel—or no process—a pullet . . . and that was it.'' Intuition at its peak, backed up by a lot of practice.

NUMBER OF CHICKS AN HOUR

Since the advent of commercial chick sexing 60 years ago, the top sexers were, as now, 100 per cent accurate. Some could also sex up to 1100 chicks an hour.

The average commercial chick sexer did from 600 to 1000 chicks in an hour.

It is the number of chicks which can be sexed in an hour which has shown the greatest improvement in chick sexing by the vent method. Speeds of 1200 to 1700 chicks an hour are the rule rather than the exception among today's chick sexers.

Some of the contestants at the Zen-Nippon championships in Japan sex their batches of 100 chicks at the rate of 2000 chicks an hour. Whether this 2000 chicks an hour can be maintained commercially I am unable to give any opinion without seeing the evidence. But there is no argument, today's chick sexers are faster.

This increase in speed has been achieved through always having two chicks in their hands at once, but not necessarily picking up two chicks at once.

Japanese Chick Sexers in Australia 1934–1940

NEW PROFESSION

In Japan chick sexing has always been treated as a profession. The governing body is the Zen-Nippon Chick Sexing Association with its head office in Tokyo.

Some of the observations of the association are worth noting.

> 1932: Boys and girls between the ages of 18 and 24 will be attracted into this new and lucrative profession. A little calculation will show their earning possibilities, with fees at one cent a chick, and experts capable of sexing from 3000 to 5000 a day.
>
> People of 18–24 years generally have the keenness of sight and the best chances of success in learning the art, but it was older men who perfected the art in Japan. Anyone with keen senses of touch and sight may become proficient. In any case it requires much practice, the use of many chicks and continuous reference to the textbook to attain efficiency in separating the sexes.

These observations about the age of chick sexers are interesting, as they were made at a time when chick sexing had only begun. In 1994 in Australia there is at least one commercial chick sexer still sexing from 5000 to an occasional 10 000 chicks in a day. He is 67. There have also been others in Australia and elsewhere who sexed chicks commercially well into their 60s and one Japanese chick sexer still working at chick sexing one or two days a week is 73.

AUSTRALIA 1934

Three Japanese chick-sexing experts first came to Australia in 1934.

Mr Hikosaburo Yogo, the son of a Japanese hatcheryman with half-million egg capacity, came to Sydney on Friday, 15 June 1934, direct from a chick-sexing season in America. He was a director of the Japan Chick Sexing Association, and one of the top chick sexers in Japan.

Late in 1934, Mr Hideo Kataoka came to Melbourne. He had four years' experience as a commercial chick sexer. Like Mr Yogo, he was one of the most skilled in Japan. His arrival so late in the hatching

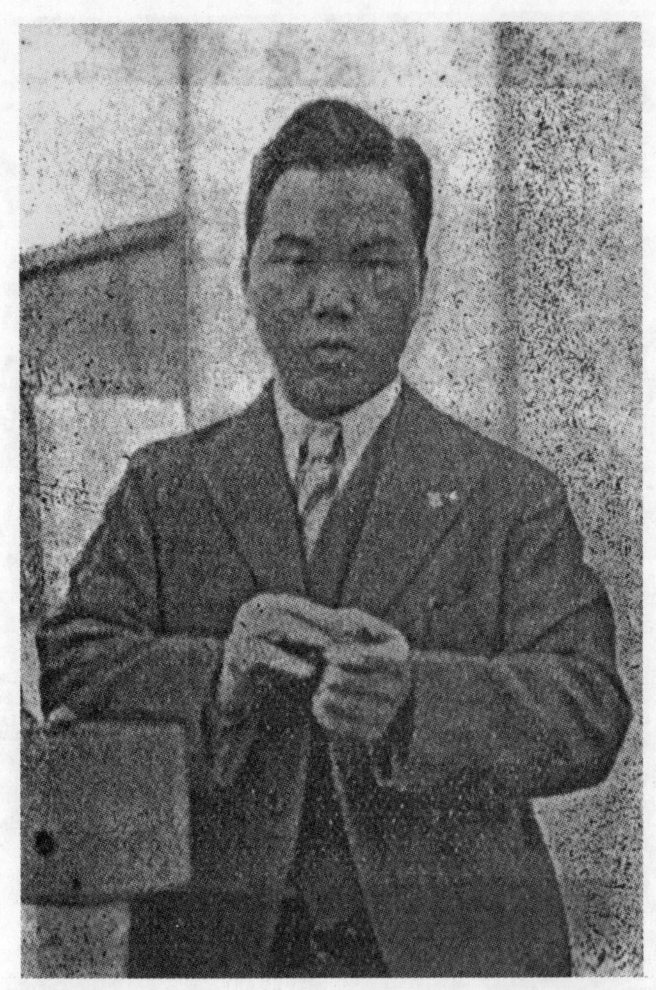

Hideo Katoaka, who held classes and sexed commercially in Melbourne from 1934 to 1940. He was the only Japanese chick sexer visiting Australia to use the Suzuki method (chick's legs away from the sexer) of holding the chick. In 1994 there are a few sexers in Japan, some Japanese-Americans, and about six in Australia who use this method. Including the Suzuki method, there are four ways of holding the chick.

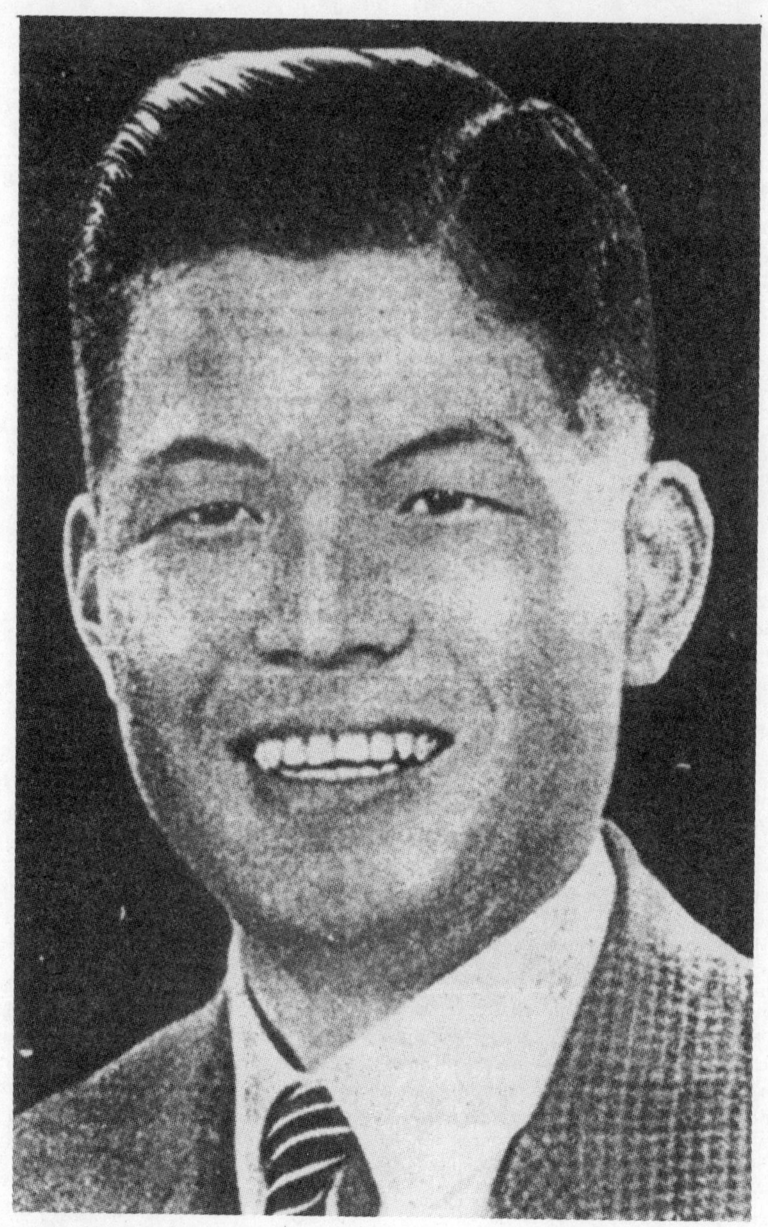

Tomeichi Furuhashi, who held classes in Sydney 1936, the year he held the world speed and accuracy record.

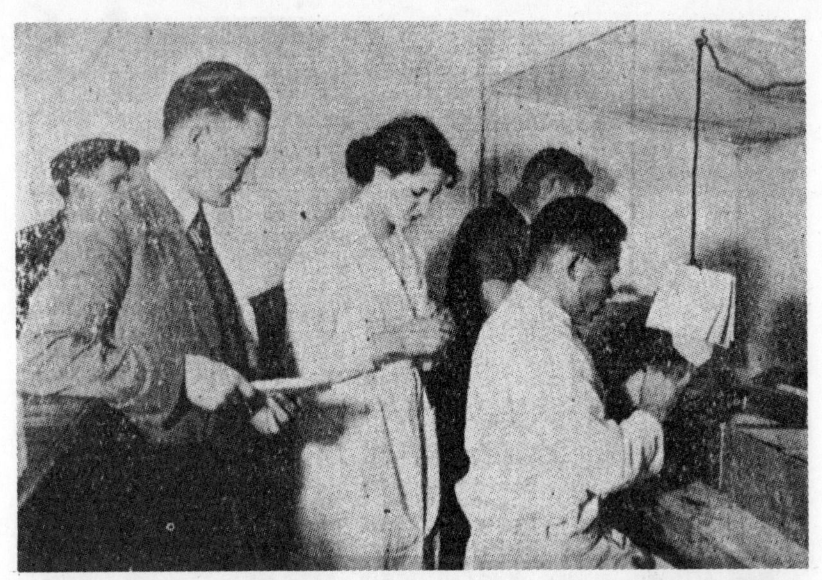

Japanese expert Saichi Hasegawa teaching in Melbourne 1935. His student is Doreen Lloyd, who was Victoria's first woman chick sexer. Hasegawa's driver is watching them.

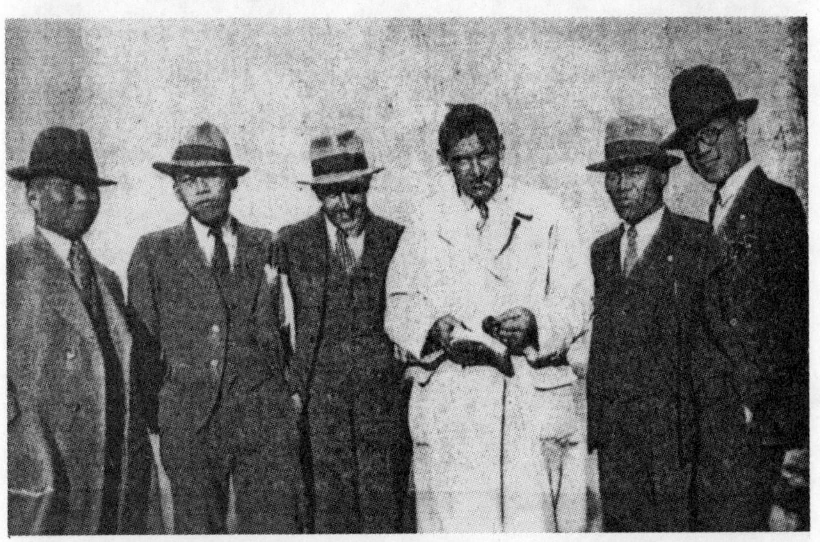

Left to right: H. Kataoka, G. Fukushima, Alf Woodman (a hatcheryman), the chick sexer's driver, S. Hasegawa and K. Kato, Melbourne 1935. The four Japanese were all members of the Japan Chick Sexing Association.

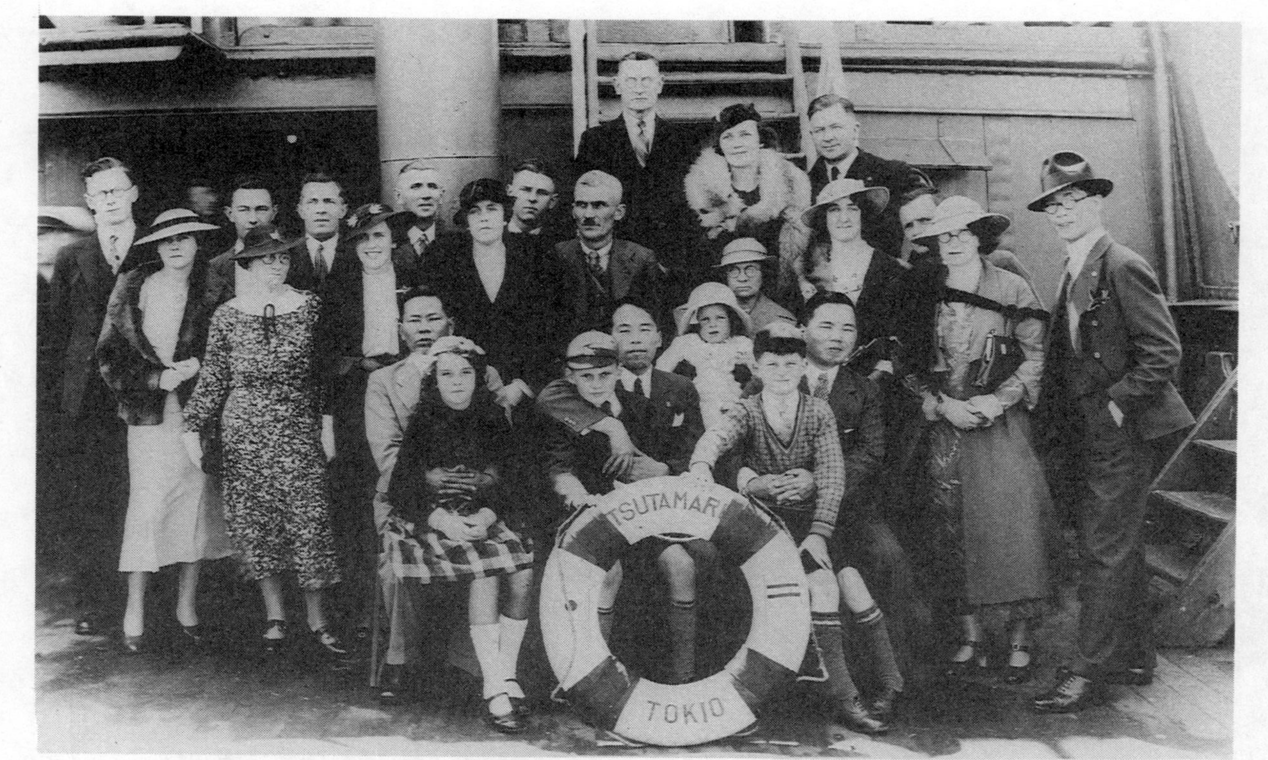

Japanese chick sexers returning to Japan from Melbourne 1935, front row from left, Saichi Hasegawa, Genbe Fukushima, Hideo Kataoka and, standing, Koji Kato. Other in the picture are George Mann, back row with glasses. The rest of the group are poultry farmers and hatcherymen from Victoria.

season was caused by the Government's slow action in allowing another Japanese expert to come out to meet the unexpected demand for their services.

In this first year they demonstrated the technique, sexed chickens commercially for hatcheries tied up with particular incubator companies, mainly Petersime Incubators, and taught Australians chick sexing.

VICTORIA

Following on the successful introduction of chick sexing in Queensland and New South Wales, Mr Hideo Kataoka was brought to Victoria on 2 August 1934. He arrived in Melbourne by the Sydney Express.

He was met by Mr Alf Woodman, a hatcheryman of Alice Street, Coburg. Mr Woodman had customers waiting for "sexed" day-old pullets. One thousand chicks were sexed that afternoon.

This was followed by approximately 5000 chickens the next day for Mr McLister, of Spotswood, Mr White, of Highet, and Mr Oliver, of Lara.

On August 4 a well-attended demonstration was held at the farm and hatchery of Mr S. T. J. Hall, of Heidelberg. The *Victorian Poultry Journal* of 1 September 1934 gives an account of the demonstration and details of Mr Kataoka's activities while in Melbourne.

"Prior to the arrival of the Japanese expert a programme of work had been laid out for him, fully allocating his time to the various hatcheries which had been responsible for supporting the scheme to bring him here. This programme is proving to be an exacting one, Mr Kataoka, also his driver, being fully taxed to cope with the demand for his services, indicating very clearly that chick sexing is proving as popular here as it has been in every other State or country which it has been introduced.

"From 2 August to 20 August over 60 000 chickens had been sexed in Victoria by Mr Kataoka. This figure will probably swell to 250 000 by the end of October, by which time the weight of the breeding season will be over.

"Mr Kataoka will remain on for a further week or two, should his services be required, after which he will return to Japan.

"Onlookers have been amazed at the ease and speed which the expert works. With a high-powered electric light suspended about a foot [30 centimetres] above the chick box, he looks neither to the right nor left, and his hand movement is no more than is absolutely necessary to pick up a chick, examine it and drop to the left in the case of pullets, or to the right in the case of cockerels.

"Some people, ignorant of the nature of the examination, claimed that 'sexing' damaged the chick. This, of course, is the usual attempt at conservative resistance to progress, and is promptly dispelled by every buyer of day-old pullets who finds, on the contrary, that not only is he saving time, labour, feed and brooder space, but that, best of all, his pullet chicks do much better by themselves, freed from the undesirable company of their greedy brothers.

"Plainly chick sexing has come to stay, and let us hope that at least by the end of next season some of the 33 young local chick-sexing students at present attending classes will reach a state of speed and efficiency which will justify their employment as first-class chick-sexing experts.

"Some of these students, both male and female, are already showing some ability with the art, one student reaching 80 per cent correct at the second lesson. True, the difficult part is beyond that figure, but at least it is a most promising start.

"DEMONSTRATION AT MR S. T. J. HALL'S HATCHERY

"A large gathering of visitors attended Mr S. T. J. Hall's hatchery, St Hellier's Road, Heidelberg, on Saturday, 4 August.

"Mr Hall arranged all details in his usual business-like manner, and visitors were given an opportunity of seeing Mr Kataoka give a demonstration of chick sexing. The crowd assembled consisted of every stage of poultry farmer in the State, from the back-yarder to the larger breeder. The NUPBA [National Utility Poultry Breeders Association] members were there in strong force, and amongst others who attended were Mr Westway, of Bendigo; Mr and Mrs Waterman, of Rochester, and Mr Kendall, veterinary surgeon.

"In introducing Mr Kataoka, who does not speak English, Captain Mann, of New South Wales, made a very nice, concise, introductory speech. In the course of his remarks about sexing Captain Mann said that, as far back as 1925, Dr Masui found the sexual eminence was pronounced in day-old chicks.

"He immediately spread the news, and experiments were at once tried out in America and England.

"The Harper Adams College was very exhaustive in its tests of two months, and it reported back to the world that it was correct, but it would be too slow for commercial work. The tiny genital eminence was too small to see, so they thought it hopeless. A little later, two Japanese poultry farmers started on adult fowls, and gradually got down to four-week-old birds.

"Then they started to kill young chicks at a day old, after which they opened up chicks in the shell and were able to trace the genital eminence in the shell.

"From then on it became an established fact in Japan. Classes were started, and it was not too long before the Japanese travelled to America to commercialise their discovery."

The expectation that by the end of October Hideo Kataoka would probably sex up to 250 000 chickens was not reached, as he returned to Japan earlier than had been expected.

The onlookers at this first demonstration, and other demonstrations which were later held at Woodman's Hatchery, Coburg, Mr Weatherhead's of Bendigo, and for members of the Commercial Poultry Farmers' Association at 18 Market Street, Melbourne, were all amazed at the ease and speed at which Mr Kataoka worked. At all these demonstrations, all the cockerels and some pullets were killed and examined and no errors found.

In the audience at the first demonstration at Hall's Hatchery was an eighteen-year-old boy who worked for a hatcheryman and poultry farmer at Research. He thought to himself: "This looks easy. If he can work like that it must be easy. It can't be to hard to learn."

Eighteen-year-old Charlie Bode had been 'hooked' on chick sexing.

The classes run by The Farm and Pastoral Supply in this first year were conducted on Saturday afternoons by Hideo Kataoka at V. Black and Co's poultry-requisite shop, at Rankin's Lane, off Post Office Place, Melbourne.

In 1935, the second year of chick-sexing classes, The Farm and Pastoral Supplies Pty Ltd held a chick-sexing examination for its students. The examinations were supervised by Mr C. J. R. Gorrie, BVSc. He was assisted by three Japanese experts, Messrs Hasegawa, Fukushima and Kataoka.

In Melbourne in 1935 another chick-sexing class was started at Carter Brothers of Werribee on Saturday afternoons, run by Hideo Kataoka. Carters had by 1935 contracted Hideo Kataoka to sex their chickens, which was a full-time job for him.

Both classes eventually produced some very competent commercial chick sexers. The classes at Carter Brothers helped break the control incubator manufacturers had over the first generation of Australian chick sexers.

The early Japanese chick sexers and also the first Australians they taught tended to be allocated to hatcheries by the incubator manufacturers who had first sponsored the Japanese visits and classes.

A chick sexer would find himself or herself sexing chickens for either all Multiplo or all Petersime Incubators owners. Mann Gamble Incubators, which were manufactured in Sydney, were tied up in Melbourne through Farm and Pastoral Supplies.

Carter Brothers

An exception to this "tied house" system was Carter Brothers, who hatched chickens in such large numbers that they could offer full-time work to one chick sexer. From 1935 till 1940 Carter Brothers engaged Mr Kataoka to sex their chickens, and to hold classes on their farm.

For many years Carter Brothers had the largest egg-producing farm in the world. Most of their eggs were exported to England.

In 1934 they were not able to engage a Japanese sexer as the incubator manufacturers had all the available Japanese chick sexers under contract.

It did not take Mr Kataoka long to work out that he would be better working under contract for Carter Brothers, which he did from 1935 until the war.

It is worth looking at Carter Brothers and their experiences and relationship with the Japanese sexers from 1935 till 1940. There were four brothers, James, Walter, Roland and John.

In the 1930s and 1940s practically all the big poultry farms in Australia carried several breeds of poultry, and many of them some ducks. Although they sold eggs for the table they also derived income from selling eggs for hatching, day-old chicks, started pullets, breeding hens, stud cockerels and table birds.

Carter Brothers differed from almost all other poultry farms in Australia: the layout of their farm and their whole operations had one object, the mass production of eggs for table use.

There were three farms within a radius of 800 metres, run under three managements. James and Walter had about 130 000 birds, Roland 60 000 birds and John 60 000 birds. They had about 250 000 birds between them, all white leghorns.

The original farm, Ribblesdale, had been founded by their parents on a five-acre (two-hectare) dry-area block bought in 1910 from the Closer Settlement Board as a workers' home.

They bought their first incubator, a "Petaluma" of 100-egg capacity, in 1911 and later several others were bought.

In 1919 they installed an Austral Mammoth incubator of 6000-egg capacity, heated by coke. Later they built two similar machines, each of 10 000-egg capacity. By this time they had increased the flock to approximately 12 000 birds and the original block was fully stocked.

Then, they set out to build the largest poultry farm in the world. They bought more land from the State Rivers and Water Supply Department.

In 1924 they bought from America a "Buckeye" Hot Water Incubator of 10 300-egg capacity, heated by kerosene and up until about 1944 it was still in use on occasions.

They built five electric machines, each having a capacity of 16 400 eggs. The coke-burning machines were discarded.

Their capacity in the mid-1930s was for 92 300 eggs. Up until about the mid 1940s the largest number of chickens hatched in a season were approximately 404 000.

From 1935 all chickens were sexed. Some cockerels were kept for breeding purposes. A few of the early hatched cockerels were sold to dealers for table purposes, but most were destroyed after they were sexed.

All pullets were kept for their own laying replacement stock. They never sold any day-old chickens or breeding stock.

In most years they exported to Britain 15 000–20 000 cases of eggs. The rest they sold in Australia. (There are thirty dozen eggs in a case.) They had a fleet of trucks to cart foodstuffs, materials and eggs. In the 1940s they again increased their incubator capacity to 190 700 eggs. This enabled them to hatch from 750 000–1 000 000 chickens in a hatching season of 13–14 weeks, starting at the end of June and finishing in September.

Carter Brothers, with their large flock of birds and large incubator capacity, were well equipped to supply as many as 10 000 partially incubated eggs a day to scientists for vaccines. It is possible that no other farm in the world could have, at that time, supplied so many.

As late as the 1936 hatching season Carter Brothers still believed that there might be some merit in an English firm's product which, it was claimed, could sex eggs. As a letter from Mr Kataoka to Carter Brothers shows, the Japanese chick sexer did not think much of this egg sexer. Mr Kataoka had a very polite way of saying this, as his letter, reproduced here, shows.

Ichinomiya,
Kagawa Prefecture,
Japan
January 12th, 1937

Dear Mr Carter Bros.

I hope you are going strong. I am also doing well.

When I was leaving your country, you told me that you bought a sexing apparatus, invented by an Englishman, which you said can sex out eggs with complete success, so that you could do without us sexers as soon as you got the machine. Well, what is the result of the test? As good as you thought?

Here in Japan, I hear that Dr Masui, the initiator of sexing and professor at the Tokyo Imperial University, is of opinion that it will be long before the apparatus can be made so perfect that with it every poultryman can do without sexers, in August last year the Doctor made a speech on sexing and was favourably commented at the International poultry farmers meeting held in Berlin.

After the meeting he went over to England to see and test the apparatus.

He seems to have found it far from satisfactory. At any rate, five Japanese sexers are now busy sexing in England and thirteen more left here a month ago to meet the demand in England. They will stay there till the spring of 1937, I hear.

I am also told that some other countries are asking the Japanese association to send some sexers.

If the apparatus you bought does not serve your purpose well, I hope you will get for me an entry permit and employ me as usual. I have refused a favourable offer from an employer as I am bound to you by contract, so please take my serious effort into your first consideration.

Expecting your favourable answer,

I am,
Yours sincerely,
Hideo Kataoka

Carter Brothers in 1941 again applied to have Mr Kataoka come to Australia to sex their chickens. Whether he came that year is not clear. However, the continuing argument between the Government and Australian chick sexers and Carter Brothers and William McFarlane of La Pollastre Mammoth Hatchery and Poultry Farm, Pascoe Vale South became academic on 7 December 1941, when the Japanese bombed Pearl Harbor.

Carter Brothers engaged three Australian chick sexers during the war: Hartley Hall, Len Lomas and Don Martin. In 1950 they again tried to engage Japanese chick sexers, but their application never got off the ground as there were ample Australian chick sexers looking for work.

Carter Brothers and William McFarlane together had more chickens sexed by Japanese experts than anyone else in Australia.

Carter Brothers contracted Hideo Kataoka for six years, and they maintained that he made only one error in each brooder of 900 chickens. Carter Brothers had an all white leghorn flock and reared all the chickens sexed each season for their own replacement stock.

It is worthwhile looking at the documentation William McFarlane used to argue for a Japanese chick sexer for the 1940 hatching season, as opposed to engaging Australians to do his chick sexing.

Attached to his letter to the Federal Government asking for approval to again bring out a Japanese chick sexer, was a summary of his experience with Japanese experts for the years 1934–1938.

The letter and the attached summary are reproduced here. In fairness to any Victorian chick sexers Mr McFarlane refers to their names have been deleted.

It must be remembered that he is comparing the skills of the Japanese experts with young Australian students, mostly teenagers or in their early twenties.

Chick sexing had been universally practised in Japan for three to four seasons before their experts came to Australia. Most would have sexed close to a million chickens. Only the very best came to Australia initially.

All the Victorian chick sexers Mr McFarlane refers to had started going to chick-sexing classes only in 1934, and, as his record shows, most Victorian chick sexers got chickens to sex only after the Japanese experts had gone back to Japan, at or near the end of the hatching season.

This takes nothing away from these early Japanese experts. Few of them ever fell below 98 per cent accuracy. Hikosaburo Yogo, Hideo Kataoka, and a later arrival, in Melbourne in 1936, Nobuyoshi Tanaka, were virtually 100 per cent accurate in their commercial sexing. All were fast, as Mr McFarlane states in his letter.

There is no record of chick-sexing speeds for these early Victorian student chick sexers.

Mr McFarlane's letter and documentation:

1st December, 1939

Mr Clinton,
Chief Poultry Expert,
Spring Street,
MELBOURNE C.1.

Dear Sir,

Hereunder please find copy of letter, which I have this day forwarded to the Department of the Interior, Canberra.

Yours Truly,
MANAGER Wm McFarlane

Minister of the Interior, COPY.
CANBERRA. F.C.T. 1st December, 1939
VIC.

Dear Sir,

I hereby make application for the admittance to the Commonwealth, Mr. Shogo Uryu a Japanese Chick Sexer, for a period of 6 months commencing from the 1st June, 1940.

I have indented the same Expert for the last 3 Seasons, and his expert ability as a Sexer, and conduct, has been highly spoken of. Nobody in Victoria can do the work in such a high and satisfactory manner as he can, as numerous local students cannot maintain the speed and accuracy required by large Hatcheries like myself, and Messrs. Carter Bros., Werribee.

I would like you to make this matter urgent, so that I may communicate the result by letter, as owing to the consent being held up, and given to me late each Season, I have been compelled to use the Cables to transact the business, and the brevity of calling does not fully explain everything, besides the additional expense.

I am,
Yours Truly,
MANAGER Wm McFarlane

Poultry Branch,
Live Stock Division.

21st June, 1939.

SUPERINTENDENT OF LIVE STOCK.

Re Importation of Japanese Chick Sexers.

Messrs. Wm. McFarlane, Manager, La Pollastre Mammoth Hatchery and Poultry Farm, 233 O'Heas Street, Pascoe Vale South, W.7, and J. Carter, Carter Bros., Werribee, called on me this morning with reference to the question of allowing another Japanese chick sexing expert to come to Victoria, and they informed me as follows:–

Chick sexing classes will be conducted at both of the above establishments, at which Mr. Kataoka, the Japanese expert will attend, and in addition he will be required to sex all the chickens at both places, probably 750,000 chickens for the season. It is considered that the amount of work involved would be too much for one Japanese expert to do, especially as he would have to travel continually between Mr McFarlane's place and Carter Bros farm. It is important that there should be speed and accuracy in this work.

Mr. Kataoka, who has just arrived at Messrs. Carter Bros, farm from Japan, is now laid up with Influenza. This has prevented him from commencing his work and the first batches of chickens will remain unsexed. If this should happen again it would disorganize the whole of the programme for the season.

Mr. Kataoka's duties for the week will be as follow:-

Wm. McFarlane, Pascoe Vale South..

Sunday afternoon and evening, until midnight.

Wednesday evening, until midnight.

Monday and Thursday evenings, chick sexing classes, from 8 p.m. to 10 p.m., and then complete the late sexing, until midnight.

He would not be able to return to Carter Bros, farm until after midnight each visit.

Carter Bros., Werribee.

Four full days.

Saturday afternoon, chick sexing class.

Mr Pederick's report on his visit to Mr McFarlane, Pascoe Vale South, on the 20th instant, is attached.

H. F. Clinton
POULTRY EXPERT.

1934: The first year of sexing introduced by Hideo Kataoka, during his visit he sexed about 5000 for me as a trial or experiment and after his return to Japan, I tried two local students xxx xxxxxx, and another lad working at Sandilands, but the results were very disappointing, both for accuracy and the number of deaths due to bad handling of the chicks.
1935: I had chicks sexed by 3 Japanese experts, Genbe Fukushima, Koje [Koji Kato], Hideo [Kataoka] and Haich [Saichi] Hasegawa, totalling about 80,000 the results would average 98% accuracy, but I think Hasegawa was below par. After their return to Japan I had about 12,000 sexed by x xxxx and his results would be under 90% accuracy. I sent 600 cockerels in one batch to the Victorian Producers from his sexing besides others that I kept on hand and sold privately.
1936: My 3rd year of sexing I had 99,000 sexed by Nobuyoshi Tanaka and his sexing was the best I have ever had, as he did not average one mistake to the 1000. When he returned to Japan I engaged H. Pettigrove of Heidelberg, and he sexed several thousand but I did not keep check on his work that year as he was servicing other hatcheries, and I sold the chickens out although I knew it was below Tanaka's accuracy.
1937: I indented Shogo Uryu and he sexed about 98,000 for me besides sexing about 122,000 for other neighbouring hatcheries, his accuracy was about 99.8 or about one mistake in 500. I reared 12,000 pullets in my yards for 16 cockerels this season. I had one lot sexed by H. Pettigrove to finish up this season. I also conducted a class and gave private tuition here besides private examinations. I gave special tuition to a young lady from Tasmania, every day for a fortnight, but she could not grasp the idea at all. I gave numerous special lessons to a young man from Sydney, who failed in the Sydney examinations and was sitting in the Melbourne examinations in which he failed also. I gave a special test to the elder, Miss xxxxxx, who showed 95% for 300 chicks, but Shogo Uryu showed her that on a certain class of chick she had no idea how to sex these difficult ones, and her accuracy would depend on the number of this class of chicks that she sexed in this grouping per 100.

Seeing that Shogo could resex the chickens which is not the easiest after a student, and pick out 15 mistakes in 300 which she killed and certified as absolutely correct in the presence of her father and myself and she remarked that his sexing was marvellous.
1938: I again indented Shogo Uryu and this season he sexed 122,000 for me besides 198,000 for 8 other hatcheries. I had about 15,000 sexed by Harry Pettigrove after Mr Uryu's return to Japan . . . Shogo Uryu also conducted a class twice weekly and gave tuition to 10

different students but none could obtain above 85%.

[The rest of the document is taken up with examples of sexing errors from other Victorian chick sexers, the errors claimed range from 27 cockerels in 200 white leghorn chickens to some Rhode Island Red chickens purchased from another hatchery and there were 10 per cent to 20 per cent errors.]

One of the names referred to in Mr McFarlane's document did become a successful commercial chick sexer, as did Mr Pettigrove. Other names he referred to who sexed chickens in other hatcheries did not last more than one or, at the most, two seasons. In the examinations conducted by Farm and Pastoral their accuracy was below 90 per cent.

New South Wales

Commercial chick sexing was launched in New South Wales on Monday 8 June, 1934. Mr Hikosaburo Yogo arrived in Sydney on 15 June, and those hatcherymen who were associated with Mann and Gamble Pty Ltd were ready and waiting to have their chicks sexed.

During the first week an average of about 2000 chicks a day were sexed. During the next four weeks the numbers steadily increased to 4000 and 5000 chicks a day. By the time another two weeks had passed, Mr Yogo was not able to cope with the demand for his services.

His time had been allocated to a particular group of hatcheries on set days each week, and at approximately the same time each week, assuring the hatcheries involved of a maximum number of chicks which could be safely booked.

Mr Yogo had sexed 10 000 chicks in one day in America, but 5000 was considered a fair day's work, and 300 000 chicks was considered the maximum for one expert in a four-month season.

A series of public demonstrations were held in and around Sydney.

This extract from an American poultry journal of 1933 could equally apply to Mr Yogo's commercial chick-sexing performances in New South Wales: ''While Mr Yogo's successful demonstrations were excellent in showing the extreme accuracy and speed with which chick sexing could be done by a first-class expert of [Mr] Yogo's calibre, the practical work done for the hatcheries was still more convincing. The star example was at the Bolivar Hatcheries, where 25 000 chicks were sexed by [Mr] Yogo in four days. A check of these birds at five and six weeks revealed only 30 cockerel chicks out of one large lot of 11 800 pullets, or an error of less than one-third of 1 per cent, or an accuracy of 99.7 per cent, which is incredibly high. In the case of cockerels, the error was less than 1 per cent. It is reported that one poultryman who purchased 2000 sexed cockerel chicks and expected to do well on the deal wasn't so enthusiastic about it when he finally counted all of the pullets which he could find.''

After 1936 all commercial chick sexing in New South Wales was done by Australian chick sexers.

Queensland

In 1934 Mr Kioshi Ozawa visited Queensland and conducted the first classes in chick sexing there. In 1935, another independent operator, Mr Suzuki, came to Brisbane to continue the classes.

In 1936 the Japan Association sent Mr Koji Kato to Brisbane to sex chicks and to conduct classes. In 1935 Mr Kato worked in Sydney. After this third year all chick sexing in Queensland was done by Australian chick sexers.

Australia

INDIVIDUAL HISTORIES

Three generations of Australian chick sexers

Historians love dividing time into different periods: the Stone Age, the Middle Ages, the Renaissance and so on. While these divisions do help to record events and people in an orderly way they have limited validity. There are always many exceptions. One period overlaps into another, and sometimes a historian's bias can blur these imposed divisions.

And so it has been here, in my attempt to bring some kind of order into these individual histories of Australian chick sexers.

Most of the men and women written about in the following pages have spread their careers over what I have termed two generations, several have even worked into part of the third generation.

Nevertheless, these divisions of the past sixty years of commercial chick sexing into three generations, I hope, have helped make clearer some of the changes which have taken place in each generation of chick sexers.

To be classified as a first generation, a sexer must have either learnt the skill from the first Japanese who came to Australia in the 1930s, or have started commercial chick sexing by 1939.

For a second-generation chick sexer label an operator needs to have learnt after the Second World War and up to the early 1950s, with most of their chick sexing done from the mid-1940s to the late-1950s.

The third generation category are those who learnt anytime from the mid-1950s onwards.

FIRST GENERATION 1934–1945

After the Japanese bombed Pearl Harbor in 1941 all commercial chick sexing in Australia was done by Australians.

In Victoria, Hartley Hall, Len Lomas and Don Martin took over the chick sexing at Carter Brothers of Werribee which had formerly been done by Hideo Kataoka. Hartley Hall spent one day a week in Bendigo sexing for several small farms, as well as sexing commercially for other farms and hatcheries around Melbourne, including his father's hatchery in Heidelberg.

Don Martin worked around Werribee and Len Lomas did work around Geelong and other country areas when not sexing for Carter Brothers.

Other first-generation commercial chick sexers were: Eric Marchant (brought down from Sydney by Clark King and Co to sex chickens for their Multiplo Incubator clients) Harry Pettigrove, Wally Millington, Charlie Bode, H. A. Jenkins, Keith McLister and Mrs D. Jeremiah.

There were other men and women who learnt chick sexing during this period and who sexed commercially for several years, but for this study only those who passed the various government chick-sexing examinations or sexed chicks for a decade or longer have been included.

Keith McLister did not sex commercially but worked at his father's hatchery at Spotswood. He later held chick-sexing classes, as did Harry Pettigrove and Charlie Bode, at their hatcheries at Box Hill and Research respectively.

Until the advent of the "machine" method of sexing in the mid-1950s only one student ever gained a special-class chick-sexing certificate in Victoria from these classes. Five others gained first-class certificates and three second-class certificates.

It was little wonder that Victoria was often short of chick sexers and this is why "machine" chick sexing was so readily adopted by new students in the mid-1950s and early 1960s, particularly to meet the demand for the sexing of broiler chicken.

FIRST-GENERATION VICTORIANS

Hartley Hall, Victoria's first chick sexer 1934

After Hideo Kataoka gave his first chick-sexing demonstration in Victoria in 1934, Seth Thomas James Hall, a true entrepreneur and proprietor of the hatchery where this demonstration was held, in St Heilers Road, Heidelberg could see the advantages of being able to offer his customers day-old pullets instead of unsexed chickens.

He had a 16 000-capacity Petersime incubator and hatched approximately 4000 chickens a week at that time, one of the largest hatcheries in the State.

Seth Hall had no doubts about the Japanese sexers' ability or the potential of being able to offer his customers day-old pullets. Seth Hall's true entrepreneur's spirit also saw the potential of sexing other farmer's chickens. Australia was still going through the Depression.

Seth's eldest son, Hartley, was attending Scots College, Melbourne. At sixteen, Hartley Hall's comfortable school days were about to end.

Hartley was brought home to work in the hatchery and learn chick sexing from Hideo Kataoka, after the Japanese expert had finished sexing his father's chickens each week. The young Hartley was one of Mr Kataoka's most successful students in that first year. Mr Kataoka could not speak English very well, but language was never a problem with any of the Japanese experts in their teaching: they showed rather than talked. Also, as their accuracy was almost 100 per cent, a student did not learn their teacher's mistakes, as well as making a few of their own.

In the 1930s the hatching of chickens was a seasonal event, starting in June and finishing in the second week of October, with peak hatchings in August and September.

Hartley Hall had been having lessons from Hideo Kataoka for six weeks when Mr Kataoka decided to return home to Japan early. In the 1930s ships to Japan were less frequent than today's aircraft.

Poor Seth Hall! He had accepted orders for thousands of day-old pullets from his customers. There were still six weeks to go before his hatching season was finished. Turning to his son, Hartley, Seth's optimism again came to the fore. "Well, mate, we'll have to do something about this."

Hartley Hall was to relate many years later: "It really put the pressure on me. In some ways it was good for me. I had to stick at it. Many times I had a quiet cry by myself. I made many mistakes. But I survived and went on. The old man was happy and so were the customers. I gradually mastered the art and in 1937–38 season sexed exclusively for a large chicken hatchery in England. I would have gone back the next season but the War prevented this."

When asked why he never obtained a government chick-sexing certificate Hartley replied: "By the time the Victorian Government started holding chick-sexing examinations in 1938 I was up and running and saw no point in sitting for the government chick-sexing exams. The Japanese didn't sit for the [Victorian] exams."

Hartley's father had had a slight disagreement with the Agriculture Ministry about some other matter and this could have had some influence on Hartley's decision not to sit for the examinations.

There is no doubt about Hartley Hall's reputation as an accurate commercial chick sexer. The fact that he sexed commercially for a little over twenty years without his name being on the government list of chick sexers speaks for itself.

It is also interesting to note that Hartley Hall and his father developed a technique where it was not necessary to evacuate the cloaca before examining the chick's vent.

He did this by placing his right forefinger across the intestine to close it off, near where it enters the cloaca. This closing of the intestine prevented the excreta from blocking his view of the folds and eminence.

Hartley Hall's first chick-sexing client after his father's chicks in 1934 was A. Schulz of Bellview Poultry Farm, 64 Bruce Street, Preston. It was a push-bike trip once a week with his light and his white coat balanced on the handlebars. On wet days or at night it was a bus trip.

Other customers from 1935 to 1938 included Hazeldeen Poultry Farm, Thornbury, Woodburne Poultry Farm, Williams Street, Heidelberg, the Allwhite Poultry Farm with owners George Hodson and son of Preston, and George Simpson's Greenway Poultry Farm, at Tally Ho.

Hall's weekly trips to Bendigo after the war broke out are stories in themselves. Most trips were made in the days of the charcoal-gas producers on cars. On several trips Hartley was forced to sleep on top of the bags of charcoal in the back of his utility—it was a cold hard night's rest before a day sexing chicks.

Many of these first-generation chick sexer's customers developed large businesses as the poultry industry grew in Australia. The now 76-year-young Hartley knows some of the big names in Melbourne's corporate world, men who were only in the "push-bike stage" as he was in the 1930s.

Frank Evans, of Sydney, another 1934 starter, also sexed for and with some of the present-day giants of the poultry industry in Australia.

In 1937, nineteen-year-old Hartley joined three other Victorian chick sexers, Harry Pettigrove, Lloyd Lawson and the "Victorian" from Sydney, Eric Marchant, and did a season's chick sexing in England.

When they arrived in England they worked in pairs: Harry Pettigrove and Lloyd Lawson, and Eric Marchant and Hartley Hall. However, they mostly worked independently.

Just as the original Japanese experts were checked for accuracy when they arrived in Australia, so it was with the four Australians. The first 300 or 400 chicks they sexed were killed and checked for accuracy before they were engaged to do the work.

Lloyd Lawson did not return to Australia. He stayed in Europe and for many years sexed in Belgium.

Hartley Hall continued on with commercial chick sexing until his early forties, when he 'retired' to his poultry farm at Narre Warren. Later, he sold the farm and renewed the Hall relationship with W. S. Kimpton and Sons (Barastoc Products, millers and stock feed manufacturers) as a technical representative, before making golf a full-time occupation.

Charlie Bode—the class of 1934—retired—1983

There at the beginning . . . there at the decline.

Interviewed in November, 1993, Charlie Bode said, "the Japanese had checked every chick I sexed at the test. They killed and examined every chicken. I obtained 97 per cent accuracy. I topped that first exam held by Farm and Pastoral, an event I'll never forget.

"The teacher and examiner was Hideo Kataoka. He was the best. He seldom made a mistake. The Japanese . . . after him were good, but they made 1 or 2 per cent errors. Hideo was the best."

RDM: "You hear how good the Japanese were, but did they make mistakes?"

"Oh, yes, most made one or two errors, even Hideo admitted that he made an odd mistake, but they were good. They made mistakes like everyone else. It's practically impossible to get a 100 per cent. Even today's "machine" sexers do not get 100 per cent accuracy."

RDM: "McFarlane used to say they were 100 per cent accurate."

"No, they made 1 or 2 per cent errors, even this bloke Hideo Kataoka missed an odd one or two in every 200 or 300 chickens."

RDM: "Incubators and chick sexing are the two great advances in the industry, Charlie."

"McFarlane of La Pollastre Mammoth Hatchery in Pascoe Vale was the first to build a big walk-in incubator. He used it in the off season as a refrigerator. Just took the inside out. He knew what he wanted, but the technology wasn't there. His hatches varied. Sometimes he would get a super hatch, other times he would only get a 50 per cent hatch. He couldn't control the humidity. Unlike the Buckeye Incubators, which had a separate hatching department, McFarlane's walk-in machine built up the humidity over the three hatches. I know as much about incubation as I do about sexing chickens.

"I first went to the classes in 1934 held at Farm and Pastoral at 500 Bourke Street in Melbourne. In the class were Lawson, Pettigrove and Jenkins. Their fathers all had hatcheries and Petersime Incubators. I was the only kid getting a quid [$2] a week.

"One of my inspirations was that I worked on a poultry farm: Brinkkotters, Research Poultry Farm. Old man Brinkkotter had a habit of watching you work. One of my tasks was to pick out the cockerels from the pullets when they were a month old.

"Old man Brinkkotter often watched me doing this job. I used to pick up the cockerels as they went past the barrier we had put up, and put them in a box.

"'You'll be an expert chick sexer one day,' he said.

"Brinkkotter was a hard old man. I thought, I must be good if he'll say that. I stuck my chest out.

"Then chick sexing came out, and he said, 'There is a demonstration at Hall's Hatchery in Heidelberg on Saturday afternoon. I'll take you along.'"

Charlie said he could always remember Hideo Kataoka sitting there at the table, with a box of chickens in front of him and an empty box each side of the box of chickens.

"I looked at him. He sexed 100 chickens to show how it was done.

"The first thing that came to my mind was, if you can do them that fast, it is not as hard as it sounds.

"I turned around . . . a penny, a penny, the bells were ringing.

"I went up to Mr J. R. Hall of Farm and Pastoral, no relation to the hatcheryman, the chap who was running the classes, and asked if I could be in the classes.

"I felt he thought: 'Here's another sucker.'

"All the other members of the class were sons of hatcherymen and Petersime Incubator owners and clients of Farm and Pastoral Supplies. I was just the boy coming in.

"I went home. I said to Mum, 'I'm going to learn chick sexing.'

"Mum replied: 'Right! Find the money and away you go.'

"Each Saturday afternoon I went along to Farm and Pastoral to learn. Hideo Kataoka couldn't speak much English.

"In England they were charging [the equivalent of] 2000 dollars to learn chick sexing. In Australia the Japanese had to teach as part of their being allowed to work in here.

"To get chickens to practise on, I rode my push bike to a couple of small farms and sexed their chickens. In 1935 I sexed chickens for McFarlane after [Mr Kataoka] left.

After the classes finished and the examinations held, by Farm and Pastoral in September and October of 1935, Millington, Pettigrove, Lawson and myself were invited in to see Mr J. R. Hall, Managing Director of Farm and Pastoral Supplies.

"Lawson did not turn up. Hall offered us a contract of $40 a week and half a cent a chicken. [The basic wage at that time was the equivalent of $8 a week.]

"They all accepted it, except me. 'What about you, Bode?' 'No thanks.'

"I'll never forget the look on Pettigrove's face, nor forgive [Pettigrove] his remark: 'Of course, we've all go swollen heads.'

"I went around to Clark King's (supplier of poultry equipment and agent for Multiplo Incubators) to buy something. Alan Clark said to me, 'Did you sign the contract?'

"When I said no, he said he would give me the same contract.

"I said: 'No, you won't. You give me the chickens from your Multiplo Incubator customers.'

"So that most of my customers were Multiplo Incubator hatcherymen.

"There was one problem in sexing for Multiplo Incubator customers: they did not have separate hatching departments in their incubators, and to run their machine to capacity they took one batch out and put the next lot of eggs in. As a result, each week the hatches would be on different days. This caused many problems for the chick sexer. Other makes of incubators with separate hatchers did not have this problem. As the industry grew many hatcherymen bought a separate incubator just to hatch in. But not in those early days."

RDM: "When sexing first came out did the hatcherymen ever hesitate about drowning the cockerels?"

"No, they just put them in a bag and away they went. Bang! Finish! That was it!

"I ended up with more business than any of them.

"Millington and Pettigrove were tied up with their contract. They suddenly realised that they were just coming behind [the Japanese] to finish the season when they went home. They weren't able to get out of their contract.

"They still earnt good money. They often only sexed 5000 chickens in a week, but they still got their $40.

"In 1936 Clark King brought down a Sydney sexer, Eric Marchant, to sex for Multiplo customers.

"Many years later another Sydney sexer came to Melbourne to live and work, Fred Wrigley.

"Fred came into a hatchery while I was sexing. Fred looked at me. I said I couldn't stop to talk at the moment as these chickens had to be finished so that they can be sent on the 7 p.m. train. I can talk but I must keep on working.

"Fred said to me, 'Do you mind if I have a look at a box of cockerels?'

"Go right ahead, there's a light down there, get into them.

"Fred was convinced that the cockerels were okay. He later said that he didn't think I was even looking at them.

"He hadn't seen too many fast sexers.

"After a five-year break from chick sexing in the 1940s I spent ten years sexing in Tasmania. Then after another five or six years away from chick sexing I started again in Victoria and retired when I was 67, which was in 1983.

"How I got started again in Victoria was Noel Hargraves asked me to sex for him while he was on holiday in England. While he was in England he died. I kept on with his clients until one by one they went out of business. The last one I sexed for was Brinkkotters of Research Poultry Farm, run by the sons and grandsons of the man who first inspired me into the art of chick sexing those many years ago.

"That's it . . . I've had a good life . . . Had four kids, two girls and two boys. They all have university degrees and I own those units out the back."

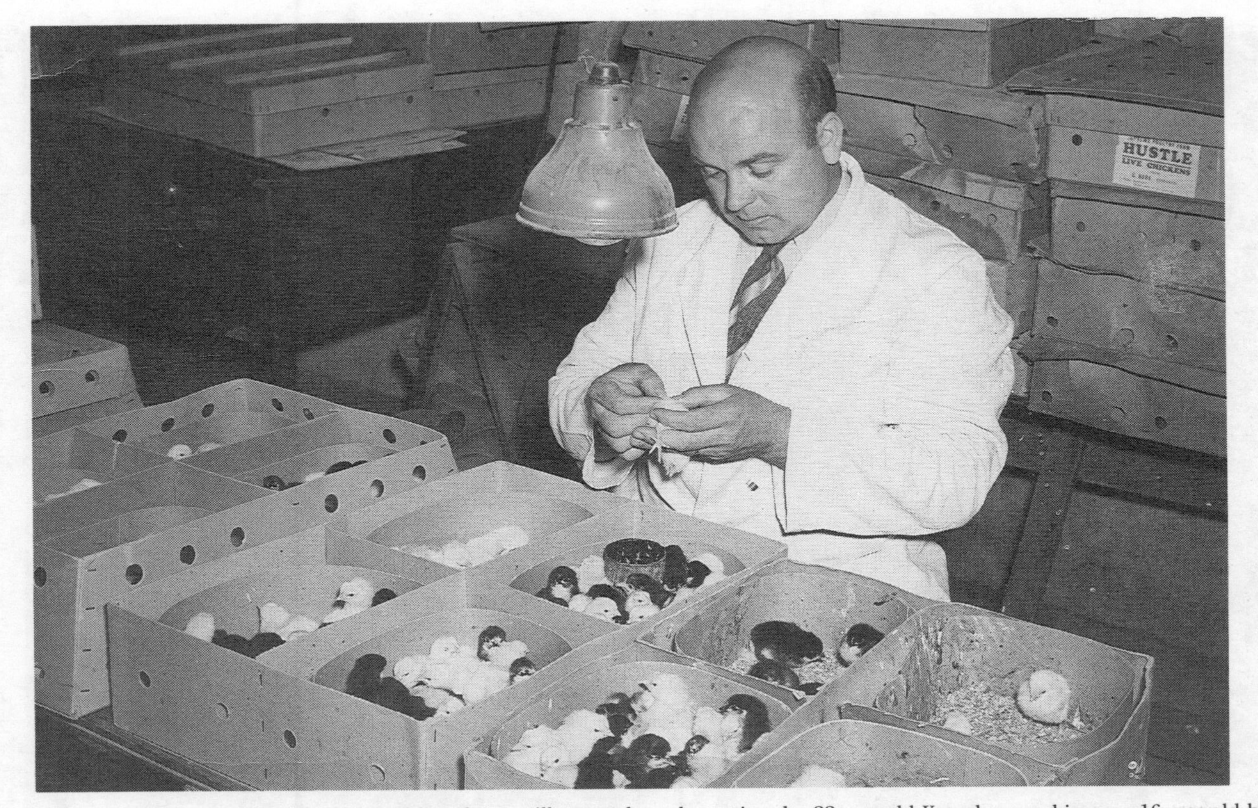

Charlie Bode, one of Hideo Kataoka's most devoted students, still remembers the praise the 22-year-old Kataoka gave him as a 16-year-old boy.

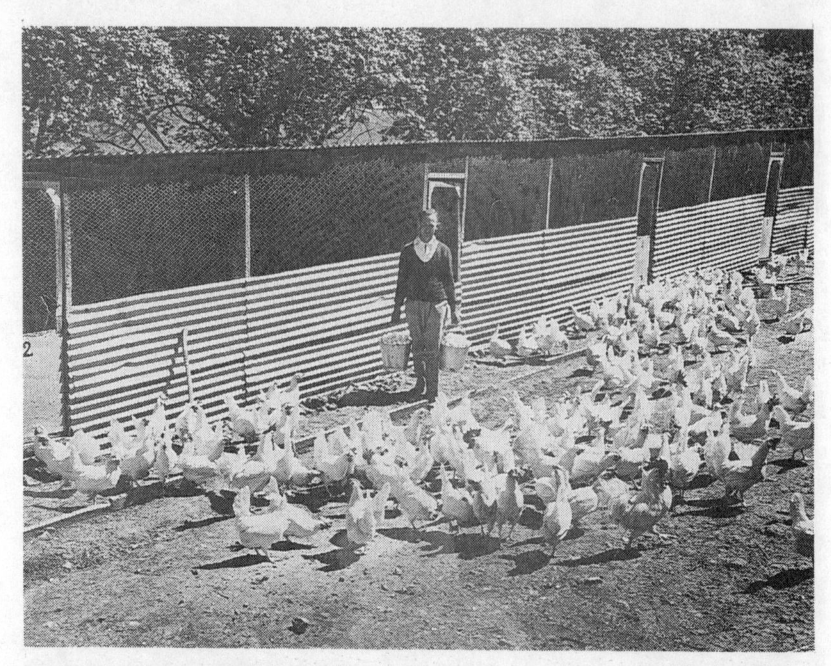

Charlie Bode's white leghorn breeders 1945.

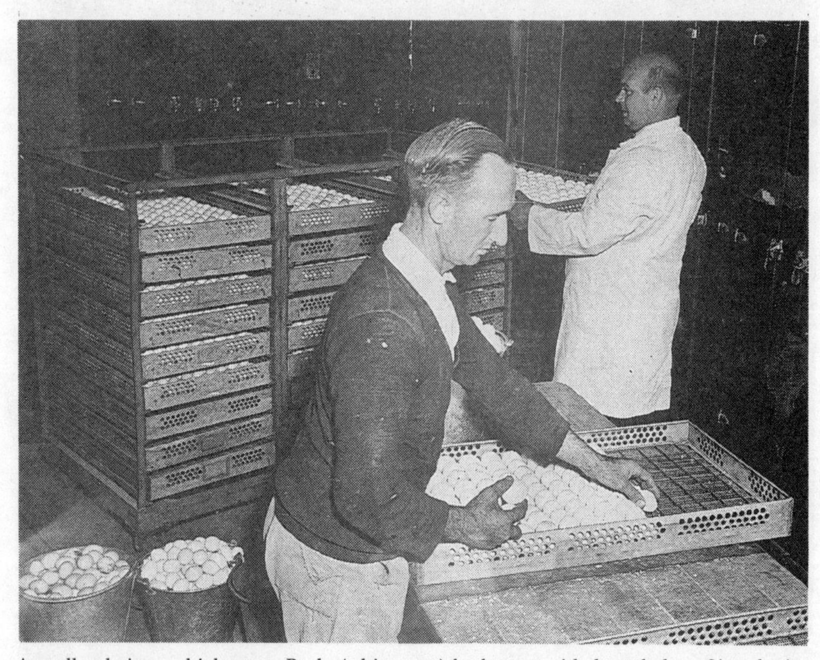

As well as being a chick sexer, Bode (white coat) had a very wide knowledge of incubation problems. Here he is loading eggs into his Multiplo incubator before chick-sexing classes begin. His helper, Les, has a handful of eggs.

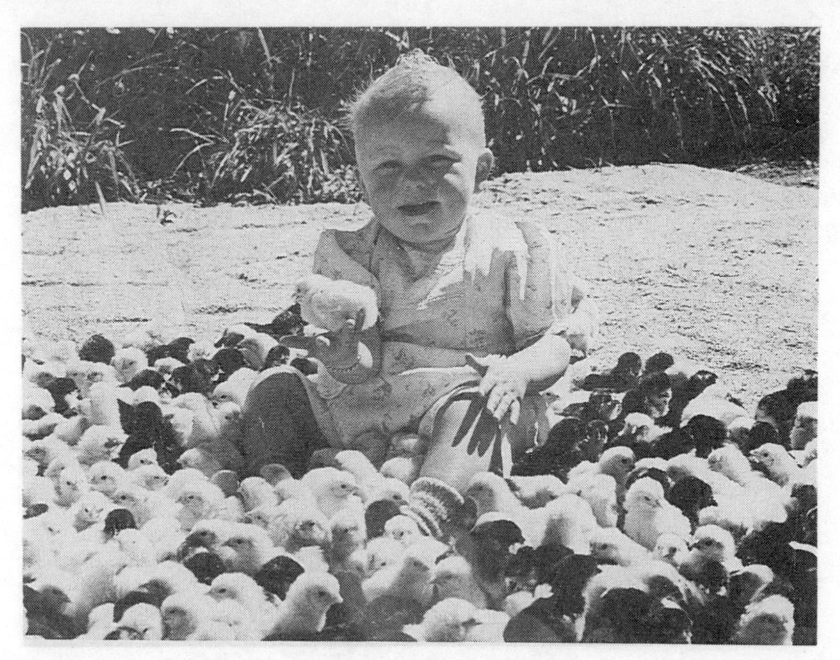

Charlie Bode's daughter, Annette, gets among the chicks.

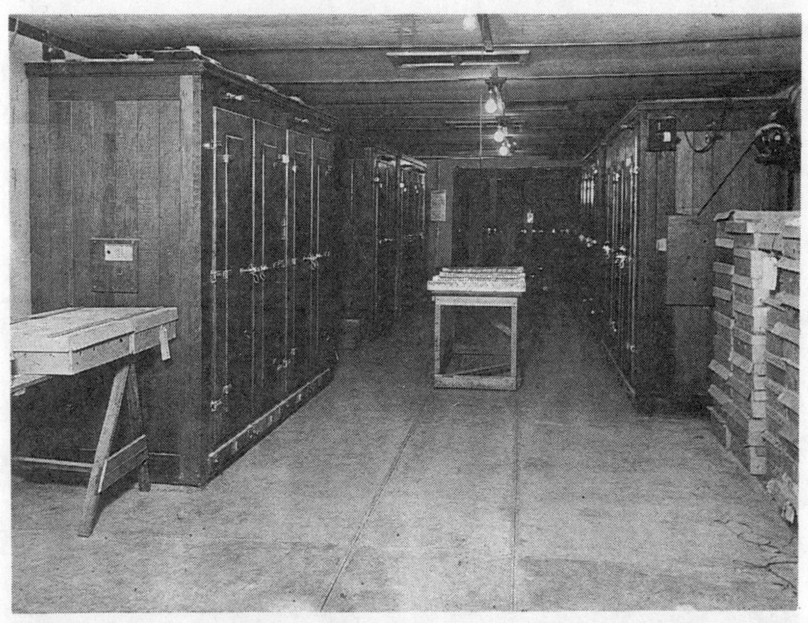

Where it all began for many second-generation Victorian chick sexers. Classes were held each Tuesday evening and Saturday afternoons from June till October, 1940.

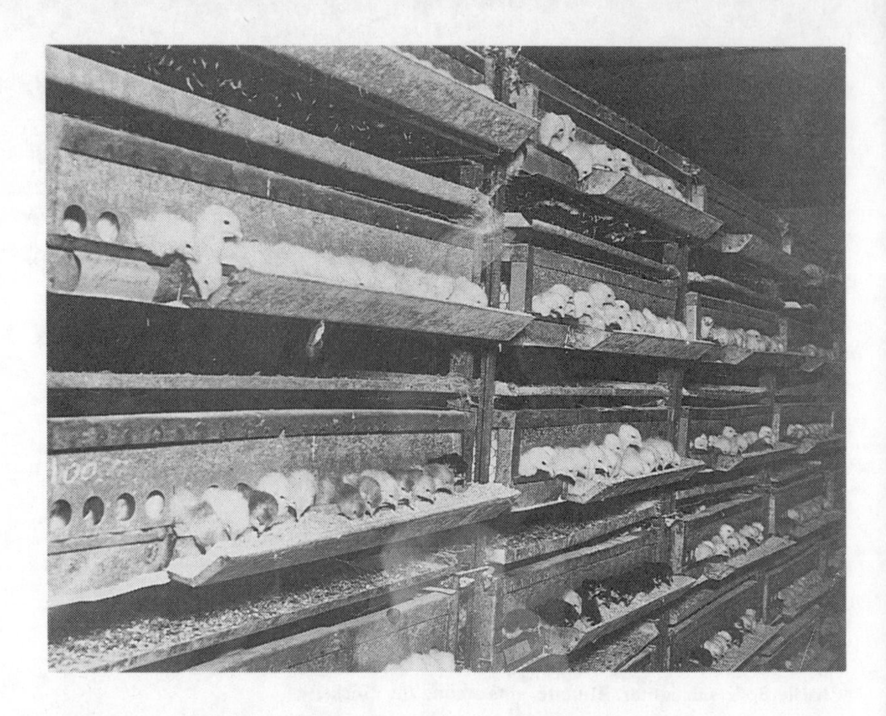

Charlie Bode, chick sexer, often said to his former student Bob Martin, ''we were ahead of our time''. Some of CB's self-made battery brooders.

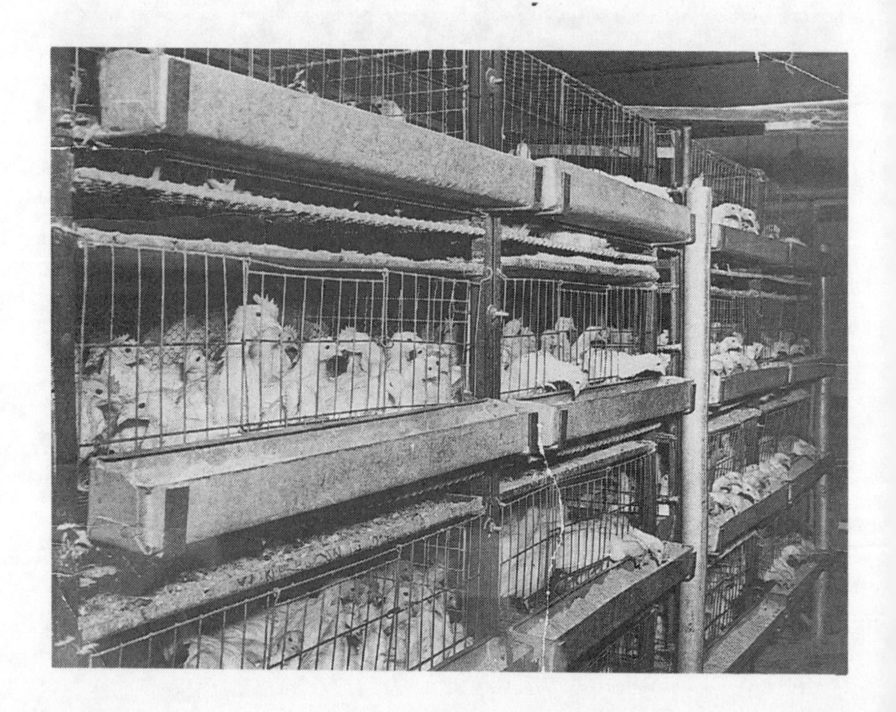

Eric Marchant 1935 Sydney to Melbourne

Another prominent first-generation chick sexer, Eric Marchant, continued to sex chickens commercially in Victoria until the late 1950s. He was a very colourful figure as well as a very accurate and reliable chick sexer. He was not above having an odd drink, but there is no documentation of this pastime ever interfering with his professional conduct or accuracy. There are many stories of his turning up at a hatchery very relaxed, at the end of a long day, but his accuracy never seems to have suffered. He was held in high regard by his fellow chick sexers as well as by his large clientele.

Most days Eric Marchant was accompanied by an assistant who fed unsexed chickens to him and counted and boxed the chicks he had sexed. The assistant also took his turn at driving.

With this first generation of commercial chick sexers several adopted this practice. Others had a counter and a boxer supplied by the hatcheryman. The only time this first generation worked alone was late at night or very early in the morning. At most farms and hatcheries the farmer was glad to help as it was a time to hear the latest news and gossip from other farms. Some chick sexers visited up to seventeen farms in a week.

When Fred Wrigley came down from Sydney in the mid 1940s to start his chick-sexing career, he used to complain that every farm or hatcheryman he approached for work seemed to have their chickens sexed by Eric Marchant.

Even Eric Marchant's exit from the ranks of chick sexers was not without its colour. He "died" several times.

One of his former customers, Gerry Grenville, of Spring Vale was in his hatchery relating Eric Marchant's death in Sydney to one of his associates when in walked Eric, very much alive.

Whenever a group of chick sexers get together the question of Eric's demise or otherwise always comes up.

The fact of his death was being accepted at a meeting of chick sexers in the 1980s, until a third-generation chick sexer claimed he had had dinner with Eric recently at a Golden Poultry Farms Reunion.

VICTORIA SECOND GENERATION 1946–1965

The Golden Age of Commercial Chick Sexing

These first-generation chick sexers were joined by a second generation in the mid 1940s. These included Fred Wrigley, a student of Frank Evans, from Sydney, Max Akam, a student of Keith McLister's, Bob Martin, a student of Charlie Bode, and Noel Hargreaves, a student of Harry Pettigrove.

As well, L. J. Smith, A. Hewett, A. Bradshaw, Miss Bruce, Ernie Bourbaud and Miss Jackson all did commercial chick sexing for several years,

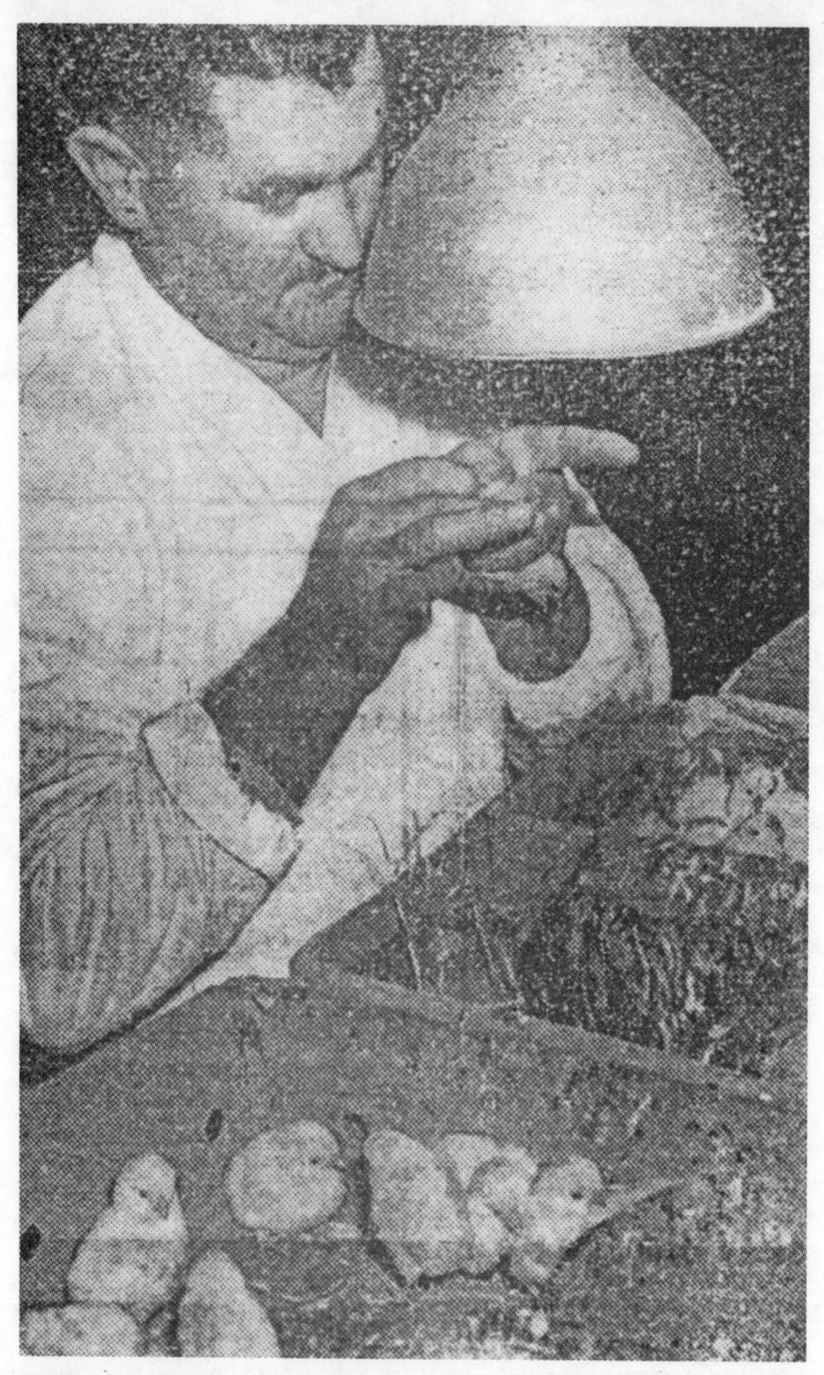

Eric Marchant, a student of the 1935 class of NSW who moved to Victoria in 1938. A leading Victorian chick sexer for many years.

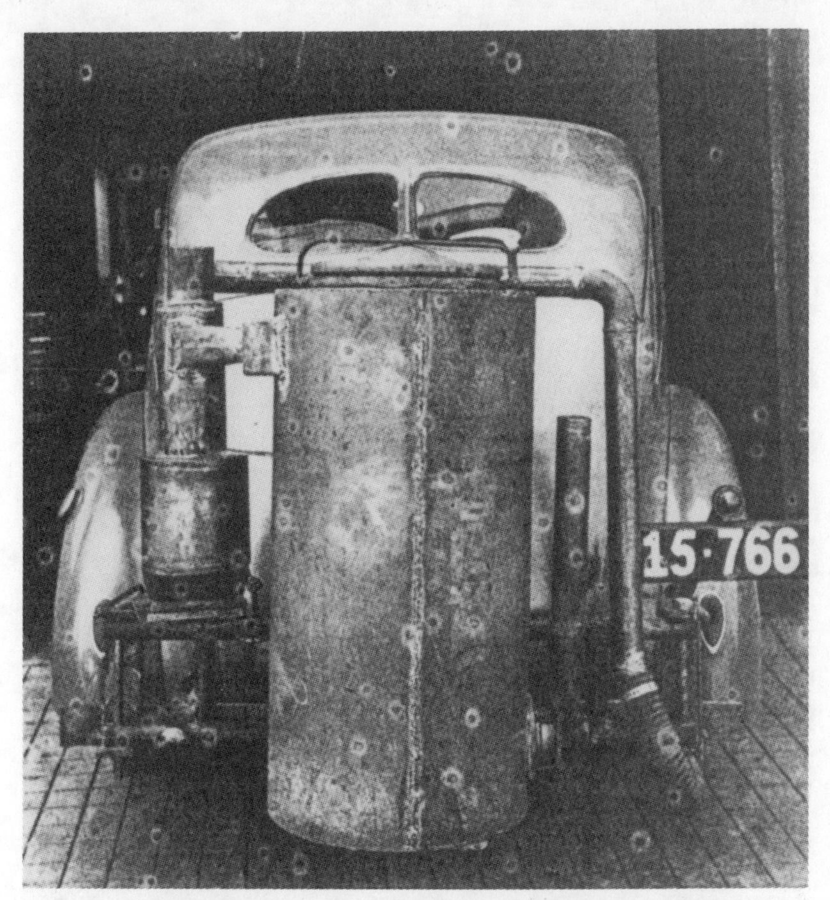

A chick sexer's nightmare: the coke gas producer, a wartime measure to save fuel.

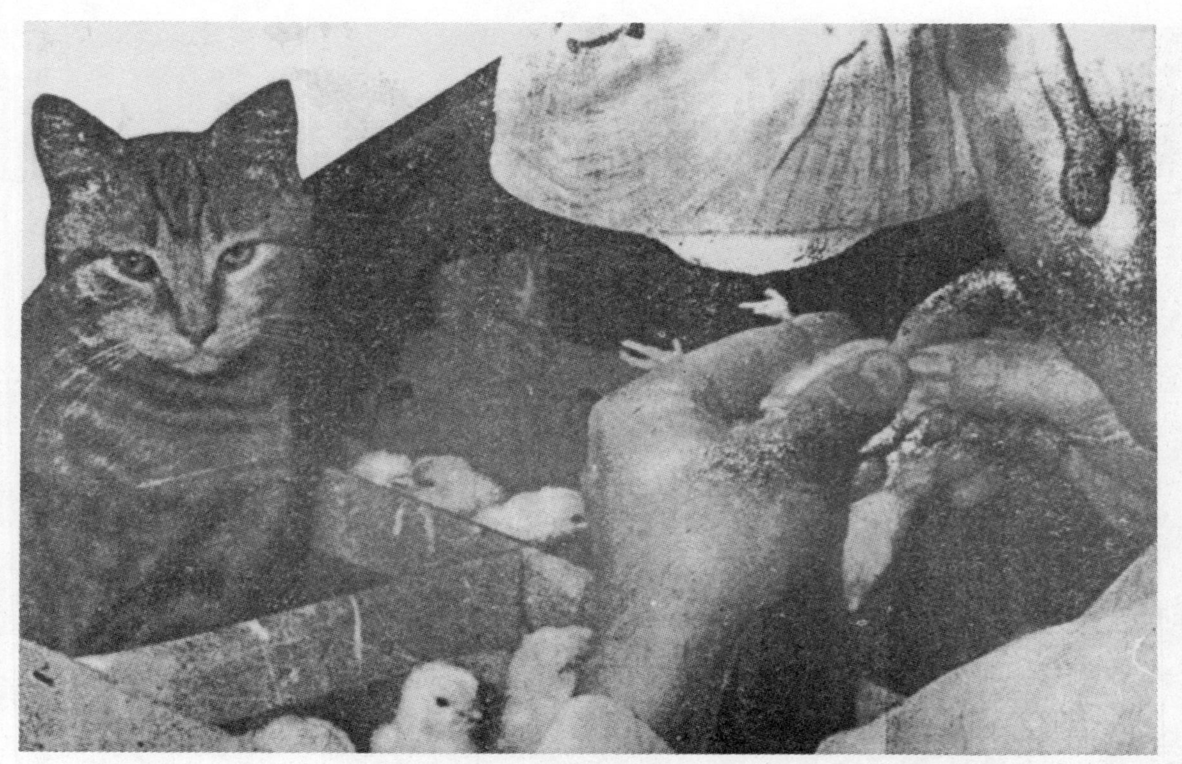

Keith McLister, a 1935 student of Hideo Kataoka, sexing chicks at his father's hatchery. The cat, Tabby, looks on.

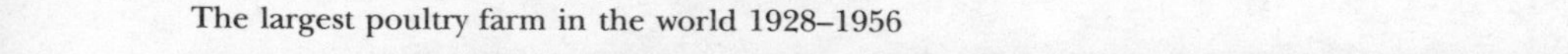

Carter Brothers of Werribee, Victoria. Australia.
The largest poultry farm in the world 1928–1956

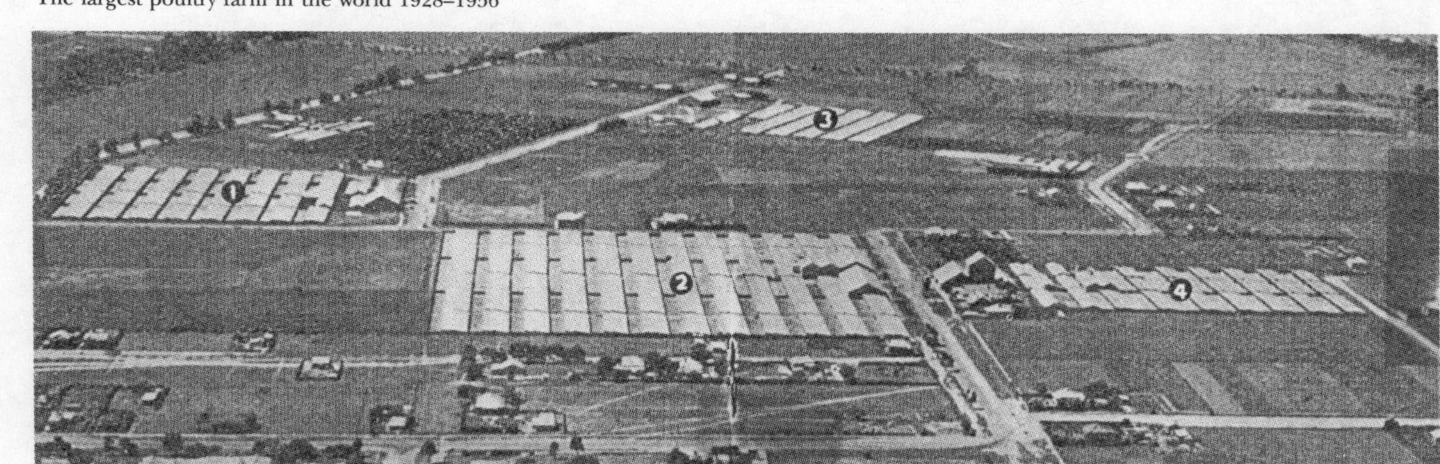

(1) Roland Carter's farm (60 000) birds (3) John Carter's farm (60 000) birds (4) the original property and (2) later extensions of the farm owned by James and Walter Carter (130 000 birds). The total number of birds on the three farms was approximately 250 000 birds, all white leghorns.

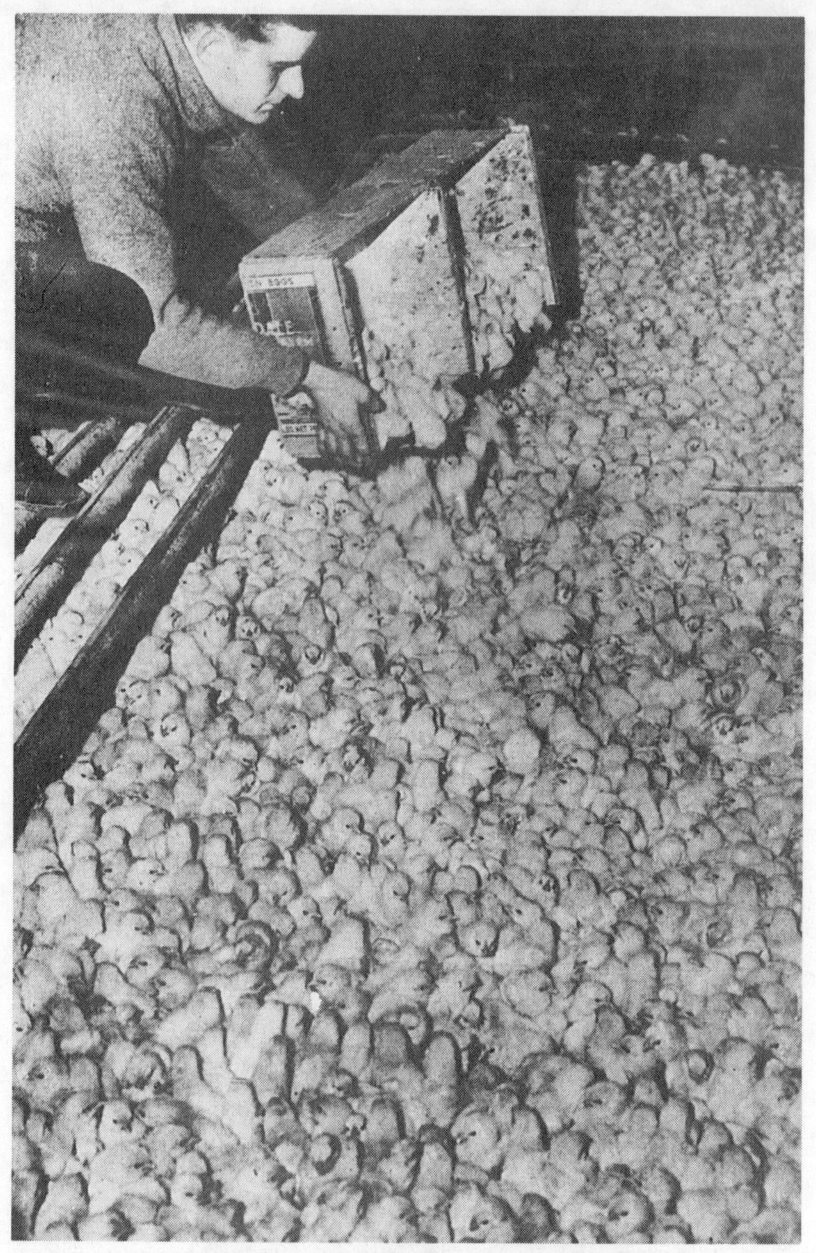

Thousands of newly hatched day-old chicks waiting to be sexed at Carter Brothers Farm, Werribee. Walter Carter Junior is assisting the chick sexer on this occasion. c 1952.

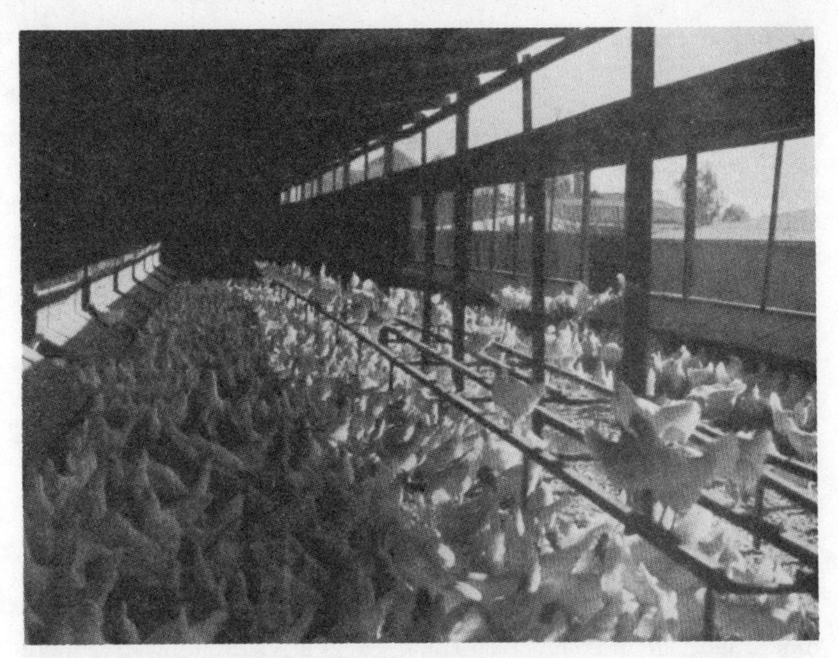

Carter Brothers of Werribee, once the world's largest poultry farms. An all white leghorn flock of 250 000 birds. Now a suburb of Melbourne.

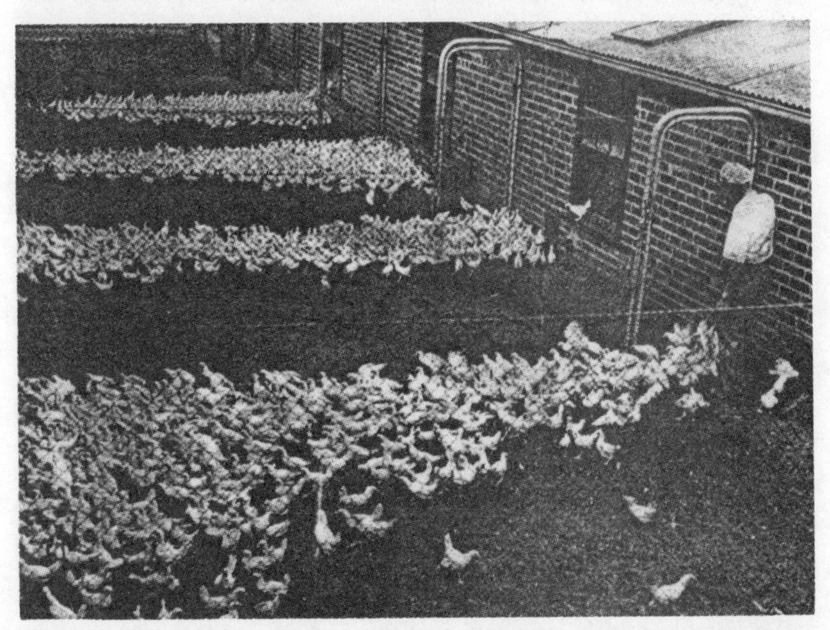

Carter Brothers' rearing yards made it easy for a chick sexer to check his accuracy as Carters kept good records of everything and did not sell any chicks hatched. The cockerels were disposed of after sexing.

but never reached the numbers of chickens sexed, or stayed at it for as many years as some of their colleagues of this second generation, or the first generation.

Jack Whyte, who learnt chick sexing when he was stationed in Japan after World War II, took on commercial chick sexing in the 1950s. He later changed to the "machine" method of sexing.

Ron Mason and Herb Burchall worked as commercial chick sexers in Bendigo.

Herb Burchall, then of Coburg, and Tony Martino, of Horsham, were the last two students to qualify using the vent method in Victoria. They both learnt from the chick-sexing classes conducted by the Victorian Hatcherymen's Society in 1955. At these classes Keith McLister was the Chief Instructor, helped by Fred Wrigley, Max Akam, Bob Martin, Noel Hargreaves and Jack Whyte.

Most of the first batch of "machine" sexers were students from this class. They decided to opt for the easier-to-learn new technique, rather than the slower, and less certain of success, vent method. Tony Martino later changed from the "machine" method to the vent method, gaining a special-class certificate on both methods. There was at that time a shortage of commercial chick sexers in Victoria. By 1970 there were only three vent sexers operating around Melbourne and eight "machine" sexers. There were others of both methods sexing commercially in other areas of Victoria.

There were other chick sexers in both the first and second generations who sexed commercially, but as they did not have government chick-sexing certificates their career paths were not as well known, nor so easy to trace. Many of them did not stay in the industry for long. An exception was Les Tait, who was a successful commercial chick sexer for over 30 years.

Herb Burchall "retired" after 15 years of chick sexing and bought a sheep property. He was always a person who knew where he was going: he learnt chick sexing when he was in his late twenties, after being a turner and fitter for a decade. He took on chick sexing, he said, because he wanted to buy a sheep property.

Ron Mason was taught by Les Tait, another chick sexer who worked in the Bendigo area. Although Tait was never successful in gaining a government chick-sexing certificate, Mason, his student, was, and is a very accurate chick sexer. He still (1994) sexes one day a week in Bendigo. Mason is one of the three chick sexers still sexing in Australia who holds the chick by the Suzuki method: the legs away from the sexer's body.

Mr Kataoka was the only Japanese sexer who came to Australia to use this method of holding the chicks. Apart from the three Australians, there are a handful of sexers in Japan and some Japanese-American chick sexers in the United States using this method of holding the chick.

Including the Suzuki method there are four methods of holding the chick.

The years 1949 to the mid 1960s were undoubtedly the Golden Age for commercial chick sexers in Australia.

Unlike most of the first generation, they were not tied to contracts by incubator manufacturers. Hatcheries were bigger, and centred around rail centres or egg-producing areas, which meant less time spent travelling.

Improvement in feeding of breeding stock, and bigger and better incubators went towards producing higher and more predictable hatch numbers. Also, all egg producers demanded day-old pullet chicks. The chick sexer was essential to the industry.

Another hazard this second generation did not have to cope with was transport difficulty. Many first generation started their careers on push bikes, but even when they graduated to motor vehicles, many had to face having a charcoal-gas producer fitted to their vehicle during the war. What monsters they were!

Second-generation chick sexers did not have Japanese chick sexers to compete against.

Hatching seasons began to be longer in many areas. All this meant more chickens could be handled in a season by individual chick sexers.

Family farms and hatcheries were still the order of the day. Many chick producers built part of their business reputations on the abilities of their chick sexer. This also of course applied to the first generation of chick sexers.

This encouraged individual chick sexers always to work towards maintaining high accuracy. It was still the age of the "Star", and they were known throughout the industry.

It was this generation of chick sexers from New South Wales, Queensland and Western Australia who went overseas to work each year.

This was the generation of independence, not only for chick sexers, but for the hatcherymen and breeders, as it was for most businessmen during this post-war golden age of growth in Australia.

Many commercial chick sexers from the first and second generation "retired" to other business ventures, some growing into large companies.

Nevertheless, many chick sexers worried about threats to their livelihood during this golden age.

The age of the "machine" had arrived—1952

Two New South Wales chick sexers on their return from Belgium were full of enthusiasm for this new faster method of sexing chickens, as far

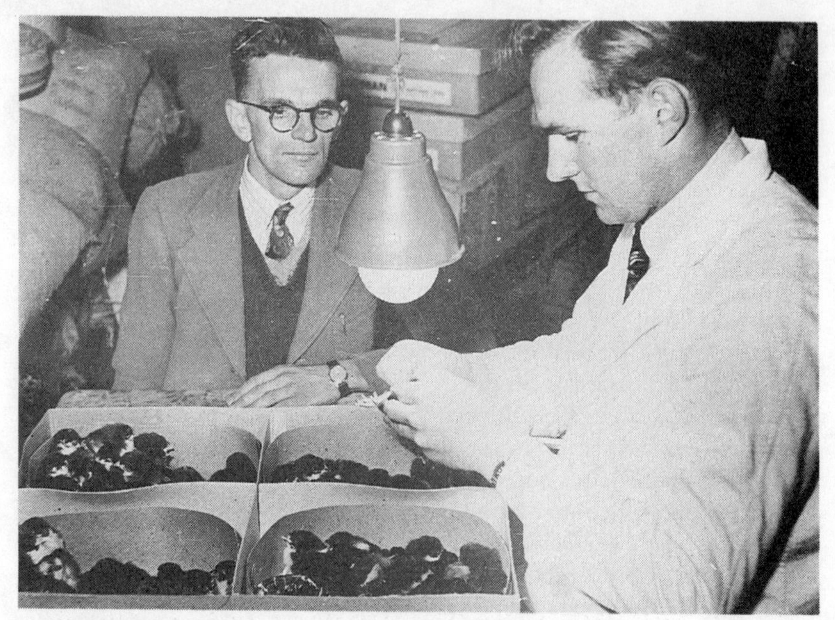

Bob Martin, right, sexing chicks for a New South Wales poultry farmer in 1952. Rod Badman watches.

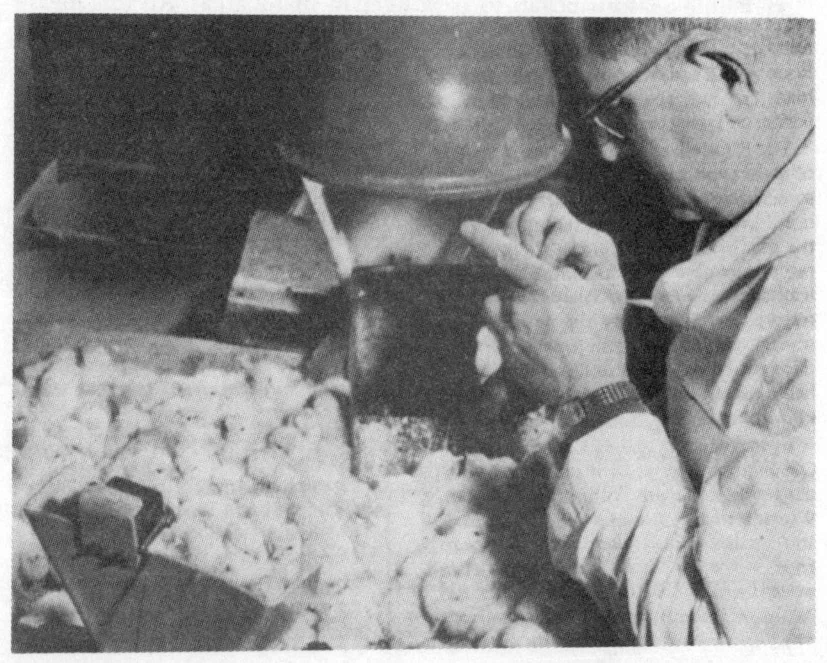

Fred Wrigley, a New South Wales sexer who moved to Victoria, working with his automatic chick counter.

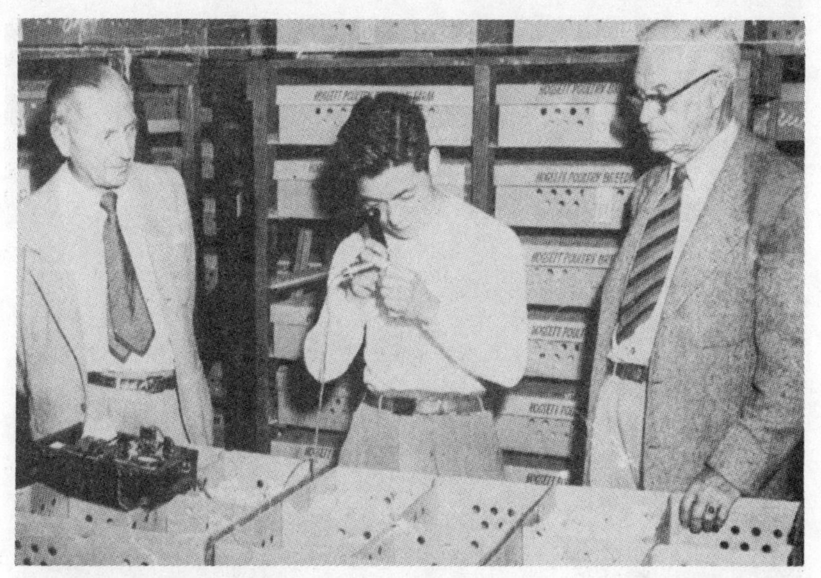

Roy M. Lynnes, publisher of *Poultry Supply World,* left and E. C. Hogsett, right, watch the "Chicktester" machine in commercial practice at Hogsett Poultry Breeding Farm, Pomona, California. The machine is being operated by Tamio Katata, twenty-three-year-old Japanese expert.

Photo courtesy of Poultry World *April 1953*

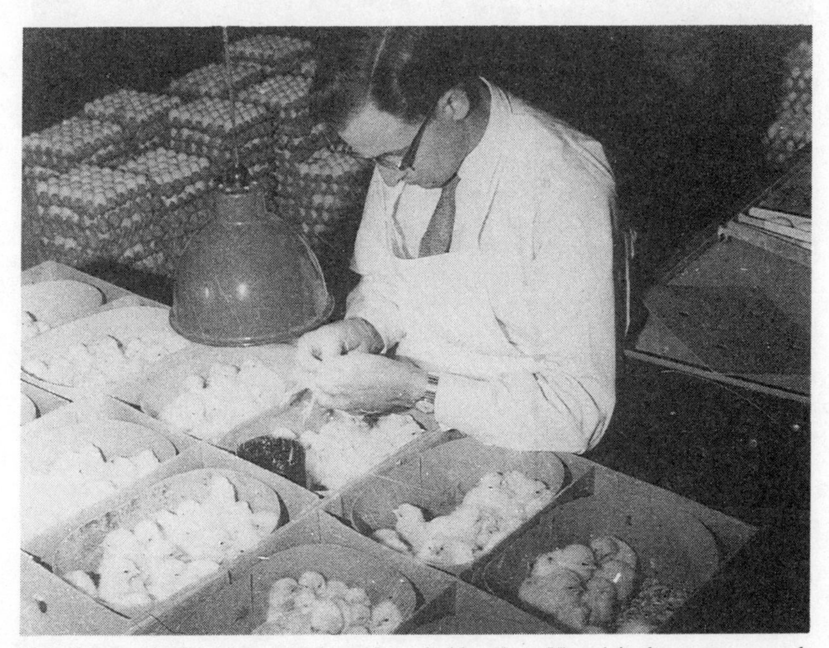

Max Akam, one of the few special-certificate holders from Victoria's cloaca sexers, works away quietly at his task.

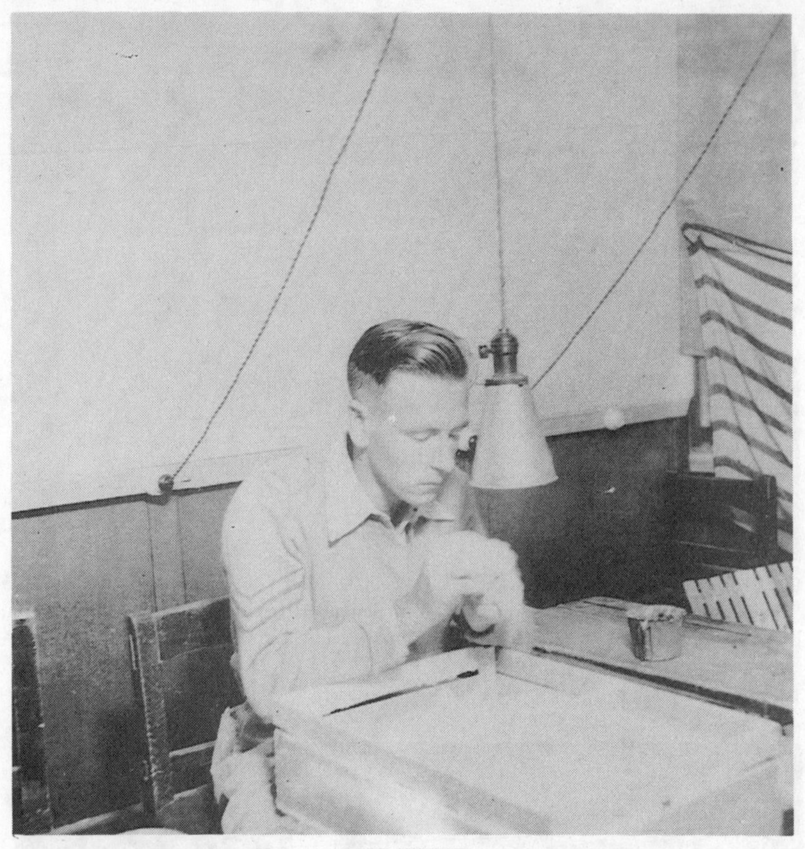

JACK WHYTE

A second-generation Victorian chick sexer learnt the art while he was stationed in Kobe with the British Commonwealth Occupation Force. He was the only commercial chick sexer in Australia who has sexed large numbers of chickens commercially by both methods. In his early forties he changed to the "machine" method and became faster at this method than he had been by the cloaca method.

When asked at an interview why he took on chick sexing he replied that as a city kid he knew nothing about chick sexing, but when stationed in Kobe the Army Education Officer had asked him if he wanted three weeks' leave to attend the chick-sexing school. And so his chick-sexing career begun. He gained 97 per cent accuracy at the final examination conducted by the School. When he returned to Australia he gained a Government first-class certificate at his first attempt.

For more than the next 30 years he made his livelihood solely from chick sexing.

He retired from commercial chick sexing at 58.

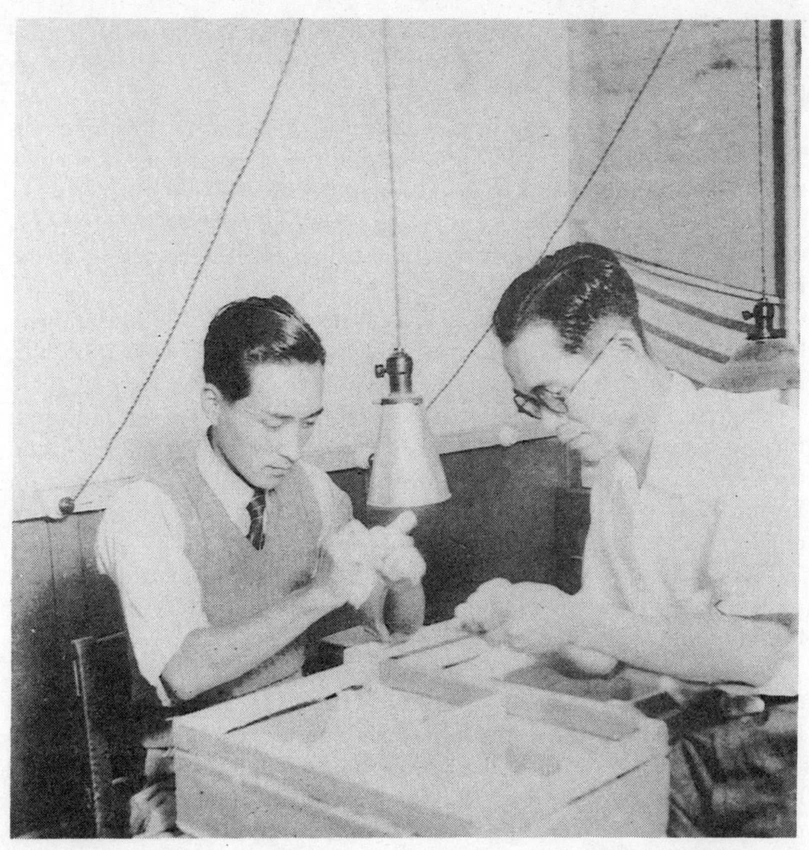

Two Japanese teachers from the Kobe School: an unnamed expert and Koji Kato.
(Both photos taken at the Kobe chick sexing school, 1948)

back as 1949. It was not until the early 1950s that the Japanese optical ("machine") method was introduced to America at Hogsett Poultry Breeding Farm in Pomona.

The Japanese operator of the "Kizawa Chicktester" machine was Tamio Katata, a 23-year-old, with just one year's experience as a chick sexer with the machine. He was compared with the vent (hand) sexer at the farm, Shiro Tanaka, who had been sexing chickens for 19 years, and was known as the dean of chick sexing. Both were sexing at the rate 900 to 1000 chicks an hour.

In Victoria, the first person to have a machine was Bob Martin, who bought a "Chicktester" from the San-ei Sangyo Ltd in Tokyo in 1952. Martin's brother was in Japan and was able to buy it for him.

After corresponding with Mr Hobo-Stepman, a chick sexer and agent for the distributors of the Japanese "Chicktester" in Belgium, Martin used the machine at the farm of one of his client's, Mr Preston, of Spring Vale, on a trial basis. Mr Preston hatched 1200 white leghorn chicks a week. All were sexed by "machine".

The cockerels were found to be 100 per cent accurate, and the pullets varied between 99 and 100 per cent accuracy. Martin never got beyond about 500 chicks an hour.

He did not use the "machine" method at any other farm, until near the time he was to "retire" to his own farm. He then used it to train his replacement chick sexer, John Hammond.

Martin says he did not change to the "machine" method in 1952 because he would have had to drop some of his clients until he could sex chicks with the "machine" at the same speed as he was doing their chicks by vent method.

By changing methods, Martin concedes that with some white leghorns his clients would have gained an improvement in accuracy of 2 to 3 per cent, but like most chick sexers who have used both methods, he would rather use the vent (hand) method.

Martin also says he was never worried about the "machine" taking over the work of the hand sexers. All it did was put further emphasis on hand sexers to increase their accuracy and speed. However, the "machine" did discourage future chick sexing students from persevering in learning the harder-to-learn vent method.

With the introduction of "machine" sexing in the 1950s, it was generally thought that this easier to learn, and almost "guaranteed" ability to sex with 100 per cent accuracy, and its greater speed, would result in an over-supply of commercial chick sexers, and that the livelihood of hand chick sexers would be finished.

This did not happen. Most vent chick sexers were more than able to hold their own with "machine" chick sexers.

Most commercial chick sexers of this generation "retired" to other business interests, but several remained commercial chick sexers into their late sixties.

Another "worry" Fred Wrigley had was that feather sexing would finish chick sexing as an occupation. Fred was sexing chickens at a hatchery which the Victorian Principal Poultry Officer, Bill Stanhope, was visiting and the talk got around to feather sexing.

Feather sexing had been around since the 1920s, long before the Japanese developed the technique of vent sexing. Feather sexing is based on the breeding of a fast-feathering strain of bird, and a strain of slow-feathering birds. When these two strains are mated, the offspring have fast-feather pullets and slow-feather cockerels (or it can be the reverse depending on the breeding), so that at day old it is relatively easy to separate the cockerels from the pullets.

On this particular day, Bill Stanhope told Fred Wrigley that he could easily sex the day-old cross chicks which Fred was vent sexing. Bill took a box of unsexed chicks and off he went.

When he had finished, he gave Fred 20 cockerels to check, they were all correct, and among the 30 pullets Fred checked, there were only two cockerels. Fred Wrigley was really worried, until Bill showed him the box still with the 30 per cent of the chicks which he could not distinguish by feather sexing. Another worry out of the way.

Some crossbreeds have always had some trait of feather sexing, but not soundly established. It takes a large breeding program to have it firmly established.

Disease

In the 1960s in Victoria there was an outbreak of *salmonella typhi-murium* at several hatcheries. The source of the infection could not be traced by the Agricultural Ministry's scientists and veterinarians.

Bill Stanhope knew all the hatcheries with the outbreak, on a personal level. He also knew the one thing they had in common: their chick sexer.

When Bill Stanhope approached the chick sexer, the gentleman in question was very indignant, protesting that he showered every morning and had a clean dustcoat every day.

Here it needs to be noted that many vent sexers let a thumbnail or one of their fingernails grow longer, so that they could use it to manipulate the chicken's vent quickly and easily. In this particular incident, it was found that the infection was under the chick sexer's nail.

There was a similar incident with another second-generation sexer, who had switched to the "machine" method. He was easily traced, and it was found that he had not disinfected his instrument thoroughly.

As a result of these incidents, the Ministry recommended that all chick sexers leave their dust coats at the hatchery and take more care in sterilising anything that they used from one hatchery to another.

Many chick sexers brought their own comfortable chair with them. This was not an unreasonable practice when it is remembered that many worked a sixteen-hour day and often a seven-day week during the peak of the hatching season.

The hatchery had to supply the protective clothing. Later the modern, fully sterilised large company hatcheries supplied everything, as well as having the chick sexer shower and change clothes before entering the hatchery. One chick sexer complained that even his lunch had to go through the steriliser.

Fred Wrigley and Max Akam both learnt chick sexing through the Ex-servicemen and women's rehabilitation scheme.

Fred served in the Royal Australian Air Force in England and Max in the Army in New Guinea. They remained firm friends throughout their commercial chick sexing careers, and beyond.

With the growth of the chicken-meat industry and the sexing of many broiler-type chicks, Max Akam was able to go on sexing full time until he retired from chick sexing at sixty-three. Max was a keen grower and judge of orchids for over thirty years.

Max Akam was a very exacting person, who always obtained a high accuracy and reliability as a commercial chick sexer. For the first thirteen years of the second-generation he was the only candidate at the chick-sexing examinations to gain a special-class certificate.

Max Akam was foundation president, and Fred Wrigley the foundation secretary, of the Chick Sexing Association of Victoria, which was formed in 1954 with eight members, two of whom were part-time chick sexers. Until the third generation of chick sexers in the 1960s, chick sexing was essentially a seasonal occupation, starting in June and finishing by the end of October.

For many years Fred Wrigley and Max Akam drove a Sennitt's Ice Cream delivery truck between seasons.

Eric Marchant and Bob Martin were able to find employment in the poultry industry for most of the year. Bob Martin did chick sexing one day a week for ten months of the year for one large hatchery and also sexed chickens in the autumn around Melbourne for several small hatcheries.

For some years he sexed chickens one day a week in Wagga Wagga during autumn. By the end of his chick-sexing career in 1966, Martin, like most commercial chick sexers, was sexing chicks for most of the year.

In 1949, Martin was probably the first commercial chick sexer to fly interstate on a weekly basis to sex chickens. He flew to Launceston each Wednesday in 1949 and 1950 to sex chickens for two hatcheries.

Martin and Akam were two of the second-generation of chick sexers who began their chick-sexing careers on push bikes.

Martin is also one of the few commercial chick sexers of the second generation to admit that he started commercial chick sexing before he had had sufficient practice to obtain the required 96 per cent to 99 per cent accuracy.

Victoria seems to have always been short of commercial chick sexers. Martin gained 94 per cent at the government examinations when he was 18. He applied for a chick-sexing position on the strength of this at one of Victoria's largest hatcheries, and also for the Tasmanian chick-sexing position. He obtained both contracts: about 400 000 chickens at the hatchery, spread over seven months, and 100 000 chickens from the Tasmanian position, plus one other farm in Melbourne of 2000 chicks a week, a full seven-day week, at eighteen.

His commercial accuracy is well documented at 94 per cent. His three main Melbourne colleagues, Marchant, Wrigley and Akam were all sexing commercially at 98 per cent or more.

Don Martin of Werribee (no relation to Bob Martin), the other commercial chick sexer who sexed chicks in large numbers, said in an interview for a weekly magazine that his sexing accuracy was 95 per cent at Carter Brothers. This was an acceptable figure. But for those chick sexers sexing chicks for hatcheries which sell all their chickens a higher accuracy is expected.

Every pullet put among the cockerels, which are usually disposed of, was a 40c loss. Multiply this by thousands and the importance of three or four percentage points can be appreciated. Bob Martin was re-engaged the following year by all his first-year clients, probably because of his reliability and speed. His commercial accuracy improved each year. After five years of commercial chick sexing, at 23 he was able to sex 10 000 chicks in thirteen hours, with an overall 97 per cent accuracy.

For half of his twenty years as a commercial chick sexer, Bob Martin sexed more chickens in a year than any other chick sexer in Victoria. This was possible through him having as a client a large hatchery which hatched and sexed all their chickens for ten months of the year. As well he sexed a few broiler chicks near the end of his chick-sexing career.

It was not until the third-generation of chick sexers and the all-year-round sexing of meat and egg strain chickens that Martin's yearly numbers faded into insignificance.

Of this second generation of Victorian chick sexers only Max Akam continued as a commercial chick sexer into his sixties.

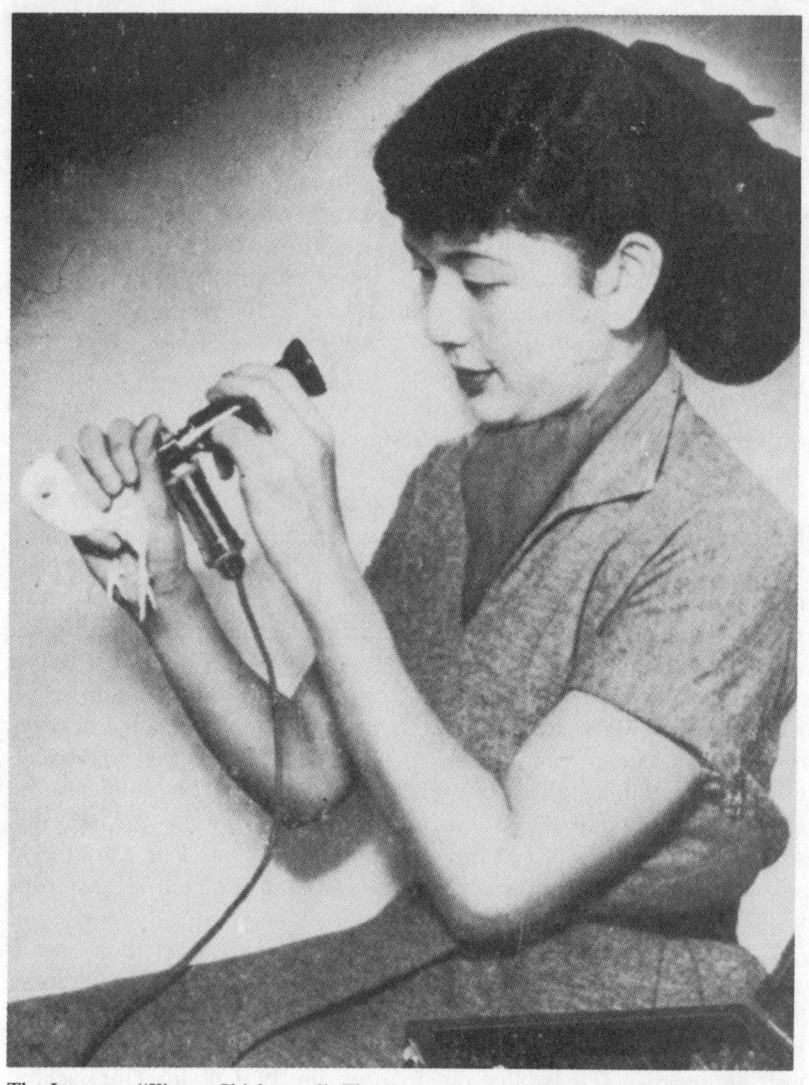

The Japanese "Kizawa Chicktester". The "age of the machine" had arrived, 1953.

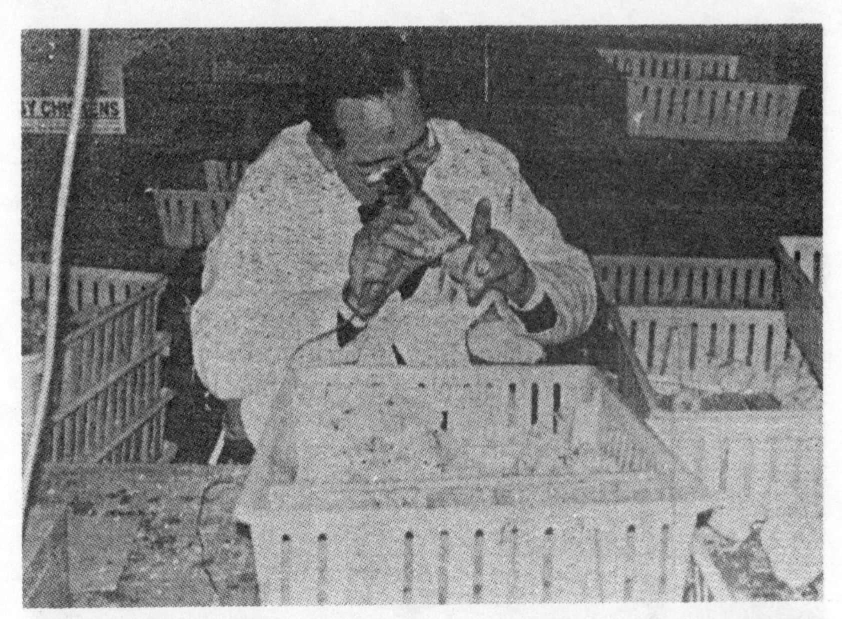

Onko Wallbrink, one of the world's most experienced "machine" chick sexers with over 40 years' commercial sexing by this method. He makes less than 0.5 per cent errors and sexes at the rate of 800 chicks an hour.

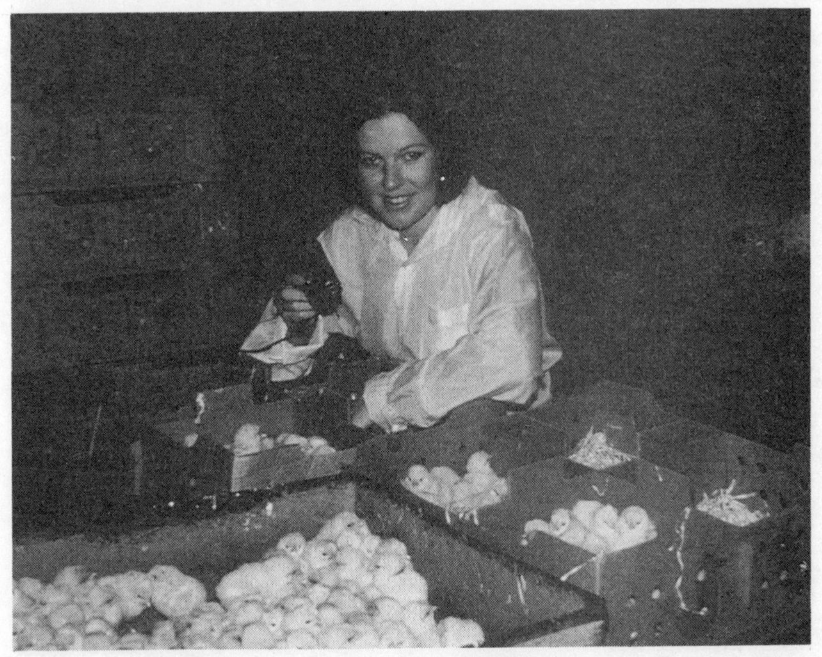

A student, and associate of Onko Wallbrink, Doreen De Carteret, one of the five full time "machine" method chick sexers still working in Australia.

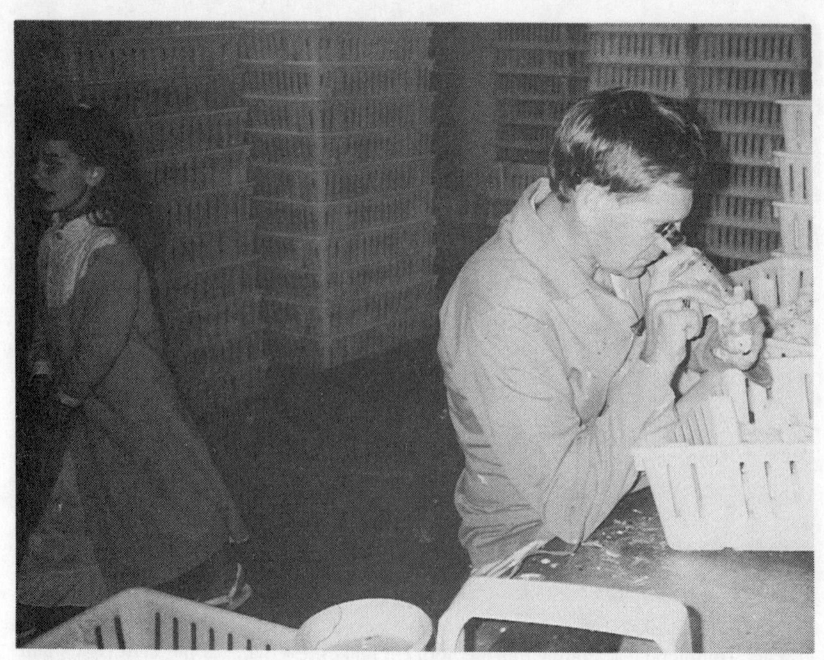

John Hammond, with help from his daughter, Fiona, sexing a 9000 hatch of chicks for a New South Wales hatchery.

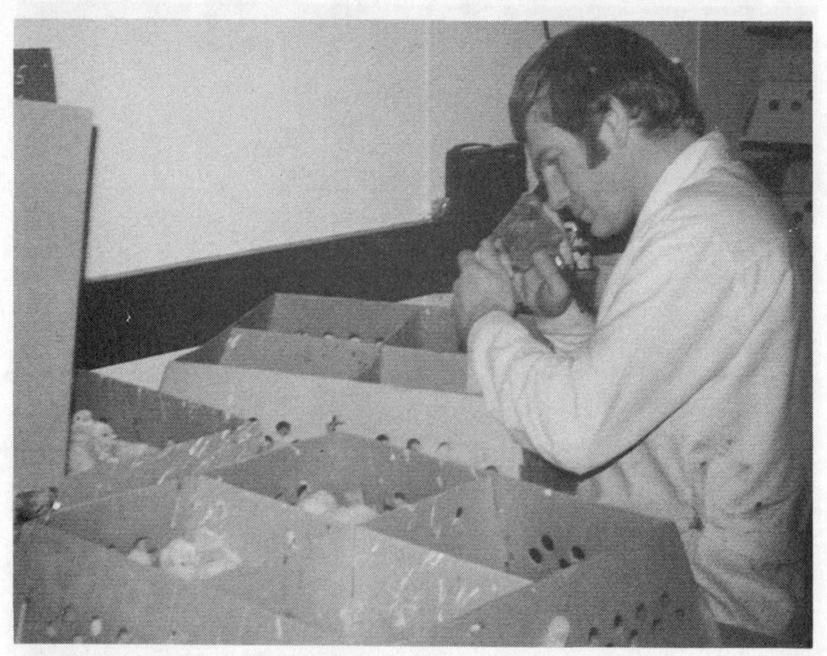

A younger John Hammond sexing at a hatchery in Victoria 1968. He is one of the fastest "machine" method sexers in Australia, at 1200 plus chicks an hour.

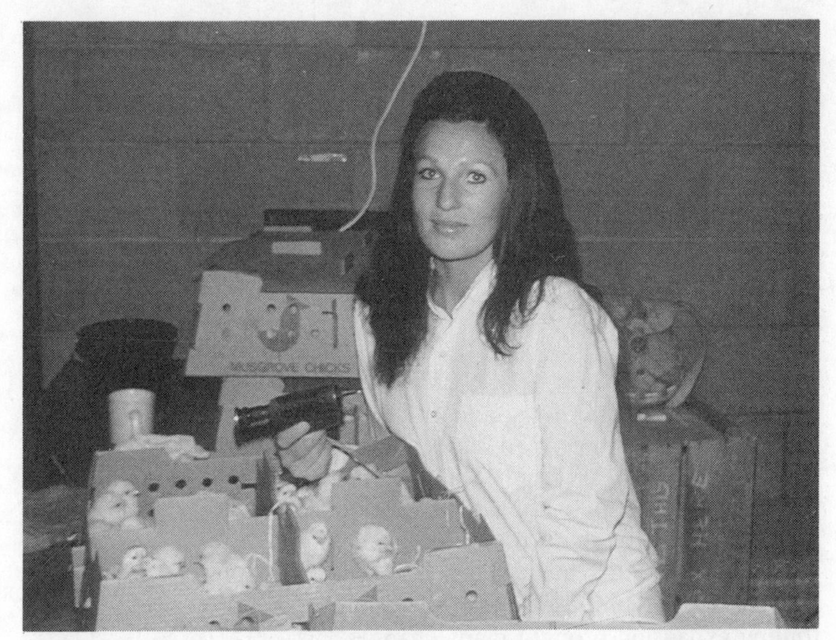

Lena Rogers, a former commercial chick sexer (''machine'' method) who also had some success using the machine sexing turkeys. Lena was a very fast chick sexer. She retired from chick sexing with the advent of feather sexing.

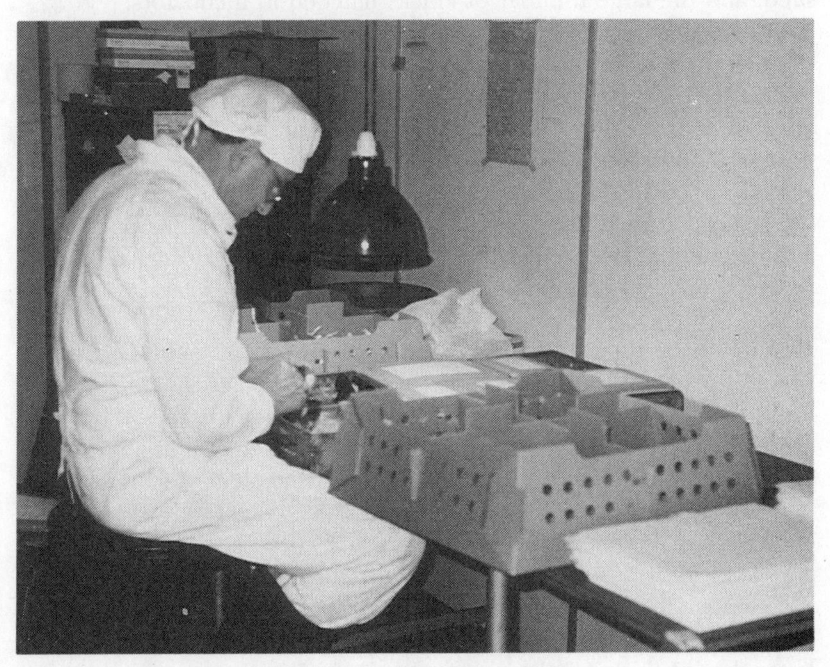

Max Akam, cloaca method chick sexer, feather sexing chicks.

The 1960s

THE TWO CHANGES: THE NUMBERS AND TECHNOLOGY

By the early 1960s both egg and chicken-meat production had started to become highly integrated and sophisticated industries.

During the 20 years from 1960 progress was extremely rapid. It was the period of greatest change in the industry's history, not only in Australia but throughout the world.

Instead of poultry meat being a by-product of the egg industry, it became a separate industry with very modern technology and its continuing expansion brought many changes.

Two outstanding changes occurred. One was the increased size of operations, such as the number of birds that could be reared in a single shed, and the large number of chicks hatched in incubators.

The other great advantage was in technology. This was necessary for the new economies of large-scale production.

The vertical integration which took place saw the rapid disappearance of individually owned farms and hatcheries. By the 1980s the poultry industry was one of the most efficient primary industries in the world.

The egg industry, with the increase in the use of the laying cage system and hatching of layer replacement stock, was no longer restricted to the spring season, but was extended to ten months of the year.

What effects did these changes have on the commercial chick sexer?

Initially, it became a second Golden Age for commercial chick sexers. From the mid 1960s many commercial chick sexers worked all the year around. The vent chick sexers from the second generation kept sexing chicks for breeding and replacement egg-laying stock. In Victoria the new wave of newly qualified "machine" chick sexers were busy sexing chickens for the meat industry. Pullets and cockerels were reared separately to meet different bird-size requirements.

The price for sexing chicks stayed the same for many years, but most full-time chick sexers earned around $1000 for three days' work in the latter days of this period.

Side effects of having broiler chicks sexed were, in some instances, a reduction in chick-sexing fees and, as broiler management was not so concerned about accuracy, there developed a practice for a while in some hatcheries of dumping a handful of unsexed chicks in the crate of sexed chicks occasionally to counteract the lower sexing fees.

As Max Akam replied when asked did he ever worry about being out of work? "No, as the family farms disappeared there was always someone there to take their place ... Frankly, I could see no end to it."

Lena Rogers, a third-generation "machine" chick sexer had similar thoughts when she said, "I never really thought chick sexing would go out ... There was so much work about you didn't worry about it."

It could be argued that this third-generation period from 1960 to the 1980s was really the golden age of commercial chick sexing, and for many it was. In Victoria, most vent chick sexers gradually "retired" from chick sexing.

Max Akam was the main exception. Noel Hargreaves also kept going, but died while holidaying in England. Charlie Bode came back into the business to replace Hargreaves, and stayed for six years, retiring at 67.

Another vent chick sexer, Les Tait, did some commercial chick sexing on a part-time basis, but this was basically an age of "machine" sexers in Victoria.

Until feather sexing made them redundant in the early 1980s, most would have done well.

But, as several have said, we earned big money, but none of us seem to have much to show for it.

Comparisons

Some comparisons between the methods and the people who took on hand sexing and the people who took on "machine" sexing need to be made here.

A large majority of vent sexers came from families of poultry farmers or hatcherymen, or had an interest in the poultry industry.

Vent sexing was difficult and costly to learn. In Victoria, there was, over the years, a success rate of less than one per cent, according to Department of Agriculture records.

No vent chick sexer in Victoria other than three Japanese experts in the 1930s reached 100 per cent accuracy at a test.

A commercial chick sexer using the vent method must concentrate, otherwise his or her accuracy will slip. Laughing and talking as you work is not conducive to accurate chick sexing. Many will argue this applies to both methods. Many argue the vent method requires a greater degree of concentration than the "machine" method, but not everybody would agree with this.

It was claimed by one manufacturer of the chick-sexing "machine", when it was first introduced, that it required no more concentration than typing. But even a good typist needs to concentrate to avoid errors.

Most chick sexers always have a subconscious fear of making errors, and even though they are sure of every chick they sex, mistakes do occur. He or she also has that hidden ambition to be more accurate than their peers. A vent sexer's reputation and business was built on accuracy; most "machine" chick sexers can get 98 per cent accuracy, or higher, seemingly without much effort.

A vent sexer's skill is one that is dearly earned.

Most "machine" chick sexers are able to gain 100 per cent accuracy after only a few months' practice. Many "machine" chick-sexing candidates who did not get 100 per cent in the examinations were 100 per cent accurate, but lost points because they punctured the bowels of some of the chickens.

There is no argument that the "machine' method is easier and cheaper to learn. Getting 100 per cent in a test is not too difficult.

An operator using the "machine" can usually be sure that what he or she is seeing is correct on most occasions. No great intuition is required. The skill is in the handling of the chick with gentleness and speed.

Both methods are reliable and being able to concentrate hour after hour after hour is essential. This is a merit not everyone has.

Victoria 1966 . . . 1994—The third generation

In 1955 the Victorian Hatcherymen's Society held chick-sexing classes to try to overcome what they saw as a pending shortage of chick sexers in the State.

Initially only one, Herb Burchall, was successful as a vent chick sexer. Later, others from this class took on the "machine" method, and one, Tony Martino, later changed back to vent sexing and became successful sexing turkeys.

Eventually five students from this (cloacal chick sexing) class graduated and obtained government certificates as "machine" sexers. Many were helped by Harry Pettigrove, hatcheryman and former first-generation chick sexer, by being able to practise at his hatchery in Box Hill. The five were Olga Shaw, Onko Wallbrink, Rolf Scott, Graham Lilley and Tony Martino.

Tony Martino was the only sexer in Victoria to gain a special-class certificate by both methods.

Burchall and Martino were the last two chick sexers in the State to learn and use the vent method commercially. Olga Shaw was the first student in Australia to gain a 100 per cent accuracy with the "machine" method at a government examination, but she did not continue as a commercial chick sexer.

Onko Wallbrink, Rolf Scott and later Graham Lilley all did commercial chick sexing. Later they were joined by a new batch of "machine" sexers, to cope with the sexing of broiler-type chicks.

The third generation 1966–1994

FOUR VICTORIAN PROFILES

Here we look briefly at four Victorian "machine" sexers, two women and two men, from the third generation.

Lena Rogers

As a fourteen-year-old girl on a farm collecting eggs, Lena Rogers, sees the chick sexer working with the newly hatched chicks. She wants to learn. At first the chick sexer does not want to teach her. But eventually the chick sexer, John Hammond, takes the young Lena Holol with him on his chick-sexing round and she later joins him as a fellow commercial chick sexer at two of Victoria's largest hatcheries.

Later, the married Lena Rogers flies to Anderson's hatchery in South Australia each weekend to sex chickens. While she was there she taught a couple of people to sex chickens with the "machine".

She also developed the skill to sex turkeys. The only "machine" chick sexer in Australia to have any success in this area, for many years she sexed poults for turkey growers all over Victoria, as well as poults flown from Sydney.

Later when chick-sexing opportunities declined in Victoria, she accepted an invitation from Steggles to shift to Sydney and sex chickens for them. She stayed there for eighteen months before returning to Melbourne.

In the early 1980s New South Wales seems to have been short of chick sexers. Several other Victorian chick sexers also shifted to Sydney. Andrew Buchan, and husband-and-wife team, Robert and Julie McKinnon, were three others to go. Only Andrew Buchan stayed there permanently. He now has a business there, and still does some commercial chick sexing.

According to Lena Rogers, there was much arguing between the chick sexers at the hatchery in Sydney. While there, Lena Rogers used to fly back to Victoria two days a week to sex poults.

Lena Rogers worked at feather sexing for awhile and became very fast at it, but the hatcheries began using their regular staff for this work.

As a ''machine'' sexer, she found 5000 chicks a comfortable day's work. The most she ever did in a day was 11 000.

Lena Rogers sexed commercially for 25 years. She now has a successful landscape-gardening business.

Onko Wallbrink, the dean of "machine" chick sexers

Onko Wallbrink has sexed chicks commercially continuously since 1955. He is Australia's most experienced ''machine'' sexer. He has sexed more chickens by ''machine'' than any other chick sexer in Australia. He has also taught more students the ''machine' method than anyone else in Australia.

When the Keeler Instrument Company of England stopped making the ''Chixexer'' chick-sexing machine, they gave the plans and specifications and permission to manufacture to Onko.

He is one of the few ''machine'' chick sexers with the documentation to back up his claim that he is close to 100 per cent accurate in his commercial chick sexing. He is Australia's dean of ''machine'' chick sexers. Several of his fellow chick sexers became upset when he used to stay back after they left to check their work for accuracy. Such is the way of people working together as a team of separate contractors.

Onko Wallbrink was secretary of the re-formed Chick Sexing Association of Victoria for several years.

He did for a while have several chick sexers he had trained working for him, but this does not seem to have worked particularly well. Nor did it in the 1930s when Farm and Pastoral Supplies had a similar scheme with their Chick Sexing Company of Australia (Victorian Division). Its stated aims were to establish chick sexing in Victoria, to train Australian students in the art and to provide highly qualified experts to hatcheries.

The fact that Onko Wallbrink was given the plans and specifications of the ''Chixexer machine'' when they went out of production illustrates the high regard in which he is held, in an even wider area than his own working environment in Australia.

According to Onko, there were a couple of years during his thirty-nine years as a commercial chick sexer when he had very little work, and had seriously considered another occupation. But his chick-sexing business had once again picked up and he was able to continue his unbroken record as a full-time commercial chick sexer. It could be said that he is a loner who endured.

John Hammond, entrepreneur

Another early ''machine'' chick sexer was John Hammond, who learnt from Bob Martin in 1964. He sexed full time for several years, but as his other business ventures grew he tended to sex commercially for only one to two set days a week.

John Hammond's chick-sexing career could well be a pattern for commercial chick sexers of the next generation, in the 90s and beyond. He has well-established business interests apart from his chick-sexing business, which leave him available for chick sexing when required. He does not depend solely on chick sexing. He is skilled in another area. Chick sexers in the future could well need a back-up business or occupation.

Some have suggested that hatcheries will have their own resident chick sexers who will work at other things at the hatchery when not sexing chickens. This is not new. South Australia, with its limited number of hatcheries, has had mostly residential chick sexers for most of its family-farms era, that is from the 1930s through to the 1950s.

John Hammond would probably be the fastest "machine" chick sexer in Australia.

He can sex chickens at the rate of 1200 chicks and more an hour. He takes ten hours to sex 10 000 chickens, much to the annoyance, at times, of the other members of the team of chick sexers working with him.

His hobbies include flying and acting. He complains that they usually give him the part of a policeman. He was in the police force for a couple of years, and, for awhile, a stand-up comic. His business and commercial chick sexing have been the two constant occupations in his professional life.

He has been a friend of Hartley Hall and Bob Martin for over thirty years. They look upon the youthful fifty-one-year old John Hammond as a kind of young new bloke to the chick-sexing fraternity.

Such is the nature of chick sexing at present in Australia, with no new chick-sexing students entering the field. As John Hammond has said, with twenty-two chick sexers in Australia in 1994, you have to wait for someone to die to get work.

John Hammond, Onko Wallbrink, Doreen De Carteret (all "machine") and Ron Mason (vent) are the only four commercial chick sexers still operating in Victoria in 1994. All except Mason fly interstate regularly to work.

Doreen De Carteret, a quiet achiever

Doreen De Carteret and Julie Mitchell both gained a special-class certificate in 1973. They were the last candidates to get a certificate at the government chick-sexing examinations in Victoria.

Doreen De Carteret learnt from Onko Wallbrink and has worked with him for twenty years. During this time she has flown to Adelaide one day a week. At another time she flew regularly to Tasmania to sex chickens there. Most of her current work is around Melbourne, at Bendigo and an occasional interstate trip.

When asked what she considered a comfortably day's chick sexing, she replied that it used to be 7000 a day but now she feels more comfortable doing 5000. Like most commercial chick sexers she agreed that 10 000 in a day is a very long day. She sexes the chicks at the rate of 800 an hour.

She took on the occupation when her neighbour, Janice Grant, a commercial chick sexer, asked her if she would like to learn chick sexing. Doreen De Carteret originally came from a farming background.

Like her colleagues of this third generation, she knew feather sexing would eventually reduce the demand for her services. But she did think her chick-sexing career would go on, and that when one place closed another would take its place. There were times when she wondered what she would do next, but something always seemed to turn up.

Currently she works all the year round. Some weeks it may be only one or two days a week.

Before feather and colour sexing reduced the demand for the specialist chick sexer, Doreen De Carteret worked in a team with Onko Wallbrink, Julie Mitchell, Max Akam and the twins Janet and Ray Lawardorn. This was a team which seems to have worked well together for many years. They were happy to check each other's work for accuracy. They took it in turns each day. One would yell out, "check" and they would all then move and check the work of the person next to them.

When Doreen De Carteret was interviewed there was also a second-generation vent chick sexer present. Both agreed fear of making mistakes was their greatest worry as commercial chick sexers. Even a "machine" chick sexer has some difficulty in identifying certain chickens. Both methods have the same fear as a driving force.

A commercial comparison

To sex chicks with the machine the chick needs a drying off period after it hatches, otherwise puncturing can occur.

In hatcheries employing both hand and "machine" sexers, they sometimes get the vent sexers to sex the late-hatched "green" chickens to avoid this problem.

Generally, the "machine" sexers were faster in Australia. This can be a big plus. In one hatchery employing eight chick sexers, a mixture of both hand and machine operators, the management divided the number of chickens to be sexed equally to overcome arguments. Otherwise the "machine" chick sexers were always ahead of their vent colleagues, and this tended to cause ill feeling.

The division of the hatch caused other minor problems for the hatchery staff. They had to wait around for the vent sexers to finish so that they could box up the sexed chicks.

A wider and more objective commercial comparison can be when we examine the experiences of other highly advanced poultry-industry countries, where, almost without exception, the vent method is used because it proved over time to be faster and more accurate. But again there were exceptions.

Commercial accuracy of the "machine" method

In Victoria the only "machine" sexer who could justify being able to claim he is nearly 100 per cent accurate commercially most of the time is Onko Wallbrink. There is documentation of his accuracy from the Random Sample Laying Test hatchings. Also, several of the hatcheries where he is the only sexer employed can verify his accuracy. Most of Onko Wallbrink's colleagues whether friend or competitor, would acknowledge that he is close to 100 per cent accurate.

The Farm and Pastoral Certificates (First Generation 1934 . . . 1945)

Examinations were held in 1935, 1936 and 1937. In 1938 the Victorian Agricultural Ministry Examinations began.

(Hartley Hall was a commercial chick sexer from 1934 till 1955 but never sat for an examination of any kind.)

These commercial chick sexers passed the chick-sexing examinations conducted by 'The Farm and Pastoral Supply Pty Ltd' held in 1935, before the Government started holding examinations. Most continued to sex commercially for many years.

Special Class: 95% accuracy required. 200 white leghorn chicks in 30 minutes

Bode, C.	97.0%
Pettigrove, T. H.	95.5%
Millington, W. J.	95.0%
Lawson, L.	95.0%

First Class: 90% accuracy required. 100 white leghorn chicks in 20 minutes

Lomas, L. P.	97.0%
Marsden-Steel, Miss	92.0%
Young, L	90.0%
Jenkins, R.	91.5%
Rogers, E. A.	91.0%
Steel, Miss D.	91.0%

" Machine Method "
Instrument

" Hand Method "
Cloacal

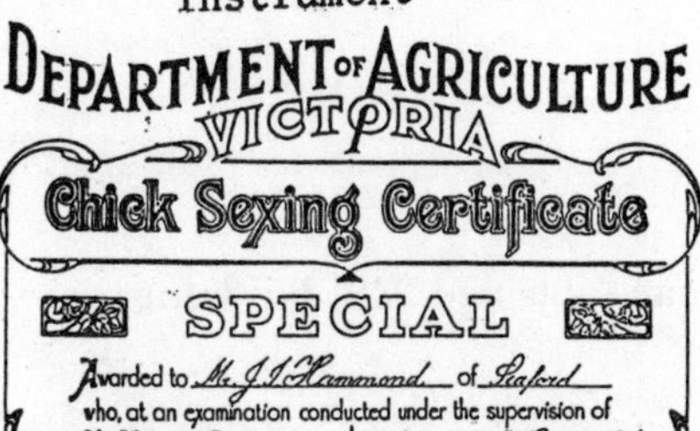

DEPARTMENT OF AGRICULTURE VICTORIA

Chick Sexing Certificate

SPECIAL

Awarded to Mr J. T. Hammond of Seaford
who, at an examination conducted under the supervision of
The Victorian Department of Agriculture on 10th November 1964
sexed 300 chickens in 25 minutes
with an accuracy of 100 per cent.

Director of Agriculture

Senior Poultry Officer

Examining Officer

DEPARTMENT OF AGRICULTURE VICTORIA

Chick Sexing Certificate

SPECIAL

Awarded to Mr R. L. Mason of Eaglehawk
who, at an examination conducted under the supervision of
The Victorian Department of Agriculture on 11th October 1961
sexed 300 White Leghorn chickens in 38 minutes
with an accuracy of 99 per cent.

Director of Agriculture

Poultry Expert

Examining Officer.

DEPARTMENT OF AGRICULTURE VICTORIA

Chick Sexing Certificate

SPECIAL

Awarded to Mrs Doreen de Carteret of Mt Martha.
who, at an examination conducted under the supervision of
The Victorian Department of Agriculture on 27. 11. 73.
sexed 300. chickens in 31. minutes
with an accuracy of 99·7 per cent.

Director of Agriculture

Senior Poultry Officer

Examining Officer

DEPARTMENT OF AGRICULTURE VICTORIA

Chick Sexing Certificate

FIRST CLASS

Awarded to R. D. Martin of Tyabb
who, at an examination conducted under the supervision of
The Victorian Department of Agriculture on 11 October 1961
sexed 200 White Leghorn chickens in 20 minutes
with an accuracy of 97.5 per cent.

Director of Agriculture

Poultry Expert

Examining Officer

DEPARTMENT OF AGRICULTURE VICTORIA

Chick Sexing Certificate

SPECIAL

Awarded to Mr R. D. Martin of Tyabb
who, at an examination conducted under the supervision of
The Victorian Department of Agriculture on 13 November 1962.
sexed 300 chickens in 30 minutes
with an accuracy of 99.3 per cent.

Director of Agriculture

Senior Poultry Officer

Examining Officer

DEPARTMENT OF AGRICULTURE VICTORIA

Chick Sexing Certificate

FIRST CLASS

Awarded to Mr. R. D Martin of Tyabb
who, at an examination conducted under the supervision of
The Victorian Department of Agriculture on 19 October 1960
sexed 200 White Leghorn chickens in 18 minutes
with an accuracy of 97 per cent.

Director of Agriculture

Poultry Expert

Examining Officer

Second Class: 85% accuracy required. 100 white leghorn chicks in 20 minutes

Rogers. E. A.	89.5%
Jenkins, H. A.	88%
Filmer, W. S.	87%
Cook, –	85%
Fethers, G.	87%

Another candidate in 1935, G. Freeman, obtained 93% but went over the allowed time.

In 1936 and 1937 the following candidates obtained certificates from Farm and Pastoral (In 1938 the Government Examinations commenced.):

Special Class 95 per cent	*First Class 90 per cent*
Mr E. A. Rogers	Mr Eric K. Mason
Miss Doreen Lloyd	Miss J. Benham
Miss Deliah Benham	

Victoria

List of Qualified Chicken Sexers — "First generation"
Department of Agriculture — 1934–1945
First Examination 1938

Special Class 98 per cent accuracy required. 300 chickens in 45 minutes.

Name	*Address*	*Year*	*Accuracy*	*Method*
McLister, K.	176 Hall St. Spotswood	1939	99.0	Hand
Jenkins, H. A.	Queenscliff Rd, Moolap	1939	98.7	Hand
First Class: 95 per cent accuracy required. 200 chickens in 30 minutes				
Marchant, E. J.	56 White St. Mordialloc	1938	98.0	Hand
Pettigrove, T. H.	159 Hawdon St. Heidelberg	1938	97.5	Hand
Millington, W. J.	1 Lyne Gve, Wst Brunswick	1938	96.5	Hand
Bode, C.	Research Post Office	1939	96.0	Hand
Martin, D.	9 Glenluss Ave, Werribee	1946	96.0	Hand
Jeremiah, D. Mrs.	Cranhaven Rd, Frankston	1948	96.0	Hand
Smith, I.	Cotterell St. Werribee	1945	95.0	Hand

Victoria

List of Qualified Chicken Sexers — "Second generation"
Ministry of Agriculture — 1946–1965

Special Class (98%). 300 white leghorn chicks in 45 minutes

Name	*Address*	*Year*	*Accuracy*	*Method*
Martin. R. D.	4 Frank St, Box Hill Sth.	1962	99.3	Machine
Mason, R. L.	58 Victoria St, Eaglehawk	1961	99.0	Hand
Akam, M. A.	4 Koala Court, Frankston	1949	98.0	Hand
First Class (95%). 200 white leghorn chicks in 30 minutes.				
Martin, R. D.	4 Frank St. Box Hill Sth.	1961	97.5	Hand
Wrigley, F.	Pound Rd, Berwick	1949	96.5	Hand
Hargreaves, N.	7 Maldon St. Footscray	1951	96.5	Hand
Hewett, A.	Central Ave. Bayswater	1945	95.0	Hand
Bradshaw, A.	Valley Rd. Highton	1946	95.0	Hand
Bruce, E. Miss	Glenormiston Sth. Terang	1947	95.0	Hand
Whyte, J.	34 Rose St. McKinnon	1949	95.0	Hand
Second Class (95%). 45 minutes for 200 chickens				
Whyte, J.	31 Rose St. McKinnon	1954	96.5	Machine
Bourbaud, E.	3 Watkins Gve, Mordialloc	1946	95.0	Hand
Jackson, E. Miss	4 Monash St. Box Hill	1948	95.5	Hand
Williams, E.	North Wangaratta	1947	95.0	Hand

Victoria

List of Qualified Chicken Sexers — "Third generation"
Ministry of Agriculture — 1962–1994

Special Class (98%). 300 chicks in 30 minutes

Name	*Address*	*Year*	*Accuracy*	*Method*
Shaw, O. Miss	406 Albert Rd. Mt Albert	1955	100	Machine
Wallbrink, O.	32 Glenvale Rd, Ringwood	1956	100	Machine
Hammond, J.	270 Baxter-Tooradin Rd. Baxter	1964	100	Machine
McKinnon, R.	30 Yarrinup Ave. Chadstone	1969	99.7	Machine
De Carteret, D. Mrs	2 Moomba St. Mornington	1973	99.7	Machine

Rogers, L. Mrs	30 Remington Dr. Glen Waverley	1968	99.3	Machine
Van Mierlo, I. Miss	Orchard Gr. Blackburn	1956	99.0	Machine
Jansen, N. P.	139 Junction Rd. N'Wading	1963	99.0	Machine
Martino, T.	37 Darlot St. Horsham	1955	98.7	Machine
Martino, T.	36 Darlot St. Horsham	1960	98.7	Hand
Russell, J. Miss	Brysons Wonga Park	1956	98.7	Machine
Lawardorn, R. Miss	Fairbairn Ave. Mt. Martha	1968	98.3	Machine
Eley, R.	7 Inga Pde. Mt Martha	1966	98.0	Machine
O'Hara, P.	12 Duke St. Ballarat West	1968	98.0	Machine
McKinnon, J. Mrs		1973	98.0	Machine

First Class (95%). 200 chicks in 30 minutes

Lilley, G.	Clarke Rd. Spring Vale	1957	100	Machine
Lawardorn, J. Miss	Fairbairne Ave. Mt Martha	1964	100	Machine
Close, R.	Kennewell St. White Hills	1959	99.0	Machine
Barnes, R.	Wireless Rd. Mt. Gambier	1962	99.0	Machine
Calligari, T.	50 Holyrood St. M'Borough	1956	98.0	Machine
McLeod, T. Mrs	Moyston West	1960	98.0	Machine
Grant, J. Miss	Volitane Ave. Mt Eliza	1964	97.5	Machine
Cole, I.	Carisbrook	1961	97.5	Machine
Buchan, A.	4 Lyndel Close, Soldiers Pt. N.S.W	1969	97.3	Machine
Hills, N.	Athel Park P/F Mooroopna	1969	97.3	Machine
Burchall, H.	2 Portland St. W. Coburg	1955	96.5	Hand
Tyack, A.	Marungi	1963	96.5	Machine
Heinhelt, E.	103 Station St. Norlane	1963	96.0	Hand
Flack, J.	Williams Rd. Horsham	1957	96.5	Machine

Second Class: (95%). 45 minutes for 200 chickens

Scott, R.	66 Virginia St. Mt Waverley	1956	99.5	Machine

Feldtmann, R.	Goorambat	1963	99.0	Machine
Overmaat, H.	5 Jardine St. Mt Gambier	1956	97.0	Machine
Davidson, K.	Daybreak Hatchery, Horsham	1958	96.0	Machine

1994: Commercial chick sexers still working in Victoria:

Mr Onko Wallbrink	Machine	100%	1956
Mr John Hammond	Machine	100%	1964
Mrs D. De Carteret	Machine	99.7%	1973
Mr Ron Mason	Hand	99%	1961

Government examinations continued to be held in Victoria until 1983, mainly for one or two students, both machine candidates. No candidates passed after 1973.

Summary: 53 candidates have obtained Certificates in Victoria during the 46 years the Ministry held examinations.

Special Class	19	5 Hand	14 Machine	(1 both)
First Class	27	16 Hand	12 Machine	(1 both)
Second Class	7	3 Hand	4 Machine	(1 both)
	53			

First Generation:	2 Special class 7 First class (all hand)
Second Generation:	3 Special class 6 First class 3 Second class (all hand/2 both)
Third Generation:	14 Special class 14 First class 4 Second class (2 hand/1 both/30 machine)

New South Wales 1934–1994

THE DOMINANT STATE

From the 1930s to the late 1940s Victoria had the world's largest egg farm, but New South Wales always had Australia's largest hatcheries and poultry breeding farms. By the 1990s all of Australia's egg and poultry meat genetic breeder companies were based in New South Wales. The other States have mainly multiplication farms reproducing offspring of these companies, or their overseas franchise genetic stock.

By 1994 there are twenty-one commercial chick sexers working in Australia, eleven full time. The rest work either two or three days a week or on a casual basis. Nine of the full-time chick sexers work in NSW. The other full timers are based in Victoria. Two of them fly interstate to work for one or two days each week.

Victoria, the second largest poultry-industry State, was the first State to send commercial chick sexers to Europe to sex chickens in 1937–38, but NSW has dominated the profession. It has produced the most commercial chick sexers, and the most with special-class certificates. It had a strong chick sexing association. There was never a shortage of chick sexers, as there were in some of the other States, particularly Victoria.

New South Wales trained chick sexers for South Australia, New Zealand, Western Australia and Victoria.

It has been argued that during the early 1950s there was an acute shortage of chick sexers in Japan, and so a quick "stop-gap" alternative was decided upon, and the optical sexing ("Chicktester/machine") method was introduced.

This method could be learnt in three to four months, compared with the three to four years of the vent method. A similar situation occurred in Victoria in the 1950s and again "machine" sexers were trained by one hatcheryman to overcome the shortage, particularly in the broiler industry. For the next two decades Victoria had only four vent sexers operating commercially. Two of the vent sexers worked into their sixties.

This did not happen in NSW. Vent sexing, in spite of early expectations for the machine, was always mostly preferred, mainly, it can be argued, because of the high professional basis on which the skill was based in that State, and the Chick Sexing Association of NSW aim of ensuring that there are always sufficient chick sexers to cope with the needs of the industry.

Two of Australia's most experienced "machine" sexers are from Victoria, one with 33 years' commercial experience and the other with 40 years' teaching and commercial sexing using this method, and both are still working.

Some militancy by chick sexers in NSW did result in one hatchery training a batch of "machine" chick sexers, but not with a great deal of success. However, some of those taught did continue to sex commercially. Of the nine full-time chick sexers in NSW in 1994, three are "machine" sexers, and so is one of the part timers. The last three chick sexers taught in NSW, in the 1980s, used the vent method. There is no doubt that all future students of chick sexing in Australia will be taught the vent method.

These last three chick sexers taught in NSW were the kin of second-generation commercial chick sexers—two lots of parents and an uncle.

The NSW Government held chick-sexing examinations up to 1991. The last successful candidate in these examinations was in 1983. All candidates used the vent method.

Almost all the candidates at the examinations since 1983 in NSW have been of ethnic Korean origin. None were successful.

The easing of examination conditions in NSW in 1952 did not help more candidates to qualify. Crossbred chickens have been used in the examinations since the change. They are usually easier to sex than the white leghorn chicks used previously. Also, to gain a special-class certificate the candidate now has to sex only 200 chicks, not 300 as in the pre-1952 era. The 98 per cent accuracy or more requirement is the same.

It would appear that in Australia there will always be a need for some specialist commercial chick sexers in the industry. Australia now uses about 30 per cent of the number of specialist chick sexers who were used in the peak years of the 1950s to 1970s. However most chick sexers now work throughout the year, a situation that did not apply for many chick sexers in the peak years. Future prospects are discussed later in this study.

More so than in other States of Australia, the NSW chick-sexing community has a strong kinship base. There have been at least four husband-and-wife teams. One of these partnerships also taught their daughter to become a successful commercial chick sexer. There has also been two uncle-and-nephew combinations. One of the most recent vent sexers to be taught is the son of one of the State's top commercial chick sexers.

Because New South Wales always had the largest number of hatcheries, the State's chick sexers worked in teams much earlier than in most of the other states. This has brought about cross checking for accuracy, which has been to the benefit of both the hatcheryman and the chick sexer.

New South Wales **1934**

The first class **The First Generation**

Frank Evans. The dean of Australian chick sexers

The 18-year-old boy had only to walk up the road from his father's hatchery and poultry farm in Leamington Street, Dundas to the first chick-sexing classes held in NSW, at the hatchery and farm of G. N. Mann and Son in Pennant Hill Road, Dundas.

The Japanese teacher was 19-year-old Hikosaburo Yogo. Mr Yogo had previously worked in Canada and the USA and later spent a season in England.

This first instruction class in Australia, ahead of Victoria and Queensland by several weeks, had twenty students. The twenty students in this first class were:

K. Jacobs
W. Norrie
A. (Oscar) Johnson
J. Robertson
J. A. Newton
A. A. Tegel
Miss M. Munday
S. Kilborn
D. O'Donnell
Miss M. Smith
Miss M. Heath
F. D. Evans
W. A. Sewell
J. A. Hazlett
S. Martin
C. R. Badman
Miss Mackenzie
B. A. Weir
K. Rogers
Miss Meili

When the course was completed an examination was held at G. N. Mann and Son's hatchery. Each student had to sex 100 day-old white leghorn chicks. The chicks were killed and the sex determined by post-mortem examination. The two most successful students were Frank Evans with 98 per cent accuracy and A. A. (Bert) Tegel with 93 per cent accuracy.

Of the members of this first class four later became successful commercial chick sexers. One, Mary Mavis Heath, later married Frank Evans.

This first class was open to anyone. Most of the students came from hatcherymen and poultry farmer establishments.

Frank Evans was working on his father's poultry farm for five shillings (50 cents) a week, and saw chick sexing as a golden opportunity to advance. The basic pay for an adult male during this Depression period was £2 ($4) a week.

Frank found that chick sexing came reasonably easy to him. But as his wife was to say many years later, "Frank was dedicated. He knew what he was after and he kept at it."

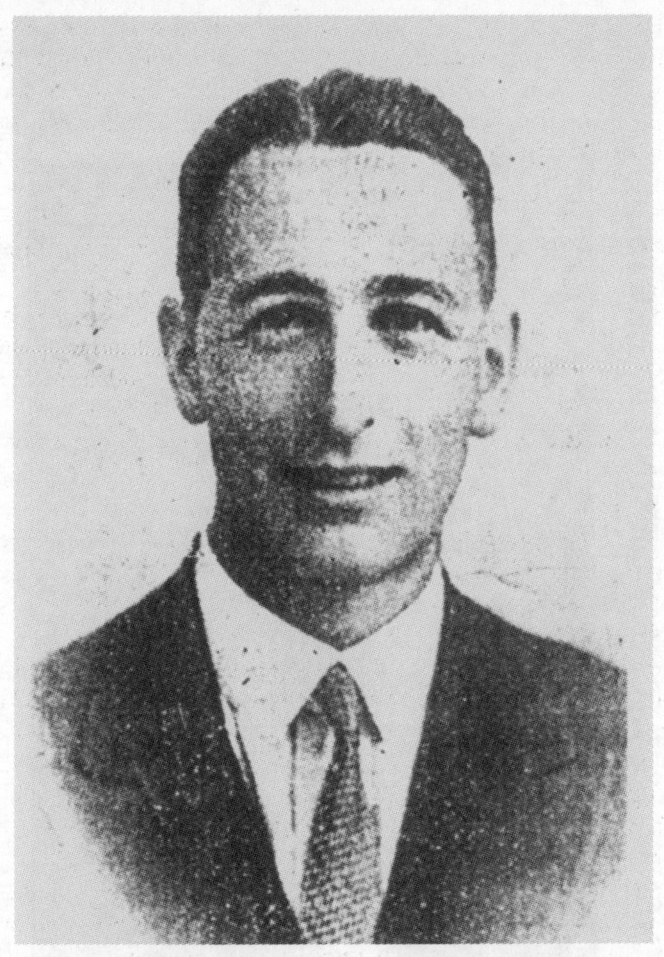

A. (Bert) A. Tegel, who with Frank Evans, was a successful student from Mr Yogo's first class of 1934. He later established one of the largest poultry organisations in Australia.

Saturday, July 11, 1936. **POULTRY**

SOME PROMINENT N.S.W. CHICK-SEXING EXPERTS

Miss M. Heath (left), of Toongabbie, who is at present engaged in sexing chicks commercially, was the first young woman in Australia to obtain a certificate of competency in public examination. Miss Heath is 19 years of age, and last year was awarded a second-class certificate by the NSW Dept. of Agriculture, after having sexed 100 chicks in 17 minutes, with an accuracy of 93 per cent. Mr Frank D. Evans (right), of Dundas, is Australia's first and only Special Class chick-sexer, whose certificate, gained last September, shows that he sexed 300 chicks in 27¾ minutes, with an accuracy of 98.6 per cent.

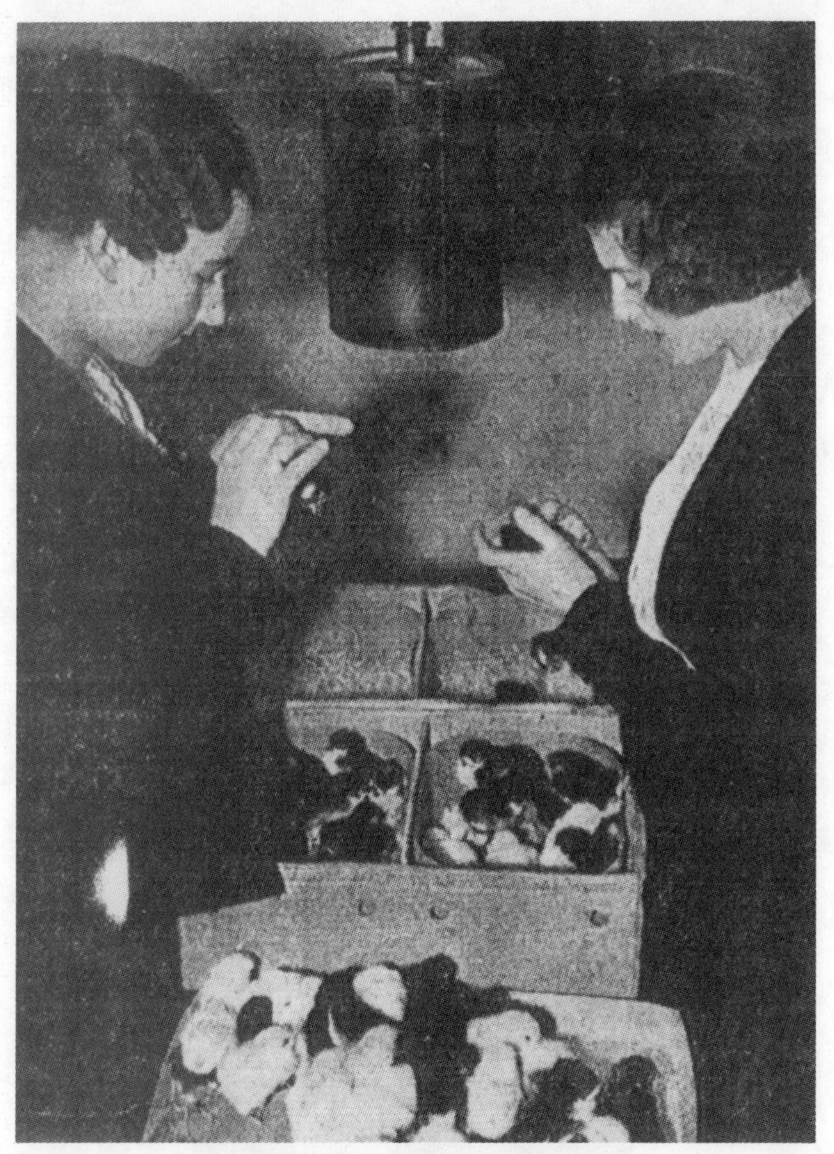

Two students of the New South Wales chick sexing class of 1935 run by Frank Evans. Dora Ranch (left) and Mrs M. Jeans practising on day-old chicks.

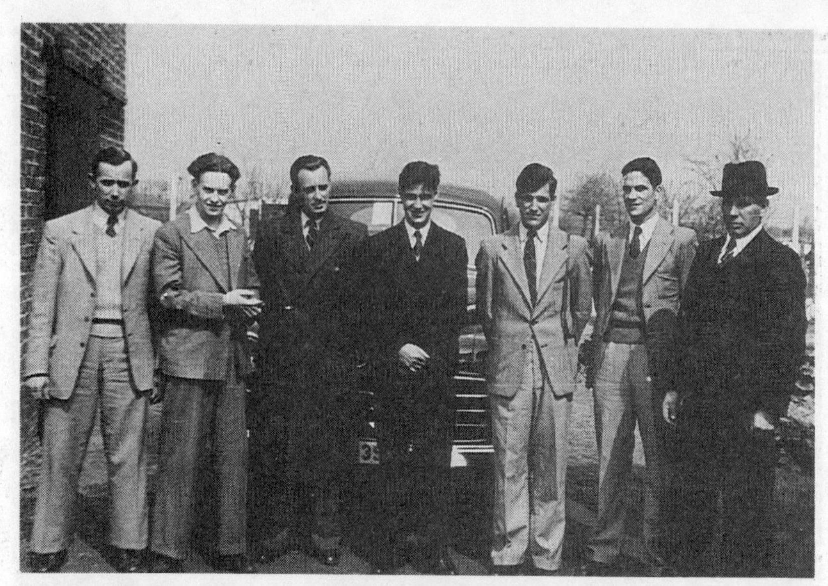

Monsieur Dambre's chick sexing team (Belgium 1946) from left: Frank Evans (Australia), an English sexer, Vic Mahon (Aust), an English sexer, Bob Mayjor (Aust), Jack Edwards (Aust) and sexing contractor Monsieur Dambre.

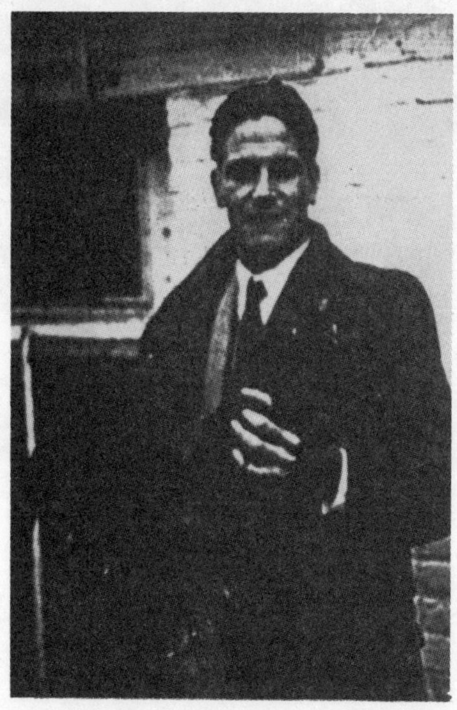

Jack Edwards, from New South Wales, sexed chicks commercially until he was 71.

CHICK SEXING ASSOCIATION
OF AUSTRALIA

21 VALENTINE STREET, SYDNEY, N.S.W.

Chick Sexing Certificate

FIRST Class

Issued to FRANK DARCY EVANS

of DUNDAS. N. S. W.

In an examination held under standard test conditions, the holder has determined the sex of one hundred day-old chickens with an accuracy of NINETY-EIGHT *per cent.*

Date FIRST JANUARY, 1935.

for Chick Sexing Association

Signature of Holder F. D. Evans.

The first chick-sexing certificate issued in Australia. It was awarded to Frank Evans by George Mann of Petersime Incubators-Mann Gamble Poultry Equipment. By 1936 all chick sexing examinations were conducted by the various agriculture ministries in each State.

When looking through the many tests and examinations which he sat for in the 1930s, it is seen that Frank Evans' accuracy was never less than 98 per cent. Many times in the first chick-sexing class it was 100 per cent. In the 1937 government chick-sexing examinations he gained a special-class certificate with 99⅔ per cent accuracy, that is, one mistake in 300 chicks. He sexed 300 white leghorn chicks in 12 minutes 30 seconds, still an Australian record for 300 white leghorn chicks. This is at the rate of 1000 chicks in 65 minutes. This was his second government special-class certificate. The other was in 1936. Frank Evans was 23 years old. His teacher, Hikosaburo Yogo, had sexed chicks at the rate of 1000 an hour with 99 per cent accuracy.

Frank Evans' performance was a remarkable achievement by any standard. Many years later, after sexing millions of chickens, other Australian commercial chick sexers were to equal his accuracy, but not his speed.

At least one other NSW chick sexer, Arthur Pamment, equalled Frank Evans' accuracy of 99⅔ per cent, at the 1950 examinations. He took 30 minutes to sex the 300 white leghorn chicks. Arthur Pamment had previously gained three first-class and one special-class certificates.

Cliff McDowell gained a Japanese chick-sexing certificate with 100 per cent accuracy in 1948. The test at this examination was on 100 white leghorn chicks. In 1950 McDowell gained a special certificate with 99 per cent accuracy. Several other NSW chick sexers have gained 100 per cent accuracy on the first 200 chicks at the government examinations.

Frank Evans, commenting on his performance fifty-six years later in November 1993 said: "When I sat for that examination I just looked at the vent. It either had a cockerel eminence or not, and that was it. I was like an athlete, I was at my peak, I had sexed over a million chickens.

"When I first took on the game, I thought chick sexing would be easy and that chick sexers would be two a penny."

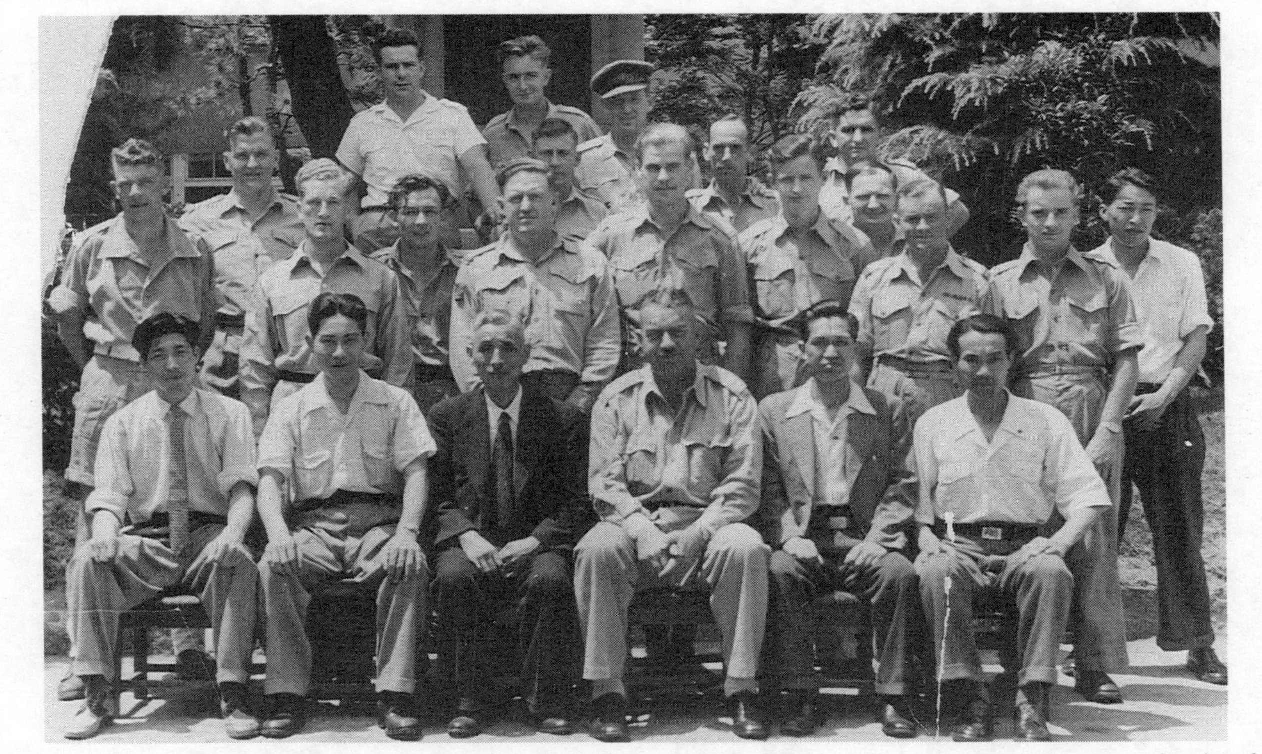

A group photo of the AASC Training School, Japan, October 1948, conducted for Australian and New Zealand military personnel stationed in Japan. Front row, left to right: Koji Kato, Japanese teacher, Doctor Masui, Major Brandwood, Sakai, and another Japanese teacher. C. J. McDowell is second from left, second back row. Bill Kilgour, another successful student is in the same row, third from the right.

BRITISH COMMONWEALTH OCCUPATION FORCE

A.A.S.C. TRAINING SCHOOL,
CHICK SEXING COURSE.
CS 45

4 Aug '48.

ubject :- SCHOOL REPORT ON NX181165 CPL McDOWELL C.J.

TATION CMD
TA JIMA

opy to :- DDST HQ S&T BCOF

The following report is submitted on NX181165 CPL McDowell C.J. who attended the No.1 CHICK SEXING COURSE of the AASC TRAINING SCHOOL at BRIT COM SUB AREA, KOBE 20th May to 30 June '48.

RESULT. 86.8%

POSITION IN CLASS. 1st of 17.

CONDUCT. Excellent.

REMARKS. Nothing too good can be said of this excellent student. His enthusiasm and diligence gained him first place in the school. He also gained first place in 3 of the 5 intermediate tests.

He spent many hours additional to his school hours at study and was of great assistance to O.C. school, the other students and the tutors.

In order that he may reach the 98% standard required as a teacher in Australia and to assist the students of the second course it is requested that he be permitted to attend that course commencing 29 Aug '48 and ending 23 Oct '48.

Copy for approval to Cpl McDowell

HD 17/8/48

OK

OK

E.P. Brandwood .... Major
(E.P. BRANDWOOD) O.C.

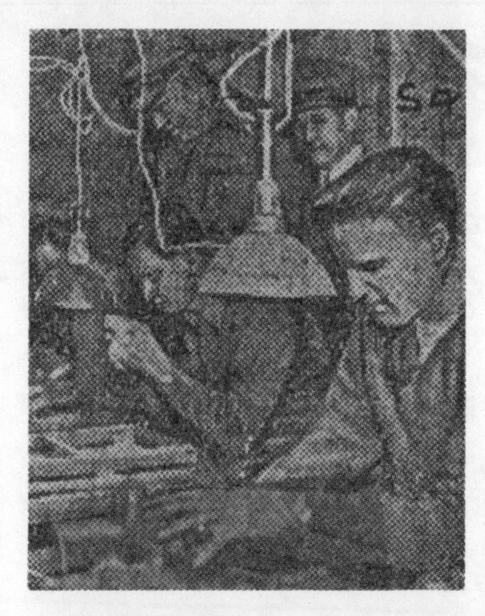

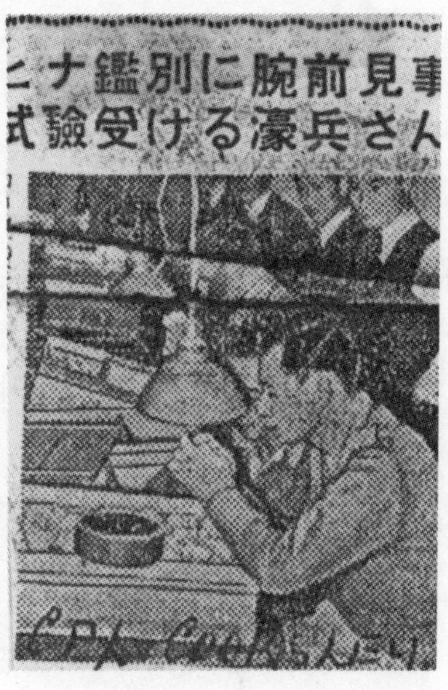

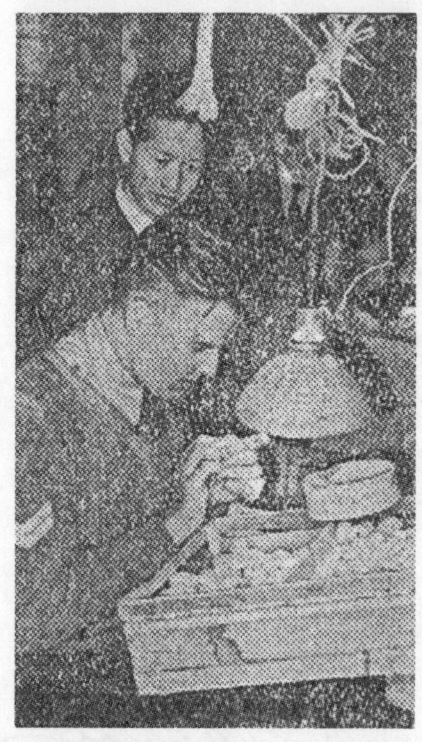

1) Cpl. Cliff McDowell and others, learning chick sexing at the Australian Occupation Army Training School Japan 1948. Major Brandwood and a Japanese teacher look on.
2) Cpl. Cooksley at the school watched by his teachers.
3) Cpl. McDowell and one of his teachers.

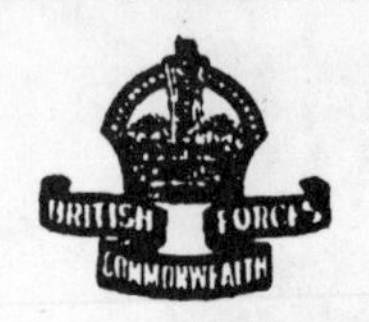

A.A.S.C. Training School

Japan

This is to certify that

NX181165 CPL McDOWELL C.J.

of

STATION COMMAND, ETA JIMA.

attended No 2 Chick Sexing Course

Period from 30 Aug 48 to 23 Oct 48

STANDARD REACHED

100 birds in 13.40 minutes

100 %

Major
Officer Commanding

Brigadier
Principal Administrative Officer

The above course was conducted under my supervison and instruction, assisted by Mr. MATAICHI SAKAI and other leading members of the Japanese Chick Sexing Association.

Dr. KIYOSHI MASUI
Professor of Genetics
Imperial Tokyo University.

The teachers

HIKOSABURO YOGO 1934

Mr Yogo was a gentleman, highly respected by all who had dealings with him, both in class and at the hatcheries where he did commercial chick sexing. He spoke some English, enough to be able to successfully teach a large percentage of the first Sydney class. Six of the twenty who kept at the class for the full four months eventually became chick sexers.

TOMEICHI FURUHASHI FRANK EVANS 1935

In 1935 there were two chick-sexing classes held in Sydney. One was conducted by the Japanese expert, Mr Tomeichi Furuhashi, who held the world's championship for speed and accuracy. Mr Furuhashi's classes were held at Messrs Mann and Gamble Pty Ltd, Berry Street, Clyde. Mavis Heath assisted Mr Furuhashi in this class.

The other class was conducted by Mr Frank Evans at his father's hatchery in Leamington Street, Dundas. A student from this class was to become the second Australian to obtain a special-class certificate: Syd Leach, who sexed 300 chickens in 24 minutes with an accuracy of 98⅔ per cent. Another successful student of this class was Mr C. C. Green, who gained a first-class certificate.

The Japanese experts came to Sydney for the last time in 1937. There were then enough NSW chick sexers to handle all the work in that State. The teaching was carried on firstly by a partnership of Frank Evans and Bert Tegel, and then solely for the next ten years by Evans.

The NSW Government examinations have always been held at the Parramatta School of Arts.

Frank Evans taught more successful commercial chick sexers than anyone else in Australia.

In the November 1993 interview he said he had looked only for the cockerel eminences during his record-breaking examination in 1937 and had not worried about the pullet eminence at all. His wife Mavis chipped in: "Did you tell your students that?"

Frank's reply was a prompt, "No."

So much for jest, but the records show a great majority of the students he taught gained special-class certificates. Mainly as a result of Frank Evans' teaching, NSW was never short of accurate commercial chick sexers.

Up to 1960 NSW had 26 special-class certificate holders, all by the vent method. Victoria, the next biggest poultry State, with three people holding classes, had three special-class certificate holders, one first-class certificate holder with 97.5 per cent and another with 96.5 per cent. All the rest were 95 percenters.

The European Excursions: 1946–1952

In 1945 the 'Secura Incubator Company' of Carlisle, England, advertised in *The Poultry Farmer*, NSW, for chick sexers for the 1946 season. The seasons in Europe were from December until May. In Australia it ran from June until October. Initially, many Sydney chick sexers were interested in going, but eventually only four went from Sydney in 1946: husband and wife team Phyllis Johnson (nee Jarman) and Oscar Johnson, Bob Mayjor and Mayjor's uncle, Jack Edwards. Two Western Australians Norm Bell and Ted Harris also went. They travelled by ship and returned to Australia by Qantas flying boat.

In 1948 and 1949 Frank Evans joined Jack Edwards and several other Australians to work in Belgium and France through a Belgium contractor, Monsieur Dambre, who arranged their work and transport.

Monsieur Dambre had a big American Ford sedan, very unusual in those early post-war austere days. Frank Evans recalls one moment of embarrassment when his entrepreneur hatcheryman turned chick-sexer contractor parked his flash car outside a church. Frank waited outside. By the time Monsieur Dambre reappeared Frank was surrounded by a crowd of curious and admiring onlookers.

In one of the hatcheries in Belgium in the 1948 season Frank Evans worked with a very fast English chick sexer. However, the owner was greatly concerned about the Englishman's accuracy, which was about 85 per cent. He asked Frank to give the Englishman some lessons, which he did. The Englishman slowed down to about 500 chickens an hour, but with a great improvement in accuracy. The extra chickens had to be sexed by the now overworked Australian.

Another of the hatcheries on Frank Evans' weekly round was just over the border in France. All of Europe, with the exception of Belgium, had rationing of food, clothing and fuel. Belgium was fortunate in that the Belgium Congo had uranium, which the Americans bought, so Belgium was not short of anything: Monsieur Dambre's American car, plenty of fuel and food.

On their weekly visits to the hatchery in France, Frank Evans and Jack Edwards were instructed to always fill the tank at the last petrol station in Belgium. While they were sexing at the French hatchery the owner would empty the tank, leaving just enough fuel to get back to that first Belgium petrol station just over the border. This was a weekly occurrence.

In his first year in Belgium, Frank Evans was billeted with an old couple who lived at Vlamatinge, about three miles from Ypres, one of the main battlefields during World War I for Australian soldiers in Europe.

In Frank's second season in Belgium he came to see how resourceful his entrepreneur contractor was.

Most of the Australian chick sexers in Monsieur Dambre's chick-sexing team were owed money from the previous season's sexing. Because he had travelled by Qantas flying boat, Frank Evans had arrived in Europe several weeks ahead of his chick-sexing colleagues from Australia.

Monsieur Dambre crossed the English Channel by ferry in his big Ford to pick Frank up. On the way back, he turned up a side road, much to Frank's surprise. Mr Dambre jacked up the car, removed two tyres and removed pound notes, which had been placed between the car tubes and the tyres. Some of the money had been damaged because of the friction.

When they pulled up at an inn, Monsieur Dambre sent Frank in to see if they had a double room for the night. Frank Evans thought this a little strange, but was not greatly worried.

When they got to the room, Mr D. had Frank sort the damaged money out and match up the numbers of the torn notes. He also got Frank to bundle the notes into lots of £400, which was the amount owed to each of the Australian chick sexers from the previous year. It goes without saying that F.E. made sure his bundle of 400 notes was undamaged. When paying the others, Monsieur Dambre made allowances for any damaged money. By their second year together there was trust all round between Monsieur Dambre and his Australian team.

When Frank Evans took the money to the bank, to be placed in an account in his name, it was the practice to explain to the manager where you got the money.

The manager happened to be an Australian and, after the happy conversation, no doubt about "home", the money source question was forgotten.

Frank had been instructed by Mr Dambre to deposit £400 in accounts for each of the other chick sexers, due in a few days from Australia. This proved too much for Frank. He kept the money and handed it to them when they arrived.

Despite all his entrepreneurial money-making ventures, the gentlemanly Monsieur Dambre was an honest man and all the chick sexers were paid in full.

In 1946 England needed Australian chick sexers because the Japanese working in England in 1939 had been interned during the War and it was not certain if they would be released for the 1946 season.

But the Japanese chick sexers in England were released in 1946, which meant that Jack Edwards, his nephew Bob Mayjor, and Oscar Johnson worked only two days a week. Phyllis Johnson was allocated a hatchery in Windsor and was kept busy. The Japanese who had been released started teaching again. In one hatchery there were Australian and English sexers working downstairs and Japanese chick sexers holding classes upstairs.

The following year, 1946, another advertisement for chick sexers appeared in *The Poultry Farmer*, this time from a chick-sexing service in Belgium. The shortage of chick sexers in Belgium was caused by the Japanese chick sexers having been sent back to Japan by the Belgian Government.

The four NSW chick sexers, now in their second year working in Europe, went to Belgium. Edwards and Mayjor worked for Monsieur Dambre and Phyllis and Oscar Johnson for an "opposition" Belgium chick-sexing service.

The first few weeks Edwards and Mayjor were in Belgium the weather was so cold the eggs froze and, as a result, there were few chicks to sex. Eventually, the work built up and they were both kept working seven days a week. Jack Edwards held chick-sexing classes in Belgium that year and again the next season.

For several years after the war there was quite a lot of chick sexing done in Europe by Australians, and chick sexers from America. The Japanese started to return also and, much later, the Koreans entered into the international chick-sexing business. Also, many English and some other European countries were starting to teach the skills of chick sexing.

There were two chick sexers from Queensland who also sexed in Europe after the war, and a Victorian, Lloyd Lawson, who had stayed on in Belgium from the 1930s.

Frank Evans did not return to Europe for a third season. As Arthur Pamment, another Australian who sexed in Denmark for a season, pointed out, sexing chickens flat out and full time throughout the year is very draining. Frank Evans taught chick sexing for ten years in New South Wales and sexed chicks commercially into his mid-sixties.

Other members of the first generation of New South Wales chick sexers 1934–1945

Syd (S. W.) Leach, the son of a prominent poultry farmer and hatcheryman was the second person to gain a special certificate in NSW (1936). He sexed commercially for many years. He was taught by Frank Evans.

A. (Bert) A. Tegel gained his certificate in the same year as Frank Evans. They held classes together for a couple of years, but eventually genetic poultry breeding took up most of Bert Tegel's time. By 1940 Frank Evans had started sexing at Tegels. A. A. Tegel Pty Ltd is now a large well-known poultry enterprise in Australia.

C. R. Badman did some commercial chick sexing but tended to sex mainly for his own hatchery. He was a member of Mr Yogo's first class in 1934.

J. R. Kilborn sexed commercially for a long time, which means he was very accurate.

Eric Marchant, another first-generation chick sexer from Baulkham Hills. He was taken to Melbourne by Clark King and Co and stayed there to become a colourful, and very successful commercial chick sexer. He retired in the mid 1960s. He was taught by Tomeichi Furuhashi in 1935, assisted by Mavis Heath.

W. Evans gained his certificate in 1936 and sexed commercially for several years, but became more involved in the poultry farm side of his business. He was taught by his brother Frank.

Miss V. Wilson Another of Frank Evans' students, she worked around Newcastle for many years.

Harold Jacobs sexed mainly for his own hatchery. He later engaged Frank Evans and Jack Edwards to do his sexing.

O. B. Johnson went to Europe each season after the war, and taught the skill to his wife, Phyllis. Did large numbers of chickens commercially for many years. Taught by Frank Evans.

Syd Martin was another successful student from Mr Yogo's 1934 class. He sexed commercially for many years. He took Ray Parkin, a young chick sexer, under his wing and helped him start off his commercial chick-sexing career in the late 1940s and early 1950s.

Ian Hazlett learnt from the Japanese, and was a commercial chick sexer with his own hatchery. Gained a first-class certificate. He introduced chick sexing in Western Australia in 1936.

Jack Edwards was a very accurate commercial chick sexer. He was among the first Australian chick sexers to go to Europe after the war, initially to England and later to Belgium. He taught his nephew, Bob Mayjor. They both went to England in 1945 and later to Belgium for several years. After Belgium he again returned to sexing in England until the early 1950s. In NSW he sexed for one hatchery until he was 71.

Jack Edwards, in a letter to Frank Evans in 1993, said, "I sexed my last chick when Harry Molle closed down. I was 71 . . . 49 years of some full-time and much part-time sexing."

J. C. H. Edwards learnt chick sexing from Mavis Heath, who was holding classes not far from where his parents had a farm. This was in 1937. In 1939 he obtained a first-class certificate with 96 per cent accuracy, the thirteenth person in NSW to gain a certificate. In 1945 he gained a special-class certificate with 99⅓ per cent accuracy.

Jack Edwards' fifth and last year working in Europe, 1951, was not a particularly successful one. To start with, some chick sexers he had taught on previous visits left to work on their own. As well, chick-sexing instruments ("machines") were introduced and the price of sexing decreased to a very low level.

Cliff McDowell, another New South Wales chick sexer, had established chick-sexing connections in Devon (England) and invited Jack Edwards to work with him. This combination was very successful.

Back in Australia Jack Edwards worked mainly by himself through the 1950s, but with the growth of the large poultry companies in the 1960s team sexing became the practice, with four to six sexers working at the one hatchery. He worked with Frank Evans, Ray Parkin, Syd Martin and Cliff McDowell.

When he first started chick sexing in 1939 he was paid a ¼ of a cent a chicken. Even at this seemingly small fee it was still equivalent to a half a day's chick sexing netting the basic male wage for a week in Australia.

In commenting in 1994 on chick sexing generally, Jack Edwards is convinced that irrespective of whether a chick sexer uses the vent method or the "machine" method, the results still depend on the skill of the person. "All chicks are different. At different hatcheries there are different types. A commercial chick sexer still needs to kill an odd chick to hold a postmortem. You are always learning. I learnt a lot after passing the chick-sexing exam."

S. G. Olsson was another student of Frank Evans. He gained a 100 per cent accuracy on the first 200 chicks in his special examination.

His speed was 40 minutes for the 300 chicks. He did not do much commercial chick sexing.

Miss B. B. Brown was another Frank Evans student from his first class. She worked commercially around Newcastle for many years. A special-class certificate holder.

C. (Charlie) R. Sims was another special-class certificate holder taught by Frank Evans. Said to have a very strong constitution, he probably sexed a greater number of chickens than anyone in New South Wales.

Other chick sexers from this first generation included Mr A. L. B. Newton, Mr N. B. Davies, Mr R. W. Druce, Mr R. A. Percival, Mrs O. B. Johnson (nee Jarman), Mr H. D. Brown, Mr G. A. Lee and Mr C. C. Green.

There were four other commercial chick sexers from this first generation period who were also taught by Frank Evans. Three were New Zealanders: Mr K. Gibson (1938), who was a very good chick sexer (he missed out on his special certificate by one chicken in his first year as a student) and who stayed with the Evans' while he was learning; Mr Gordon Thomson (1938) who came to Australia to learn the skill, and another New Zealander, Mr Lionel Doughty, who learnt in 1936.

The fourth member from outside NSW of this generation taught by Frank Evans was Mr Tom (T. V.) Gameau from South Australia, who introduced chick sexing to that State. He gained a first-class certificate at the first government examination held in South Australia in 1936.

New South Wales ... the second generation 1946–1961

Ray Parkin

Another very young student to take on chick sexing, Ray Parkin was a member of the Boy Scouts and one of the Scout leaders was a poultry enthusiast. Among the stories he related to the young Raymond was the money to be made as a chick sexer.

The boy was a student of Frank Evans. The two other students in the class that he remembers were a wrestler, who did not go on with chick sexing, and Arthur Pamment, a student from the previous year and who later became one of the State's most prominent commercial chick sexers.

Ray Parkin recalls those early days, the late 1940s and the early 1950s, when he first started as a commercial chick sexer. "I was a bit shy. It took me awhile to get involved. I took what they gave me. NSW always had plenty of chick sexers. Those early days were a dog-eat-dog situation."

In NSW, as in other States, an experienced chick sexer could also often help the hatcheryman with incubation problems. Many came from hatchery families, and after sexing for a few years at so many hatcheries there were few problems and solutions the experienced commercial chick sexer had not heard of. By observing so many day-old chicks, he or she could often tell what was lacking in the hatcheryman's incubation management.

As the young Ray Parkin was to find out, for a new young student, not one from a chick hatchery background, entering the overcrowded commercial world of chick sexing with only his sexing skills to offer, they were not always enough.

One incident in particular he remembers well. He asked a hatcheryman why he had engaged someone else to do his sexing the following season. "What's wrong? Wasn't I good enough?"

"Yes, you are the best we have ever had. It's just that this other chap has helped us with our incubator problems, and he needs the work."

Eventually, Syd Martin, a well-established first-generation commercial chick sexer, got the young Ray Parkin into Inghams. This gave R. P. a big boost to his chick-sexing career.

Ray was also a poultry farmer for several years. Then instrument "machine" sexing came along, followed by feather sexing. He then went into taxis for five years. He always had an ambition to have his own fishing trawler, and he has now achieved this with his fishing company at Wisemans Ferry, Rayjon Prawns Pty Ltd.

Ray Parkin still sexes commercially, one day a week, sometimes less. This arrangement suits him, as it gives him a chance to see his son, Peter, who is a full-time commercial chick sexer at the hatchery. When the hatchery needs extra help they call him.

Apart from teaching his son, Peter, the vent method of sexing chicks and turkeys, he also taught Peter Walker and Les Solomns, all full-time commercial chick sexers of the third generation.

A second-generation chick sexer, Ray Parkin, now in his mid-sixties, claims he is probably the oldest chick sexer still working in Australia.

When questioned about the practice of picking up two chickens at once, which some NSW sexers say helps speed things up a little, his reply was: "I pick up two at once, sex one then throw it, and then sex the other. It doesn't always make you faster, but instead of picking up 5000 times, you cut your movements by half."

When asked about standing up to sex chickens, as some chick sexers do, he said, "When I am at Newcastle I stand up all the time, not because I want to, but because I cannot seem to be able to adjust the chair, to meet the focus of the light. So there, I decided to stand up."

Ray Parkin is an experienced poult sexer. The vent sexing of turkeys requires a slight adjustment to the opening of the vent. If you are not careful you can push both sides and make a female look like a male. If you are doing a lot you can get speed up, but when you are not doing them all the time, it takes 200 to 300 poults to get back into the way of handling them.

Currently (1994) all turkeys sexed in Australia, are sexed by the vent method. Most full-time turkey sexers are very accurate.

To the author's knowledge there has only been one commercial chick sexer in Australia able to sex turkeys by the "machine' method, a Victorian. Many have attempted to sex with the "machine" but without any success. Turkeys are difficult to sex with the "machine", because of the dark pigment of the turkey's bowel wall.

Bob Mayjor—certificate at sixteen

Bob Mayjor learnt from his uncle, Jack Edwards, and later had some lessons from Frank Evans. He went with his uncle to England in 1946 for a season's chick sexing there. As he observes, there weren't many chick sexers around in those days.

Bob Mayjor found working in Belgium a bit rugged at times when compared with Australian conditions: the general way of life, eating in

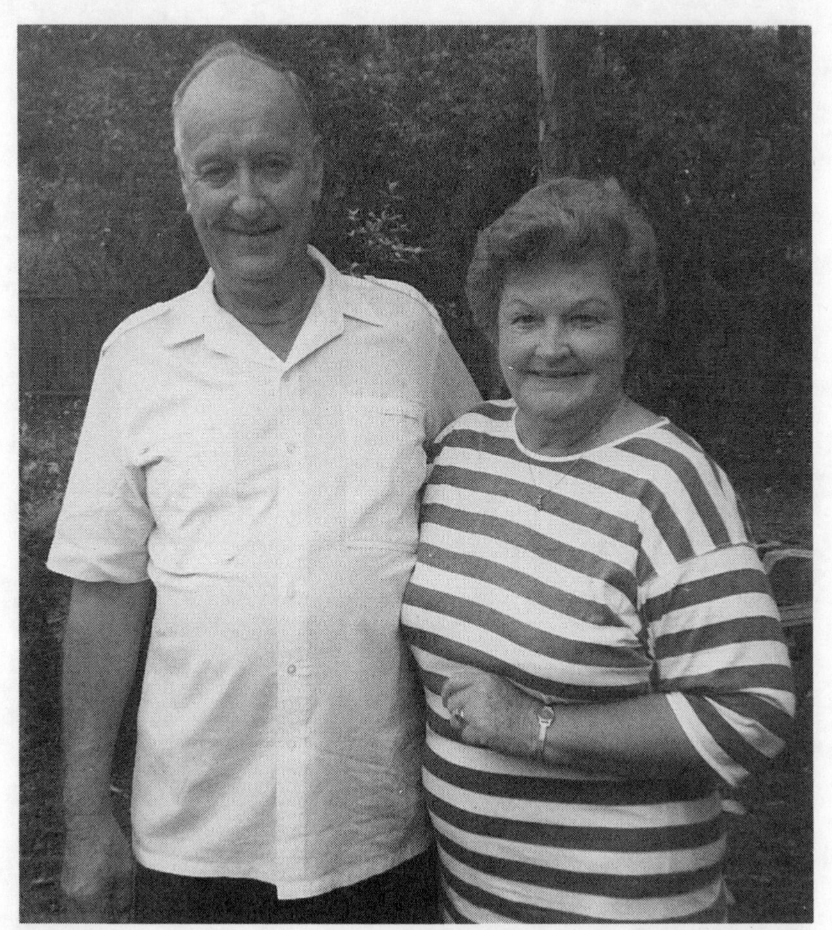

A husband-and-wife chick sexing team. Arthur Pamment, special class certificate 1950, 99.9 per cent accuracy, equals his teacher, Frank Evans' 1937 accuracy. Aileen Pamment, special-class certificate 1953, 98.5 per cent accuracy. Daughter, Amanda, is also a commercial chick sexer with a special-class certificate 1988, 98 per cent accuracy.

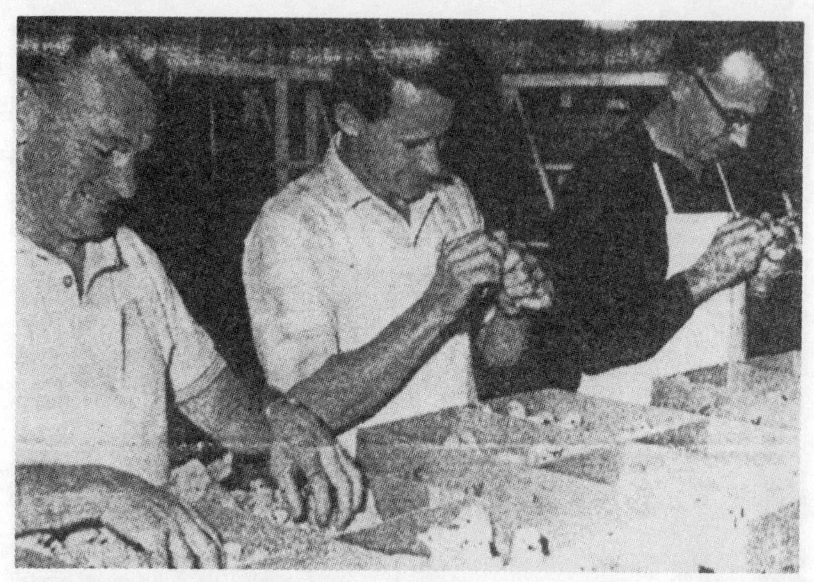

Posing for the photo are three prominent New South Wales chick sexers from left: Ray Parkin, Phil Hill and Frank Evans. They are at the Inghams-Tegel organisation of NSW.

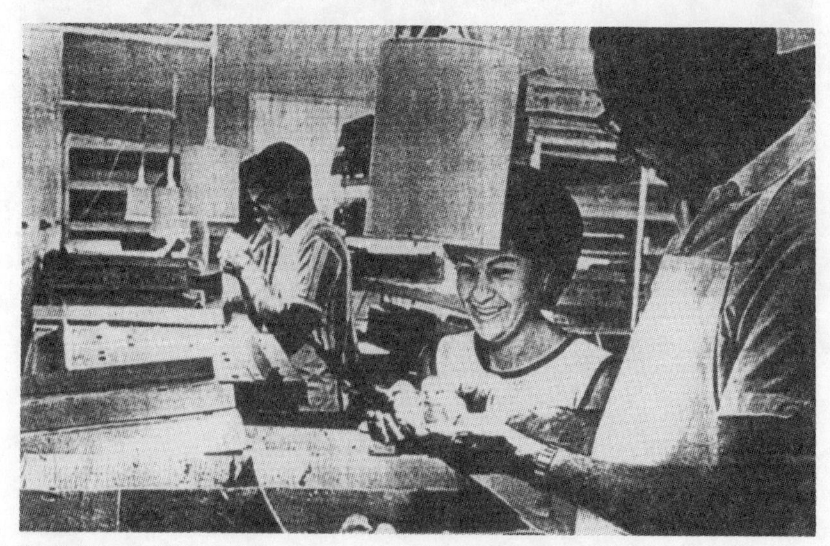

Frank Evans talking to the secretary, Lyn Allen from Inghams. The other members of the chick-sexing team are Ray Parkin, Phil Hill and Cliff McDowell.

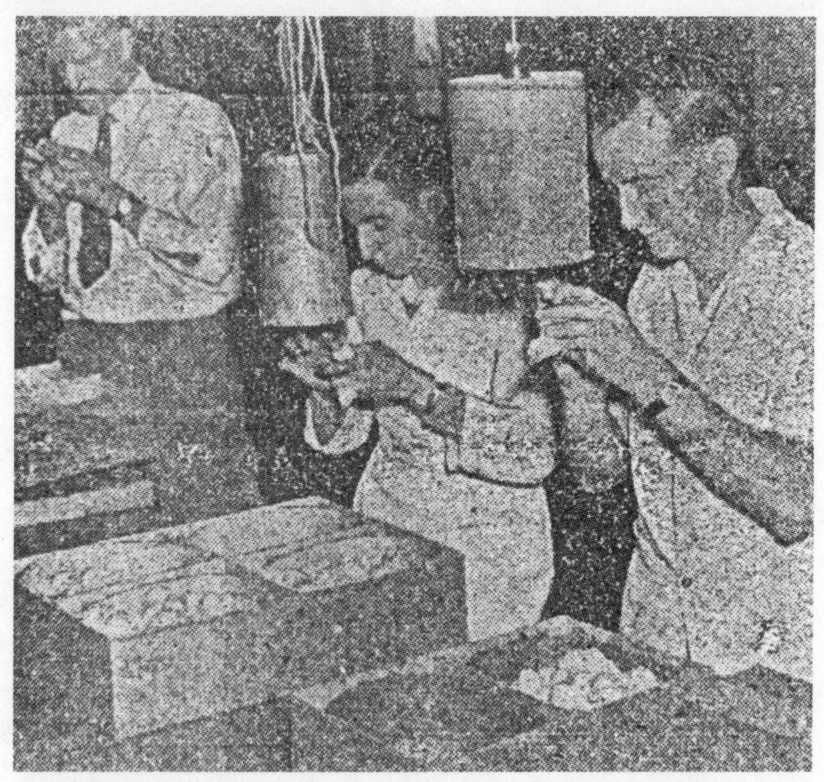

Left to right: Cliff McDowell, R. L. Watson and Arthur Pamment ''sitting'' for a chick-sexing examination run by the New South Wales Agriculture Ministry 1950.

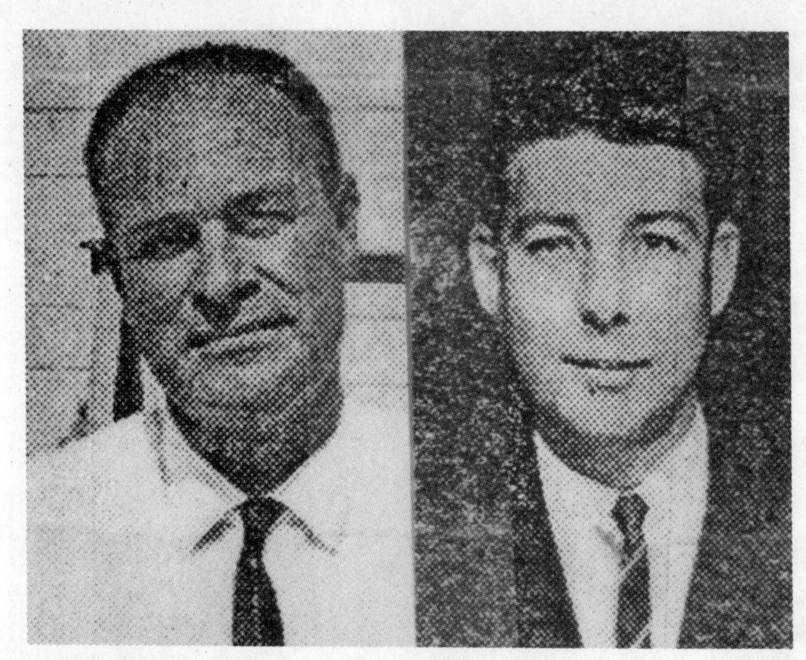

Charles Sims
New South Wales

Bill (Warren) Dewberry
New South Wales

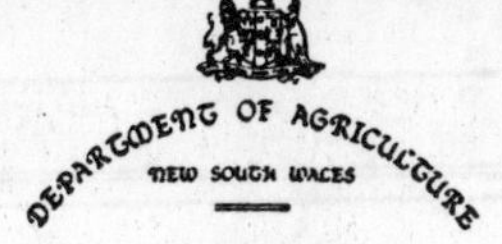

DEPARTMENT OF AGRICULTURE
NEW SOUTH WALES

Chick Sexing Certificate

SPECIAL CLASS

At an examination conducted under the supervision of the New South Wales Department of Agriculture on 30th Sept. 35 Mr Frank Darcy Evans of Dundas sexed 300 White Leghorn Chickens in 27½ minutes with an accuracy of 98·6 per cent in accordance with the prescribed conditions and is therefore granted a "Special Class" certificate.

Examiners:

[illegible]
Poultry Expert.

[illegible]
Veterinary Officer.

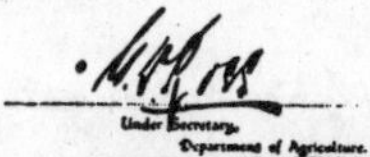

Under Secretary,
Department of Agriculture.

Two firsts: below Australia's first chick sexing certificate and left the first Government chick sexing certificate awarded in Australia. Both awarded to Frank Evans of NSW.

CHICK SEXING ASSOCIATION OF AUSTRALIA
21 VALENTINE STREET, SYDNEY, N.S.W.

Chick Sexing Certificate

First Class

Issued to FRANK DARCY EVANS

of DUNDAS, N.S.W.

In an examination held under standard test conditions, the holder has determined the sex of one hundred day-old chickens with an accuracy of Ninety-eight per cent.

Signature of Holder F. D. Evans

Date FIRST JANUARY, 1935.

for Chick Sexing Association

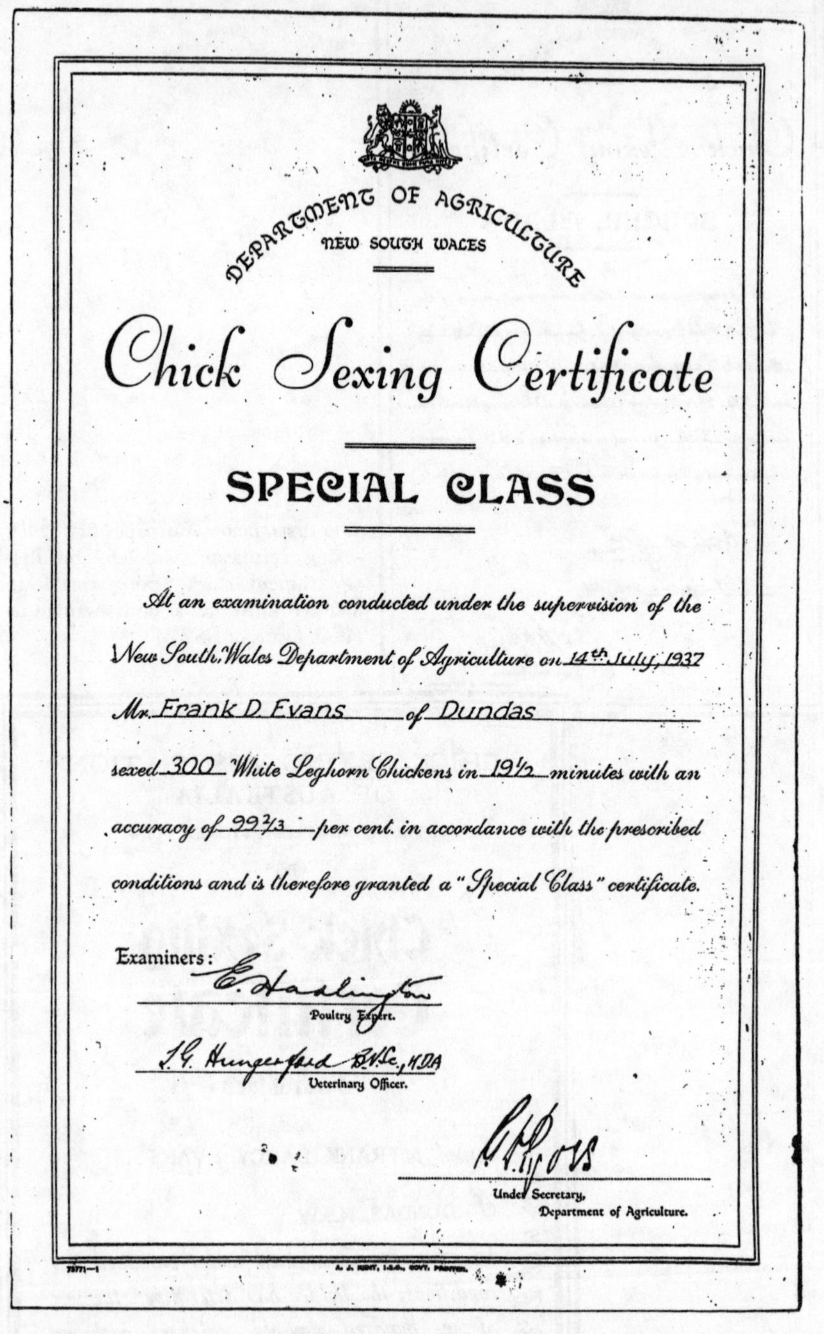

DEPARTMENT OF AGRICULTURE
NEW SOUTH WALES

Chick Sexing Certificate

SPECIAL CLASS

At an examination conducted under the supervision of the New South Wales Department of Agriculture on 14th July, 1937 Mr. Frank D. Evans of Dundas sexed 300 White Leghorn Chickens in 19½ minutes with an accuracy of 99⅔ per cent. in accordance with the prescribed conditions and is therefore granted a "Special Class" certificate.

Examiners: E. Hadlington
Poultry Expert.

T. G. Hungerford B.V.Sc., H.D.A.
Veterinary Officer.

Under Secretary,
Department of Agriculture.

Australia's top award to a cloaca-method chick sexer. Others have equalled and, on 200 chickens, obtained 100 per cent accuracy, but none have equalled Evans' speed.

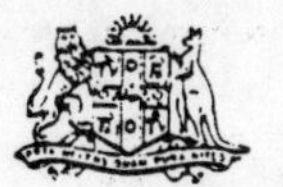

DEPARTMENT OF AGRICULTURE

NEW SOUTH WALES

Chick Sexing Certificate

SPECIAL CLASS

At an examination conducted under the supervision of the New South Wales Department of Agriculture on 27th Sept 1950 Mr. J. C. Pamment of 75 Harris St. Guildford sexed 300 White Leghorn Chickens in 30 minutes with an accuracy of 99 2/3 per cent. in accordance with the prescribed conditions and is therefore granted a "Special Class" certificate.

Examiners:

____
Poultry Expert.

____
Veterinary Officer.

____
Under Secretary,
Department of Agriculture.

23771—1

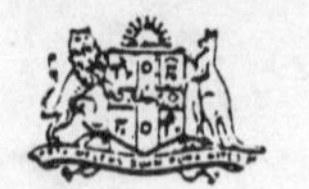

DEPARTMENT OF AGRICULTURE

NEW SOUTH WALES

Chick Sexing Certificate

SPECIAL CLASS

At an examination conducted under the supervision of the New South Wales Department of Agriculture on 23rd June 1953 Mrs A. R. Pamment of Guildford sexed 200 White Leghorn Chickens in 22 minutes with an accuracy of 98½ per cent. in accordance with the prescribed conditions and is therefore granted a "Special Class" certificate.

Examiners:

V. H. Brann
Poultry Expert.

J. J. [illegible]
Veterinary Officer.

[illegible]
Under Secretary,
Department of Agriculture.

73771—1

A. J. KENT, I.S.O., GOVT. PRINTER.

Department of Agriculture
New South Wales

CHICKEN SEXING CERTIFICATE

awarded to

Amanda Pamment

200 DAY-OLD CROSS BRED CHICKENS IN 24 MINUTES
WITH ACCURACY OF 98%

Chief, Division of Animal Production

Director-General, Department of Agriculture

008 11.81 D. West, Government Printer

The last chick sexing certificate (1983) awarded in Australia. New South Wales and Victoria, the last two states to hold chick-sexing examinations, ceased examinations at the end of the 1980s. In both States no-one passed the examinations during the last five or six years they were held. In NSW all candidates used the vent method. In Victoria they used the "machine" method.

hatcheries, sometimes with 20 or 30 other people, and the cold weather causing problems for the farmers: dead birds, frozen eggs and disease. The second year in Belgium was much better. By their second year Jack Edwards and Bob Mayjor had learnt the language and Monsieur Dambre had bought a car for each of them. Bob Mayjor has worked with English chick sexers who could do up to 1200 chickens an hour. How accurate they were is difficult to gauge as it is many weeks before this can be checked.

When Bob Mayjor first went to Europe he could sex at the rate of only 400 an hour, but with help from his uncle checking his accuracy, his confidence soon allowed him to get up to 600 an hour. He was fortunate in having such an accurate teacher. His uncle had the reputation of being 99 per cent accurate.

Bob Mayjor and his uncle had been working in one hatchery in Belgium from 4 a.m. to 2 a.m. the next day when the hatcheryman came to test their accuracy. The hatcheryman just started tearing the chickens open without killing them first.

'Jack Edwards got a bit cranky and told the bloke off,'' Bob Mayjor recalls. ''He said, 'We don't mind you bloody well checking but wring their necks first. Go into the next room and do it.'

''Funnily enough, we were 97 per cent, even at that stage . . . It had been a long day. We'd driven a couple of hundred miles as well.''

Bob Mayjor went on to recall other memories of his time in Europe: ''We were only paid for the pullets. They didn't trust anybody . . . Slipping across the border into France we smuggled petrol many times. Once on our return journey to Belgium we had to be pushed across the border into Belgium. Belgium came out of the war well, American cars, no rationing.''

When asked how European hatcherymen treated their chick sexers Bob Mayjor replied: ''In England they treated you like a labourer. They paid their sexers a basic wage. Yet the English chick sexer who worked with me was okay. We were so busy travelling from one end of Europe to the other that Dambre couldn't keep up with the business. He trusted us and let us collect the fees from the hatcherymen. They had to pay on the spot. Nobody trusted anybody over there.

''There were money restrictions between countries. Dambre had four Australians to pay, their airfares and accommodation. Once he put all the money in a spare wheel but then got worried near the ferry and put the spare wheel on the car and drove onto the ferry. Poor old Frank Evans was there a week before us and he copped it. Had to sort all the damaged money out before we arrived. Dambre was fair. He gave us extra money to cover the damaged notes.''

In Belgium hatcheries, the sexers insisted that they have someone to help them so that they did not have to get up while they were sexing.

Each time before he went to Europe to sex chickens, Bob Mayjor had his eyes tested. On his last trip, he claims they made a mistake with his glasses. As a result, in Belgium he had trouble with his eyes. At 27, Bob Mayjor retired from chick sexing. By the time chick sexing "machines" came on the scene he had retired.

Aileen Pamment

Aileen Pamment, a New South Wales second-generation chick sexer, shares the record of having sexed more chickens commercially than any other woman in Australia with Dorothy McCulloch, of Queensland, a first-generation chick sexer.

Aileen Pamment and her husband Arthur have together sexed well over 30 million chicks in the 40-plus years they have worked together as a commercial chick-sexing team. Aileen and Arthur always worked together. This is one of the reasons she was able to rear two daughters. She was able to drop them off at school and pick them up afterwards, having sexed her 5000 to 6000 chickens in between. The largest number of chickens she has sexed in a day was about 10 300, but like most commercial chick sexers she found 5000 to 6000 a comfortable day's work. Aileen gave up sexing large numbers of chickens in her early 60s, but still does 2000 to 3000 chickens some weeks. She also sexes guinea fowl.

When one of her daughters was born, she worked up until two days before the birth.

Aileen Pamment recalls: "I had her on the Thursday and I was back at work on the Tuesday, although I didn't resume regular work for three weeks."

Like most commercial chick sexers she did not think the demand for chick sexers would ever diminish. While there is less demand now for specialist chick sexers, because of colour and feather sexing, she thinks the specialist chick sexer will come back. The industry will want more chick sexers.

When asked how she had endured so long in a very demanding occupation, her reply was: "If you have an interest in the job . . . a curiosity about learning ... keep on looking for the different types [of eminences] . . . learning is what keeps you young.

"If I got to the stage where I thought I knew everything, I think I would die.

"If you are not interested you give up."

Aileen Pamment recalls some advice she was given, not by anyone in the industry, "but by a guy who never made it": "I tried it and it worked. It came to me like a flash."

One of Aileen and Arthur Pamment's daughters is also a commercial chick sexer. Amanda Pamment was the last student to gain a certificate from the NSW Agriculture Ministry in 1983. Their other daughter is a dental therapist.

Sexing chickens has not prevented Aileen Pamment pursuing one of her other loves, horses. As well as doing the things that keen horse people usually do, she entered a 1200-kilometre ride from Sydney to Melbourne, something she had always wanted to do. Aileen commented at the time, "It was something I was glad I took part in."

A remarkable woman, from a remarkable family.

Stewart McKenzie . . . another second-generation chick sexer . . . champion Olympic sculler

Stewart McKenzie's achievements as a commercial chick sexer are over-shadowed by his sculling successes and his alleged "wild boy" personality. His father had a hatchery at Seven Hills. He sexed chicks commercially around Sydney and overseas. Comments about him include: "A good bloke, one of the world's best scullers, ex-King's School boy."

One story goes that when McKenzie was rowing at Henley he got so far ahead of the other scullers that he stopped rowing, opposite where the Queen was sitting, doffed his hat to her, and then continued rowing.

He now lives overseas and was not available during the research period. There is no doubt that he was a successful commercial chick sexer. His sculling record is well documented in other places.

Cliff McDowell 1948
Japanese certificate 1948, 100 per cent accuracy
New South Wales certificate 1950, 99 per cent accuracy

It is often interesting to hear why people take on a career such as chick sexing.

During the war, Cliff McDowell was training to be a metallurgist. One day in the laboratory he had a disagreement, and he walked out.

He tried to join the Air Force as a fighter pilot, but as it was late in the War they did not want any more fighter pilots. Then he tried the Navy, but here there was a six months' delay, so young Cliff settled for the Army.

Six months after the Bomb was dropped on Hiroshima, Cliff McDowell found himself in the Commonwealth Occupation Forces in Kobe, Japan.

McDowell's father was an engineer with the Sydney Council, and he also had a 2000 bird poultry farm in Greystanes Road, Prospect. Cliff McDowell knew what chick sexing was: the Japanese chick sexers had come to the district in the 1930s, when he was a boy.

When he was stationed at Kobe he wrote to the Japanese Chick

Sexing School at Nagoya to ask if it would teach him chick sexing. They replied that they would be happy to teach him. But the Army would not let only one person learn. There had to be a full school.

Cliff McDowell was instrumental in getting the Army to run a chick-sexing school for the Australian and New Zealand Military Forces personnel in Japan.

When Cliff McDowell first approached his C.O., Colonel Craig, of B Coy Headquarters, the colonel's reply was, in part: "What a bloody good idea. We'll get something out of it etc. etc."

However, it still took two years before the school eventuated. The school cost the Japanese Government 2 000 000 yen. There were 47 students in the class. Three were successful in learning the skill. Two became commercial chick sexers.

As reported in *The Mainichi* (English-language) daily newspaper, on Wednesday, 10th November 1948:

> Nagoya: Nov. 8. Selected as excellent students among some 50 soldiers who finished this year's training in the chick-sexing course of the AASC Training School of BCOF at Kobe, five corporals took the formal examination of the Japan Chick Sexing Association with its office at Mizuho-ku, here.
>
> They were Corporals Clifford James McDowell, William Kilgour, Lloyd Leonard, Kevin Cooksley and Jack Whyte.
>
> They were led by Major P. Brandwood, officer commanding the course.
>
> Although the speed is slow compared with a Japanese sexing expert, Corporal McDowell sexed 100 chicks in 11 minutes and 30 seconds with a 100 per cent accuracy. Ninety eight per cent accuracy was displayed by others.
>
> The examination was at the Hattori Poultry Farm at Ishibotoecho, Showa-ku, here, with Dr Kiyoshi Masui, president of the Association and professor emeritus of Tokyo University and Mataichi Sakai, director of the Association, as examiners.
>
> Certificates will be issued to the five soldiers by the Association.
>
> Trained for 14 weeks in two courses starting May and September, respectively, the five soldiers have made excellent progress in a comparatively short time.
>
> Corporal McDowell said to the reporter: "The Japanese sexing method is fine. I had some difficulty at first as there are many types of chicks. I'll secure a job as a chick sexer in Australia when I am discharged there.
>
> "Some of the soldiers will return to Australia within this year to be discharged there as the first soldiers trained in the Japanese chick sexing method."

Another extract from a Japanese-language newspaper, *The Tokai Mainichi* of the 23rd November 1948 had the following item:

They Beat Us in Chicken Sexing

Led by Major Brandwood, a party of 7 BCOF NCO's who have been learning the Japanese art of Chicken Sexing visited Yamamoto Hatchery at Yagiubashi in Toyeoka on the 1st November for more practical exercise. They represent the best of 47 who went through the course, and they impressed the Mayor of Toyeoka, Mr Otake, and the Director of the Sexing Association Mr Sakai by successfully identifying over 500 chicks in one hour with 95 per cent accuracy.

Major Brandwood said: "Due to the untiring effort of Dr Masui of Tokyo University, and Mr Ohayashi, 47 personnel completed with great success. These seven soldiers have been picked as the best among those who finished the course, and we have come to Toyeoka, the centre of poultry farming, to get a further practical experience. I expect they will do fine work in this line when they go back to Australia."

On their return to Australia, Cliff McDowell, of NSW and Jack Whyte, of Victoria became successful commercial chick sexers. Given the 47 candidates, this was a four per cent success rate, about the usual rate since the introduction of chick sexing in the 1930s. The cost of training the two chick sexers is about what it would cost if a student had to buy all his chicks for practice. A third successful student, Bill Kilgour, of South Australia, did not take on commercial chick sexing. South Australia, a much smaller poultry-industry State, may not have afforded him the same opportunity as the larger States, but here again experience has shown that not all who are capable of mastering the skill in class or examinations become commercial chick sexers.

One of the Japanese instructors at the school, Tadashi Sakai, looked at all the students' hands, and when he came to McDowell, said: "No good, too big, damage the chicks."

McDowell went on to gain a 100 per cent in the final examination, the only student to that time to do so. When he returned to Australia he was almost as successful in the NSW examinations, making only three errors in 300 white leghorn chicks.

This myth about needing small hands is an old one and one that many people still cling to. Another one is that Asian people have some magical ability that enables them to be more successful at the skill than others. As Mr Hitoshi Miyata, Executive Director of the Zen-Nippon Chick Sexing Association, himself a 100 percenter, said at an interview with Bob Martin, "there is no secret: it's just practice, practice, practice and more practice."

The Japanese expert and former managing director of the Association, Mr Nobuyoshi Tanaka, another 100 percenter of the 1930s, said the same thing. He went on to say that a student really needs to sex 250 000 cockerels before starting on mixed chicks.

Cliff McDowell, unlike most of the chick sexers from Australia who went overseas in the 40s and 50s, went to England privately, not engaged by a chick-sexing contractor. He placed an advertisement in an English poultry magazine and started from there.

When he arrived in England there were fifteen replies. He decided on the one that was in the part of England near where his new fianceé, Patricia Pritchard, lived, at Amesbury, Wiltshire, near Stonehedge. Cliff McDowell and Patricia met on the Orion on this first trip to England. They became engaged before the ship reached port.

When McDowell rang the hatchery the reply was: "Bad luck, old fellow, the hatchery just got burnt down."

McDowell managed to earn enough to pay fares working for a subcontractor.

Cliff McDowell made successful trips to England for the next four years, eventually starting his own contracting business, which he sold when he finally returned to Australia to stay. He went on to sex commercially around Sydney until he bought a car agency and he now deals in caravans.

He taught his nephew, David McDowell, the skill. David McDowell, a third-generation chick sexer, now sexes chicks full time at Newcastle and occasionally interstate.

A discussion between Arthur Pamment (A.P.), Ray Parkin (R.P.), and Bob Martin (B.M.) 12 November 1993 (An edited version)

A.P. After 1953 the Government (NSW) examination conditions were changed. Instead of pure white-leghorn chickens they had crossbred chicks, and for a special-class certificate you now had to sex only 200 chickens instead of the former 300 chickens. The accuracy requirement at 98 per cent was the same.

R.P. I was the last to get a special certificate with 300 chickens. I asked to have 300 chickens, to be the same as my former colleagues.

A.P. At Leach's Hatchery the sexers and owners had a monthly conference. The management decided to sack the only "machine" sexer on their team. I had to go back in after the meeting and ask why did you put X off? The reply was, "I don't want to go through all this again. I spent ten years working on this!"

A.P. My daughter [Amanda] was the last one to get a Government chick-sexing certificate, nine years ago [1983]. The last chick-sexing examination was held in NSW in 1991. As former secretary of the chick-sexing association I still get the official notification.

No "machine" candidates, all vent sexers, all ethnic Koreans, all failed on the one side. [That is, they made enough errors on the cockerel side to fail and that it was not necessary to postmortem the pullet side.]

A.P. I've got two special-certificates [300 white leghorn chickens], three firsts, more than anyone else in Australia. Each time you get another certificate you have to hand the previous one back to the department. The last certificate I got 100 per cent in the first 200 chickens and made one error in the last 100 chicks, an overall accuracy of 99⅔ per cent. I took 30 minutes to sex the 300 chickens.

A.P. Amanda [Pamment] and Ray's son [Peter] are the only young ones coming on.

B.M. What about the future for chick sexers?

A.P. As is the case overseas, all future sexers will be cloacal sexers [vent] . . . the penny has dropped everywhere but in Australia.

B.M. Have you seen the German chick-sexing machine?

A.P. Yes, its soft colour is easy on the eye.

A.P. At one hatchery we used to hold a monthly competition between the sexers. The vent sexers won every time for accuracy.

A.P. At XY hatchery, Victorian "machine" sexers came up to sex broiler chickens . . . they were sexing them at half price, because they were getting the numbers. The hatchery didn't worry about accuracy . . . 95 per cent was good enough.

Then all of a sudden the hatchery came along and wanted to look at the culls. The vent sexers had very few, the "machine" sexers had boxes of them . . . they started going through looking at the high mortality . . . the vent sexers only had a handful.

You know if you puncture them!

A.P. At Leach's they always checked a couple of hundred cockerels.

B.M. What, every week?

A.P. Not just every week, every hatch.

B.M. You could thank them for your high accuracy in the examinations.

What about your overseas sexing? Did you only sex for one hatchery?

A.P. No, I sexed for several hatcheries—all on contract [1952]. Overseas you sexed from drawers. You did not move—the chickens were fed to you—no advantage to pick up two chickens.

B.M. That set-up was the same as they had at Hockeys Hatchery in Victoria . . . you never had to move, the chickens were brought to you and the sexed ones were counted and taken away.

A.P. In America, a chap there taught us to use each of our four fingers in case one was ever injured.

[Some discussion by Arthur Pamment about some of the changes brought about by genetic breeding and the difficulty in sexing some of the chicks followed . . .]

R.P. When you open the vent there was nothing there but you know it's a cockerel.

[The future prospects' question came up again.]

A.P. There'll be work, but you'll have to be tops. Down the track a little . . . maybe they'll get overseas sexers.

B.M. They would still have to pay them and have comfortable working conditions if they want accuracy.

R.P. 800 chicks an hour is the speed if you do it properly.

[After further discussion it was agreed that 5000 chickens a day was a fair and comfortable day's work.]

A.P. Glasses—two frames more than reading glasses will cope with sexing anytime.

[The use of prismatic glasses was discussed. Some sexers use them. Max Akam in Victoria, who sexed until he was 63, used them from about 40. They were to correct an eye fault. Generally, as Arthur Pamment pointed out, two frames above what is required for reading will do the job. This is only an opinion—see your ophthalmic surgeon and tell him or her what your needs are. Bob Martin is in his mid-sixties and he can still sex chickens at the rate of 800 an hour. He uses two frames above reading, with a slight tint. He does not now sex chickens commercially nor has he done for twenty years. This bits-and-pieces discussion also covered the effects, if any, of the chick-sexing "machine" on the DNA patterns and loss of breeding goals.]

New South Wales

List of Qualified Chick Sexers — "First generation"
Department of Agriculture — 1934–1945
First Examination 1936

Special Class: 98 per cent accuracy required. 300 white leghorn chickens in 45 minutes.

Name	*Address*	*Year*	*Accuracy*
All vent method			
Mr F. D. Evans	53 Leamington St.	1936	
	Dundas	1937	99⅔
Mr S. W. Leach	Windsor Rd.	1936	98⅔
	Baulkham Hills		
Mr A. L. B. Newton	Blacktown		
Mr N. B. Davies	Garnet Rd. Miranda		
Mr R. W. Druce	Old Prospect Rd.		
	Wentworth		

Mr R. A. Percival	135 Longueville Rd. Lane Cove
Mr S. Martin	Duggan Farms, Blacktown
Mrs O. B. Johnson	52 Dickson Ave. West Ryde
Mr B. B. Brown	Green's Ave. Dundas
Mr J. Edwards	74 Grantham Rd Seven Hills
Mr C. R. Sims	5 Millar St. Drummoyne
Mr H. D. Brown	Braeside Rd. Wentworthville
Mr G. A. Lee	60 Beaufort St. Croydon Park

First Class Certificate: 95 per cent accuracy required. 200 chickens in 30 minutes

Name	Address	Year
Mr A. A. Tegel	Leppington	1936
Mr C. R. Badman	Mackenzie St. Revesby	
Mr J. R. Kilborn	9 Denman St. Eastwood	
Mr E. Marchant	Melbourne Vic (Baulkham Hills)	1936
Mr W. Evans	Dundas	1936
Mrs F. D. Evans (nee Heath)	(Toongabbie) 53 Leamington St. Dundas	1936
Mr C. C. Green	82 Carlingford Rd. Epping	
Miss V. Wilson	Box 249 P.O., Newcastle	
Mr H. Jacobs	Vimiera Rd. Eastwood	
Mr I. A. Hazlett	Ingleburn	
Mrs A. Brakell	Church St. Carlingford	
Mr K. Gibson	Wensley House, Stanford Park Rd. Mt Roskill, Auckland N.Z.	1938
Mr Gordon Thomson	Opoho Dunedin N.Z.	1938
Mr J. H. Turner	Hotham Rd. Sutherland	1944
Mrs T. M. Brown	Main Rd. Kearsley	1940
Mr J. Herrman	86 Station St. Fairfield	1940
Mr H. Wallastre	Grantham Rd. Plumton	1940
Mr O. Van Stappen	Pacific Highway, Wyong	1940

Mrs H. M. Leach	Windsor Rd. Baulkham Hills	1940	
Mr A. M. Smith	Richmond Rd. Blacktown	1940	
Mr A. H. Baker	13 Marion St. Harris Park	1941	
Mr R. Pitt	Government Rd. Weston	1941	
Mr O. Korting	Bid-a-wee Poultry Farm, Quakers Hill	1942	
Mr R. O. Clucas	Excelsior Ave. Castle Hill	1943	
Mr K. J. Fooks	Tomah St. Carlingford	1944	
Mr R. Clark	Bay Rd. Arcadia	1944	
Mr S. G. Gibson	Richmond Rd. Marsden Park	1944	

List of Qualified Chicken Sexers "Second generation"
Department of Agriculture 1945–1965
First Examination 1936

Note: From 1952 onwards crossbred chicks were used, not white leghorns, as had been the practice up to this time, and also candidates were required to sex 200 chicks not 300 as in the past. The exception was Ray Parkin in 1953 who chose to be tested on 300 chicks.

Special Class Certificate: 98 per cent accuracy required. 300 white leghorn chickens in 45 minutes.

Name	*Address*	*Year*	*Accuracy*
Mr R. G. Amies	Windemere Ave. Northmead	1945	
Mr K. L. Moore	5 Daisy St. Chatswood	1945	
Mr A. E. Sutton	65 Bungaree Rd. Wentworthville	1945	
Mr B. J. Dawson	Withers Rd. Kellyville	1950	
Mr A. Pamment	1 Colbran Ave.	1948	
	Kenthurst	1950	99⅔
	(3 Firsts before 1948)		
Mr C. J. McDowell	Summer Hill	1950	99
Cross bred chicks used from 1952			
Mrs A. Pamment	1 Colbran Ave. Kenthurst	1953	98½

Mr R. Parkin	Chaseling Rd. Wisemans Ferry (300 chicks)	1953	
Mr Stewart McKenzie		?	

First Class Certificates: 95 per cent accuracy required. 200 white leghorn chicks in 30 minutes. From 1952 crossbred chicks were used.

Name	*Address*	*Year*	*Accuracy*
Mrs Z. Jacobs	Kildare Rd. Doonside	1945	
Mr N. Long	Fernhill St. Guildford	1945	
Mr R. Lockyear	Hurt St. West Wollongong	1948	
Mr G. E. Mahon	Kings Rd. Ingleburn	1946	
Mr R. J. Mayjor	106 Ballandella Rd. Toongabbie	1947	
Mr F. S. Wrigley	Melbourne Vic	1947	
Miss N. Hall	Herring Rd. Eastwood	1945	
Mr D. Melville	c/o Leach's Hatchery, Windsor Rd. Baulkham Hills	1945	
Mr J. R. Clucas	Old Northern Rd. Castle Hill	1945	
Mr C. M. Whitehead	Addison Rd. Manly	1946	
Mr R. L. Watson	4 West Terrace, Bankstown	1950	
Mr R. D. Martin	Melbourne	1951	W/L

Crossbred chicks from here:

Mr W. G. Savage	Oak Rd, Sutherland	1952	
Mr F. Ramsbottom	Castle Hill	1953	
Miss J. Clarke	Strathfield	1953	
Mr Phil Hill		1954	

Second Class Certificate. Second generation NSW (discontinued only a wartime measure)

95 per cent accuracy required. 200 chicks in 50 minutes.

Mrs W. J. Hanley	219 Princes Highway, Charlestown	1945

"Third generation NSW"
1964–1990

Special Certificate 98 per cent. First. 95 per cent. Both 200 chicks crossbred or meat chicks used.

Name	*Address*	*Year*	*Accuracy*	*Method*
Mr Peter Parkin		1981	Special	vent

Miss Amanda Pamment	1 Colbran Ave. Kenthurst	1983	Special 98%	vent

[Note: Miss Pamment was the last candidate to qualify for a chick-sexing certificate in NSW. Examination were held until 1991]

The candidates listed below have qualified for government certificates but there is no record of whether they obtained specials or first certificates. There were three other candidates who passed examinations (not listed here) during this period using the "machine" method but they did not continue on with commercial chick sexing for more than two years.

Mr Andrew Buchan, 4 Lyndel Close, Soldiers Point NSW qualified in Victoria in 1969. First Class 97.3 per cent using the "machine" method. [All chick sexers listed under the third generation list on this page are currently (1994) working as commercial chick sexers. Some, however, do not work full-time.]

Mr Bill (Warren) Dewberry	machine	1960
Mr Col Peek	machine	1960
Mr David McDowell Nelson's Bay	vent	
Miss Cheral Jones	vent	1980s
Mr Peter Walker	vent	1962
Mr Les Solomns	vent	1962
Mr Tom Brown	machine	1964
Mr George Apap	machine	1956

[While Mr Apap qualified during the period I have designated the second generation in this study, I have included him in the third generation as most of his commercial chick sexing would have been done during the third generation period.]

Queensland 1934–1994

Chick sexing was introduced in Queensland in 1934 with the arrival of Mr Kiyoshi Ozawa. Mr Ozawa came to Brisbane independently: he was not a member of the Japan Chick Sexing Association, as were the experts who came to New South Wales and Victoria. He did not have a working permit and was detained by the Australian authorities for his illegal entry.

George Mann and Mr Yogo came to his rescue and got him work and set up a class in Brisbane. This first class, in 1934, was held at Red Comb House, Roma Street, Brisbane.

Among the first generation of Queensland chick sexers taught by Mr Ozawa in 1934 were Miss Dorothy McCulloch, Mr W. Slawson and Mr R. Alcorn, all of whom became commercial chick sexers. Two other successful students, but who did not take on commercial chick sexing, were Mr E. Pennefather and Miss M. Coulson. All second-generation chick sexers in Queensland were taught either by Miss McCulloch or Mr W. Slawson.

During the years since 1934 many people have learned chick sexing in Queensland, but comparatively few have made it a full-time occupation, due partly to Queensland being a small poultry-producing State.

Only the vent method was used until 1961 in Queensland. Mr Eric Lehtonen was the first person to use the "machine" method commercially in Queensland. By 1965 there were six licensed "machine" chick sexers.

The price of chick sexing in Queensland has ranged from 42c a 100 to 50c a 100 in 1947, to 60c in 1949 and 84c a 100 in 1952. It was up to $1 a 100 by the 1960s.

In 1946 there were 1 884 000 chicks sexed in Queensland. By 1964 this figure had risen to 5 500 000 chicks. Approximately 8 per cent were meat chickens.

Queensland's chick-sexing industry is different in two ways: it is the only State where it is a requirement for the chick sexer to spray the cockerels when he has finished sexing them. This is under Section 22 of *The Poultry Industry Acts,* 1946 to 1965. It is also an offence for a person to sell or offer for sale day-old cockerel chickens unless they have been marked with the prescribed stain or dye.

The other unique feature of chick-sexing in Queensland is the development of a small group of part-time counters to assist the chick sexers. They were paid 10c a box.

Mr R. Nivin, a second-generation chick sexer, went to New Guinea on a two-year contract to introduce chick sexing there.

In 1965 a man from South-East Asia was taught chick sexing by the NSW Chick Sexing Association, and in early 1967 the Government of the Philippines sent two men to Australia to learn both the "machine" and the vent method of sexing. This work was undertaken by four members of the Australian Chick Sexer's Association. Queensland was involved in both of these ventures.

The conditions for obtaining a government chick-sexing certificate in Queensland were: prior to 1966, first-class certificate, 200 chicks in 30 minutes with 95 per cent accuracy; a second-class certificate, 100 chicks in 20 minutes, with 90 per cent accuracy; from 1966, first-class 97 per cent accuracy in both sexes; expert class 200 chicks in 30 minutes, second-class 93 per cent accuracy in both sexes.

A separate licence is issued to "machine" and vent sexers.

On average, during the second generation of Queensland sexers, there were 33 chick sexers. Of these only nine were fully occupied as commercial chick sexers during the hatching season.

PEOPLE INVOLVED IN CHICK SEXING IN QUEENSLAND

1st Generation taught by Mr Kiyoshi Ozawa in 1934	*Method*
Miss D. McCulloch (Commercial Sexer)	Vent
Mr W. Slawson (Commercial Sexer)	Vent
Mr R. Alcon (Commercial Sexer)	Vent
Mr E. Pennefather	Vent
Miss M. Coulson	Vent

Second Generation taught by the above	*Method*
Mr R. Nivin (Commercial Sexer) taught by D. McCulloch	Vent
Mr D. Fraser (Commercial Sexer) taught by W. Slawson	Vent
Mr H. George (Commercial Sexer) taught by W. Slawson	Vent
Mr C. Hazel (Commercial Sexer) taught by W. Slawson	Vent
Mr J. Rumball (Commercial Sexer) taught by D. McCulloch	Vent
Mr R. Slawson (Commercial Sexer) taught by W. Slawson	Vent
Mr N. Seymour (Commercial Sexer) taught by W. Slawson	Vent
Mr M. McLucas taught by D. McCulloch	Vent
Mr J. Obst taught by C. Hazel	Vent
Mr H. Stehn taught by C. Hazel	Vent
Mr A. Mangel taught by C. Hazel	Vent

Mr R. Phyall taught by W. Slawson	Vent
Mr D. Elkes taught by W. Slawson	Vent
Mrs Haseman taught by W. Slawson	Vent
Mr J. Cameron taught by W. Slawson	Vent
Mr J. Gowan taught by H. George	Vent
Mr F. Maxfield taught by D. McCulloch	Vent
Mr J. Greenland taught by D. McCulloch	Vent
Mr G. Smythe taught by J. Rumball	Vent
Mr G. Bowtell taught by J. Rumball	Vent
Mr K. Hoopert taught by C. Hazel	Vent

3rd Generation	*Method*
Mr M. Kemsley (Imported Tasmania/West Australian Chicken Sexer)	Vent & Machine
Mr T. Davis (Chicken Sexer) taught by R. Alcorn	Vent & Machine
Mr G. Grindrod (Chicken Sexer) taught by R. Alcorn	Vent & Machine
Mr R. Grindrod (Chicken Sexer) taught by R. Alcorn	Vent & Machine
Mrs G. Hosmer (Chicken Sexer) taught by R. Alcorn	Machine
Mr M. Francis (Chicken Sexer) taught by D. Fraser	Machine
Mr K. Batkin (Imported New Zealand Chicken Sexer)	Machine
Mr J. McLeod (Chicken Sexer) taught by R. Grindrod & M. Kemsley	Machine
Mr R. Moffatt (Chicken Sexer) taught by M. Kemsley & R. Grindrod	Machine
Mr R. Hodgekinson (Chicken Sexer) taught by M. McLucas & M. Kemsley	Machine

Commercial chick sexing in Queensland has always had a lot of travelling. During the war years this presented many problems with fuel and tyre rationing. To overcome this, many chick sexers travelled long distances in one car, then split up at their destinations.

The Queensland Chick Sexer's Association was formed in 1944 to help overcome some of these problems.

As well as the people listed earlier as having been involved in chick sexing in Queensland, the following people have obtained chick sexing licences:

Mr Eric Lehtonen	("machine")	first class
Mrs Lehtonen	("machine")	first class
Mr Doug Loveday	(vent)	second class
Mrs Jan Spicer	("machine")	first class
Mr G. Bond	("machine")	

Mrs J. Van Bekham	("machine")	first class
Miss G. Mills	("machine")	
Mrs G. Hosmer	("machine")	

One of the most prominent of the first generation of Queensland chick sexers, and the only one surviving, is Miss Dorothy M. McCulloch. Dorothy McCulloch was also responsible for teaching many second-generation commercial chick sexers.

Below is an edited interview between Dorothy McCulloch and Bob Martin held on 26 November 1993:

BM: Why did you take on chick sexing?

DMc: My father had a small hatchery and I was there. There were no boys so I took it on.

BM: In the first year, you were in the first Japanese class, weren't you? Could Mr Ozawa speak English okay?

DMc: No. He understood it, but could not speak it.

BM: He still taught you okay then?

DMc: Yes, he could explain it to you.

BM: How many were in the first class, do you remember?

DMc: Yes, we started off with about twenty but we dwindled down to twelve.

BM: Did the Japanese do commercial chick sexing in Queensland?

DMc: Oh, yes! Because there was no-one else who could do it.

BM: How many years did they come to Queensland?

DMc: Only the two years.

BM: What age did you give up commercial chick sexing?

DMc: I was sixty-three.

BM: Remarkable!

DMc: My eyes started to get cataracts and I gave it up.

BM: For you, what was a comfortable day's number of chickens to sex?

DMc: Well . . . 8000 to 10 000 . . . I did the old way. I did 750 an hour. I could go for hours and not get tired . . . when I did that many it was near home . . . I used to stop, go home for a meal, perhaps a few hour's sleep and start again, until I was finished.

BM: They've all gone back to the vent method overseas. Maybe we'll be able to get a job again.

DMc: No, No! My eyes wouldn't let me. I'm 81 now.

BM: You've probably heard of Frank Evans.

DMc: Yes, yes, I have.

BM: He's been my hero for over forty years. I met him for the first time three weeks ago. He'll be eighty in February. He's a very sprightly bloke too. Max Kemsley tells me you have a crook leg at the moment.

DMc: I have a bad leg, poor circulation. I'm in an old-people's home, but I look after myself and my sister. I live in a cottage. I take an interest in everything. I'm in a singing group which I conduct and I play the organ for the church ... I keep myself busy.

BM: When you were sexing, did you ever think the chicks would ever run out and there would be no more chickens to sex?

DMc: Oh no, I don't think so. There was always plenty for you to do.

BM: The "machine" didn't affect you at all?

DMc: No. I did try the "machine" but I was always frightened of hurting the chicken. I very seldom had a chicken die when they were in my hands.

BM: Overseas, they have all gone back to the vent method, not because of any damage to the chicks so much as it is claimed that putting the light inside can affect their breeding program.

DMc: I'm not surprised. I used to think something like that would happen and there's so much feather sexing now.

BM: Yes. But even there they can only feather sex either the parents or the offspring, not both.

DMc: That's right.

BM: They still need some sexers ... there're still about 25 chick sexers in Australia compared to when you and I were operating. There were about 150 at the peak.

DMc: When I started there were only four in Queensland ... Then I taught some people up the country ... I taught people in Cairns, Mackay, Townsville, Gympie and Bundaberg. Mr Slawson, Bill Slawson, taught around Brisbane.

BM: According to my research, you taught the most people in Queensland.

DMc: Yes, I would think so.

BM: Were you able to drive yourself around? There weren't many women drivers in those days [1930s].

DMc: Yes. I drove myself all the time. Some of the trips were from Brisbane to Ipswich [40 kilometres]. Three of us would go in the one car, all chick sexers. The boys would do the driving. We'd leave home about 5 a.m. We'd start work at Ipswich about 8 a.m. then we would go back to Brisbane and I'd have to work at night around the Brisbane area.

BM: Did you ever have to use gas producers on your car during the war?

DMc: No, we had an allowance, a ration, and had to keep a record of our mileage every month. We had a tyre allowance also. The department was very good here.

BM: You and a woman, Aileen Pamment, a chick sexer from Sydney, have sexed more chickens than any other women in Australia.

DMc: When we first started sexing it was only in a small way ... A lot of people didn't believe in it . . . They thought it would kill the chicks and all sorts of things. It took years, nearly until the war, before Queensland fully accepted chick sexing.

BM: Were you still sexing when they started sexing meat chickens in Queensland?

DMc: Yes, then sexing was all the year round, but I started to do less chickens then. My eyes and legs were starting to give trouble.

BM: When did you start wearing glasses?

DMc: When I was about 32. I started sexing when I was 21 and by the time I started getting into it I was 24. I remember the first time I did 15 000 chickens on my own . . . I said, listen that's too much for one person, I can't do them in one day. It will take two days.

BM; Did you get through the lot?

DMc: Yes, I did the lot. It took me into the next day. I worked from 8 a.m. It was a hatchery near my home. I went home for my lunch, then I went home for the evening meal. Then I worked until 10 o'clock . . . I came back at 6 a.m. the next day and finished them after lunch.

BM: Some people used to stand up to sex.

DMc: I stood up all the time. I couldn't get a bench that was suitable—never the right height. I carried a rubber mat with me.

BM: Some of these first Japanese only made one mistake in 900 chicks. Not bad is it!

DMc: Not bad. Someone told me once I left three pullets in 1000 cockerels.

BM: That classes as 100 per cent in my view. Those three probably changed sex.

DMc: Others wanted to learn, but it wasn't that easy.

BM: Did you take anyone with you to count and box the chickens?

DMc: Yes, at some farms I took someone with me to feed me unsexed chicks and take away the pullets and cockerels, also to count and shift the boxes. I started off just sexing my father's chicks, then after a year someone else asked me to sex their chicks. They weren't satisfied with their sexer and the business just started from there.

BM: Your business grew gradually then. I enjoyed my commercial chick-sexing career.

DMc: So did I . . . I am the only one of the first ones still alive.

[One of the hatcherymen Dorothy McCulloch sexed chickens for comes to visit her twice a year.]

Currently (1994) there are three part-time chick sexers working in Queensland. One, Max Kemsley ("machine" and vent) also works for the Ministry for Primary Industries.

The other two are Mr T. Davis and Mr Robert Grindrod. Both use the "machine" method. Feather sexing has taken over as the main method of determining the sex of day-old chickens in Queensland. Most of Australia's genetic poultry breeders are in New South Wales.

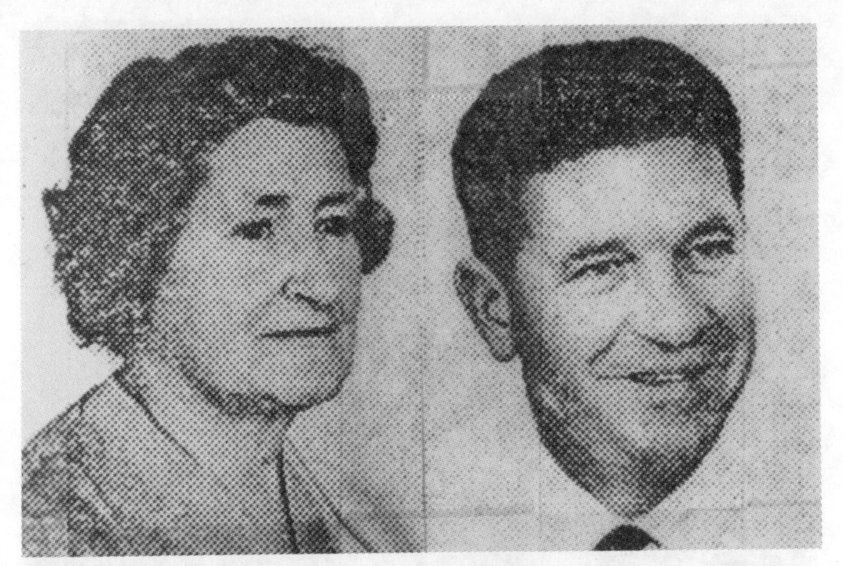

Dorothy McCulloch
Queensland

Ray Slawson
Queensland

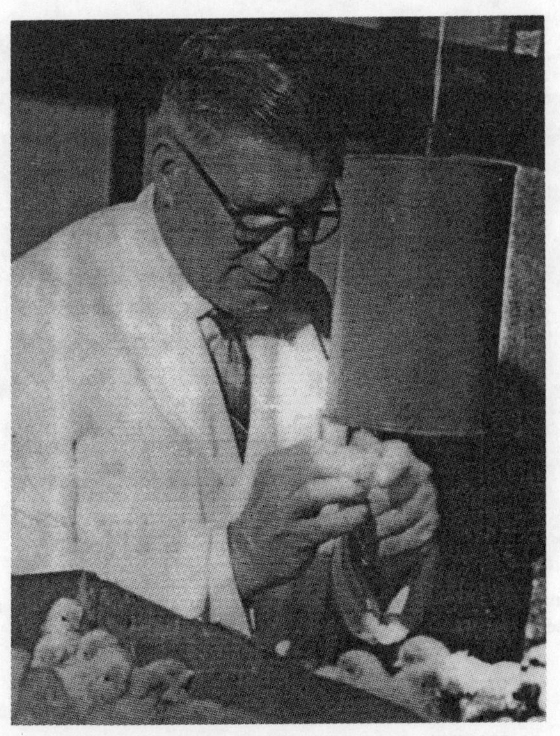

Norm Bell of Perth, Western Australia, sexing chicks in the UK 1955. Norm Bell is still actively engaged in his hatchery in Perth. (1994)

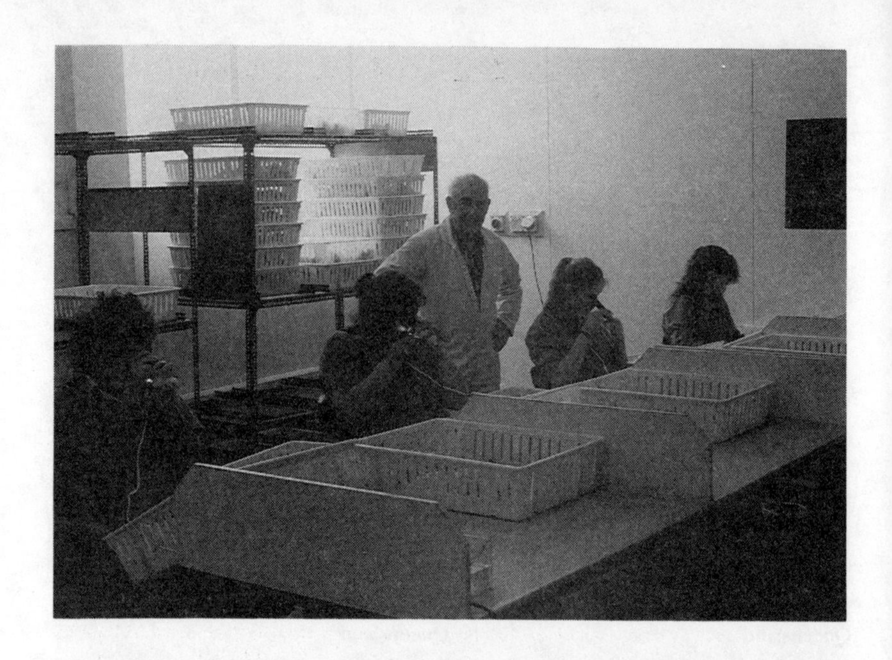

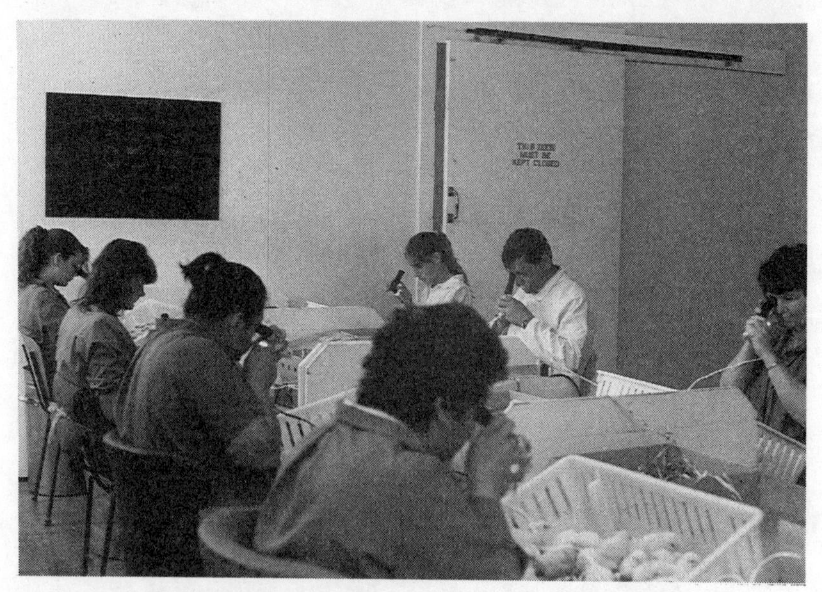

Top: Hans Enzler and his students. Bromley Park, Tuakan, New Zealand, 1992.
Bottom: Students at work. Bromley Park Hatchery. 1992.

Western Australia 1936

Chicks sexed in 1966 . . . 2 500 000. No meat chickens sexed. Ten per cent of Australia's poultry industry production comes from Western Australia.

Ian Hazlett

A Sydney chick sexer who learnt from the Japanese expert, Hikosaburo Yogo, in 1934, he introduced chick sexing to Western Australia in 1936.

He was brought to Perth by John Linton, the Western Australian agent for Gamble Incubators, and was supported by Matt Love, a prominent hatcheryman in Western Australia at the time.

Ian Hazlett came to Perth for three years. After that time all commercial chick sexing was done by Western Australian chick sexers.

Ian Hazlett in his first year in Perth taught eighteen-year-old Norm Bell and others. Norm Bell was the only student to continue on with chick sexing. During Ian Hazlett's three years in Perth he also taught Ken Harrison, Phil Pearce and one of the Castlemain Brothers. Mr Castlemain did not sex commercially outside his own hatchery.

Norm Bell, Phil Pearce, Ken Harrison, Fred Gaynor and Nick Nicholaidis sexed commercially for many years.

Norm Bell, Ken Harrison, Fred Gaynor and Nick Nicholaidis also sexed commercially in England in the late 1940s through to the early 50s.

Norm Bell 1936

In 1936 Norm Bell started sexing chicks in his father's hatchery. In 1993, at 76, he is still actively engaged in the chicken business at Altona Hatchery at Forrestfield, which he started in 1942. A lot has happened in between.

In 1938 he started sexing commercially for hatcherymen other than his father, and sexed commercially until the late 1950s, before the pressure of business took up most of his time. He had a son on the Western Australian Egg Board as well as his growing hatchery business.

Like most of the first generation and many of the second generation chick sexers, he worked on a farm and is familiar with the smell of kerosene from incubator and brooder lamps.

Chick sexers from this background of poultry farming know about cleaning sheds, growing and cutting greenfeed crops, mixing mashes and breeding your own stock, knowledge which many early chick sexers passed on to their clients.

Norm Bell's chick-sexing professionalism, both in Western Australia and England is well known. In doing research for this study, some forty years later, the researcher came across someone who remembers his professionalism and accuracy when he was sexing chickens in Cornwell, England in the late 40s and 50s.

He has a special-class certificate with 99.66 per cent accuracy.

During the war he was in the services for 18 months, but like most chick sexers at that time he was transferred back to chick sexing by the Manpower Authority, because of Australia's role in supplying food to England and the American Forces.

At the end of the war, the Australian Government set up a Rehabilitation Training Scheme for ex-service men and women, to help their re-entry to the workforce. Norm Bell was asked to hold chick-sexing evening classes at the Perth Technical College in St George's Terrace, Perth.

These courses were free. Many joined the classes, but very few kept at it. Sometimes, it was because the students did not have a supply of chickens to practise on when they went home.

One of the successful students from these classes was Noel Hummerston, who sexed commercially for many years in Tasmania as well as around Perth.

Other successful people taught by Norm Bell include Allen Uren, Nick Nicholaidis, Norm Greenway and John Foreman. The latter two did not take on commercial chick sexing.

Norm Bell was the only person to hold classes in Western Australia, mainly because he was the only chick sexer who had a ready supply of chickens from his father's hatchery for students to practise on. Classes for ten people needed at least 1000 chicks for each evening's lesson. He used cockerels and reject chickens.

When asked by Bob Martin why Western Australia never had any women chick sexers, Norm replied: "No women chick sexers in WA! An interesting question Bob, and one that had never really occurred to me. I guess it was that girls were not usually into poultry work, and as chick sexing was seen to be a task of long hours, moving from hatchery to hatchery, they did not seem to fit into the role."

In Western Australia "machine" sexing was not widely accepted. Some "machines" were bought but not used commercially to any great degree.

All chick-sexing work in Western Australia is around Perth's metropolitan area. Norm Bell in his early twenties (1938–45) used a motor bike and side car to get around in. Unlike many of his colleagues from the eastern states, he did not have to travel long distances or endure the "nightmare" of a gas producer on a car during the war years.

In 1993 there were two vent chick-sexers working at Altona Hatchery Pty Ltd, Nick Nicholaidis and his twenty-six year-old son Peter. They did other work besides chick sexing.

Most sexing is done by colour or feather sexing. But as Norm Bell pointed out, "It is handy to have a chick sexer on the premises as sometimes breeding and genetic matters can go a bit wrong and they can check things out."

When asked about future prospects, Norm Bell said, "It is regrettable that there aren't any vent sexers being trained in Australia, as far as I know.

"Peter Nicholaidis, twenty-six, who was taught by his father is the only one I know of.

"It's the old story, you must have chickens to learn on and then for practice . . . and you can't get work until you're good and you can't get good until you get the work.

"Feather and colour sexers can be trained in a few hours.

"I get correspondence regularly from the Korean Chick Sexing Association offering to send contractors here. They are working in America, they are independent of the Japanese. They're all vent sexers of course."

1936 TILL 1993

The first government chick-sexing examination in Western Australia was held in 1936. Nine students presented themselves for examination. Although none were successful in obtaining certificates, the results generally were good. The best results were several candidates getting 92 per cent accuracy. These results compare favourably with the first tests in the eastern states. There were three level of certificates: special-class, 98 per cent. 300 chicks in 45 minutes; first-class, 95 per cent. 200 chicks in 30 minutes; second-class 95 per cent. 100 chicks in 20 minutes.

The last examination was held in 1973. Most years, particularly during the 1940s and 50s, there were three to five candidates for certificates each year. Norm Bell and Allen Uren, under the supervision of department officers, carried out the postmortems at these examinations.

In the 1940s there were about 28 hatcheries around Perth. By 1993 there were four. At the peak of demand for chick sexers, 1950s to the 1960s, there were six chick sexers who did most of the commercial chick sexing in Western Australia. By the mid-sixties there were about ten qualified chick sexers, but most of the work was done by four people.

There has never been a chick-sexing association in Western Australia. The Agriculture Department, hatcherymen and chick sexers have always been a happy, co-operative family. Perth is an isolated city so perhaps unity and cooperation is more readily achieved in such an environment.

Western Australia Lists of chick sexers 1936–1993

First generation: 1936+	
Mr Norm Bell	Special class
Altona Hatchery Pty Ltd	
Forrestfield	
Mr E. O. Harrison	First class
Leederville	
Mr Phil Pearce	First Class
Bayswater	
(Mr Castlemain worked in own hatchery only)	
Second generation: 1945+	
Mr R. Vagg	Special class
Kewdale	
Mr Nick Nicholaidis	Second class
Mt Lawley	
Mr A. Uren	First class
Bayswater	
Mr N. Hummerston	First class
Murdoch	
Mr John Foreman	Second class
South Belmont	
(did not sex commercially)	
Mr Norm Greenway	Second class
(did not sex commercially)	
Mr K. Brunning	—
North Perth	
Mr Fred Gaynor	First Class
Mr R. Wells	First Class
Carlisle	
Third generation 1960+	
Mr D. Hoult	Mr Peter Nicholaidis
Maida Vale	Mt Lawley
Mr S. L. Porter	Mr Max Kemsley
Narrogin	now of (Rochedale Q.)

South Australia 1936–1969
Resident Chick Sexers

The Japanese chick sexers did not visit South Australia. There was a plan by Farm and Pastoral Supplies of Melbourne to take a Japanese expert there in 1935, but this never eventuated. A Sydney firm sent a representative who gave several lectures to prominent breeders and hatcherymen in 1935.

The first chick-sexer in the State was Mr Tom Gameau, of Why Worry Hatchery. Mr Gameau learnt from Mr Frank Evans of Sydney, as did two other South Australian chick sexers. Many of the other South Australian chick sexers learnt from Tom Gameau.

Other commercial chick sexers were Max Charlesworth, Arnold Young, Mr E. A. Lamerton, Ron Ackland, Brian Rueder, Peter (Kevin) Stone, Roy Harris, Bob Dawkins (the first candidate to get a first-class certificate, 98 per cent accuracy), and Brian Apps.

There were two brothers also who sexed chicks commercially: Michael Bressington and P. Bressington. There was also Peter Whitham, the only one to use a "machine".

There was a "machine" student from Anderson's Hatchery and Breeding Farm, who had been taught by Lena Rogers of Victoria, but he was not able to gain a government certificate to practise because at the examination he punctured the bowels of many chickens.

RESIDENT CHICK SEXERS

Many South Australian chick sexers were attached to a particular hatchery. At the Why Worry Hatchery there was Tom Gameau and later Max Charlesworth. Peter Stone was resident chick sexer at the Peter Syme Harvey Hatchery.

Roy Harris was attached to his father's hatchery.

Bob Dawkins was a freelancer. He later taught another freelancer, Brian Apps.

Before the entry of the large companies into the poultry industry in the 1960s, there were from twelve to fifteen hatcheries selling day-old chicks in the State, with about four to six chick sexers working commercially.

Most chick sexers were examined by Gordon Lowe, manager of the Parafield Poultry Station. In the late 1940s, the poultry station under Mr Lowe's management developed a crossbreed made up of a slow-feathering strain of Australorps, and a fast-feathering strain of white leghorns, the offspring of which they were able to feather sex with 100 per cent accuracy. There was little commercial interest shown at the time.

In South Australia, chick sexers had to be registered, although people could sex chicks without being registered. But it is unlikely many would employ an untested chick sexer. To register, you had to pass an examination. A registered chick sexer could be required to undergo a check examination at any time if the department received repeated reports of a chick sexer's poor performance. The department checked the complaints first.

Only one chick sexer has been asked to undergo a check examination. He had been a very accurate chick sexer for many years, but suddenly he started making up to 15 per cent errors. He did not do any better in the check test. Another chick sexer tried to help him "get back on the track," as he stated at the time, but to no avail. He retired from commercial chick sexing.

This has happened to many commercial chick sexers, vent sexers and "machine" sexers. Sometimes a successful "machine" sexer would suddenly start puncturing the chicks in such numbers that his or her chick-sexing career would suddenly come to an end.

The South Australian Department of Agriculture held the first examination in 1936. Three candidates were successful in gaining certificates. They were:

Mr R. O. Dawkins, of Gawler, 98 per cent, first-class; Mr E. A. Lamerton, of Edwardston, 94 per cent, second class; Mr T. V. Gameau of Murray Bridge, 92 per cent, second class.

Other successful candidates between 1936 and 1969: Mr Max Charlesworth, Mr Arnold Young, Mr Peter (Kevin) Stone, Mr Ron Ackland, Mr Brian Rueder, Mr Michael Bressington, Mr P. Bressington and Mr Peter Whitham (the only one to use the "machine" method).

Currently (1994), there are no resident commercial chick sexers in South Australia. Onko Wallbrink, from Victoria, flies there for one day each week, sometimes assisted by Doreen De Carteret, another Victorian.

Occasionally two New South Wales chick sexers are sent from Sydney to sex breeders for a NSW-based breeder.

Tasmania

Except for very brief periods, there has never been a domiciled chick sexer in Tasmania who has sexed chicks commercially. Tasmanian poultrymen have always relied upon engaging chick sexers from Victoria, South Australia or Western Australia.

Tasmania has always had an egg-producing industry and hatcheries both in the north and the south of the State.

During the 1940s there were years when Tasmania was not able to gain the services of a chick sexer.

In the mid 1940s Mr Power from Victoria went to Tasmania for several reasons.

In 1949, another Victorian, Bob Martin, flew to Hobart each weekend to sex chicks around the Hobart area and to Launceston each Wednesday to work for two hatcheries there. In 1950 he flew only to Launceston each Wednesday.

Later Miss Elsie Bruce of Glenormiston South, in Victoria, was engaged at 2c a chicken and handled 70 000 chickens. Tasmanian poultrymen were very satisfied with her work, stating that she was 96–98 per cent accurate. She married on her return to Victoria and declined an offer to return a second season.

Two men were engaged to replace Miss Bruce at a 50 per cent increase in costs.

A Western Australian, Noel Hummerston, also sexed in Tasmania for many years. He taught another Western Australian, Max Kemsley, who also worked there for a couple of seasons before moving on to Queensland.

Another Victorian chick sexer, Charlie Bode, a first-generation chick sexer who learnt from the Japanese expert Hideo Kataoka in 1934, worked in Tasmania for six seasons in the 1950s. The first season he flew home each weekend, but the following season he stayed there for the four months' hatching season.

During his six years there, he taught two Tasmanians the skill: Mr W. Proctor, of Kettering, and Mr F. Kitson of Port Sorell. There was another Tasmanian, Mr Foster, who passed a Tasmanian government chick-sexing examination, possibly the only Tasmanian to do so.

A Western Australian chick sexer went there to sex for a season during the time Charlie Bode was working there, but there was not enough work to support two chick sexers and he returned to Western Australia.

In the 1960s and 70s Victorian chick sexers flew to Tasmania each week to work for one or two days. Among some who went during this period were John Hammond, Doreen de Carteret and Lena Rogers.

At the peak of demand for chick sexing, Tasmania seems to have had about 150 000 chicks to sex in the 12-week season.

Currently (1994), there are no specialist chick sexers working in Tasmania.

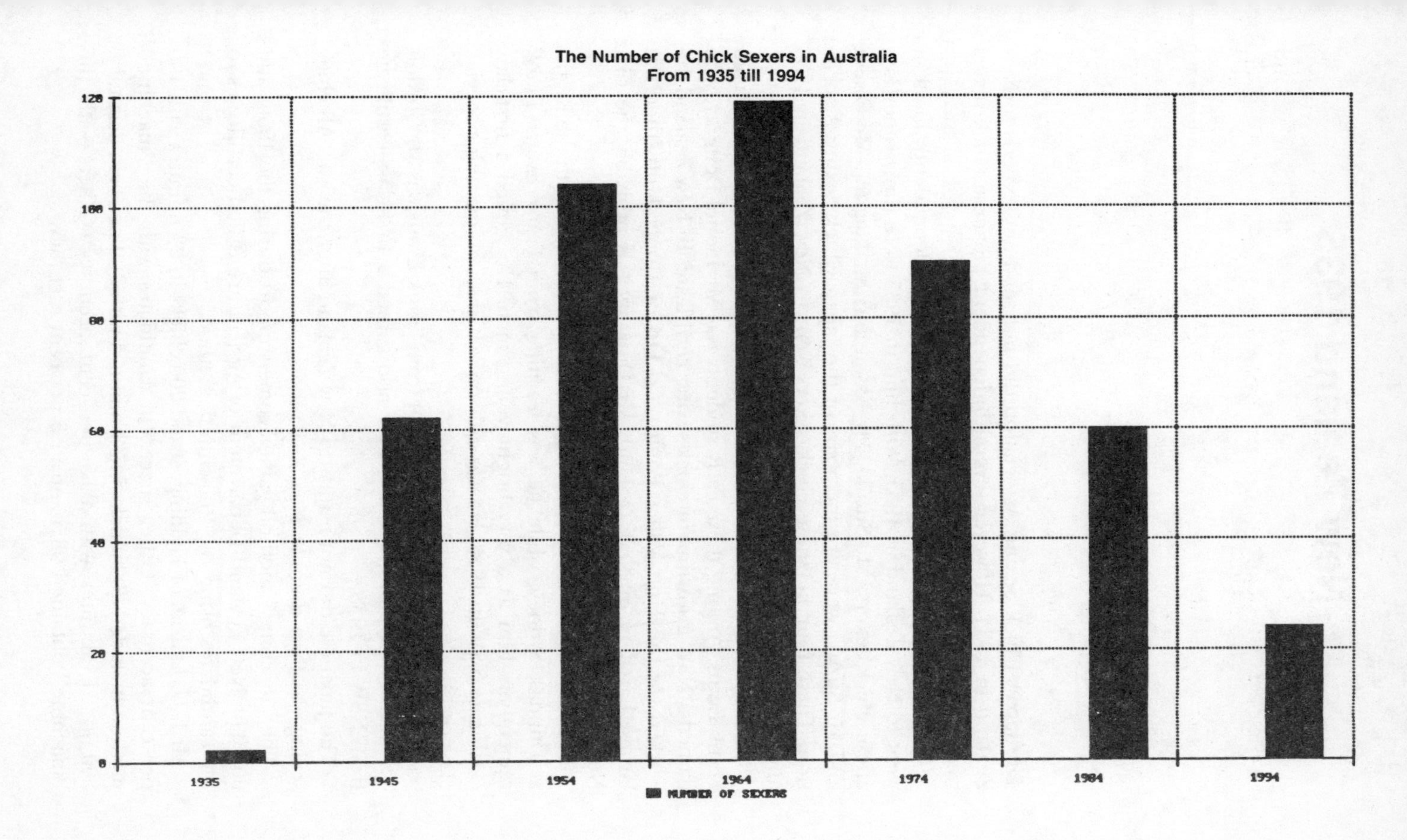
The Number of Chick Sexers in Australia
From 1935 till 1994
120
100
80
60
40
20
0
1935
1945
1954
1964
1974
1984
1994
NUMBER OF SEXERS

New Zealand 1935

The Japan Chick Sexing Association did not send any experts to New Zealand in 1934. However several independent Japanese chick sexers went to New Zealand from 1935 till 1939.

Mr Kiyoshi Ozawa, who had gone to Brisbane independently in 1934, went to New Zealand in 1935. With him in 1935 were three other Japanese chick sexers: Mr Suzuki, Mr Kawai and Mr Nagura. Mr Ozawa and Mr Suzuki were not members of the Japan Chick Sexing Association. These four Japanese chick sexers went to New Zealand in 1935 and stayed there until 1939.

Several New Zealanders went to Sydney to learn chick sexing from Frank Evans. Among these early students was Mr Lionel Doughty, who gained a NSW government chick-sexing certificate. In New Zealand, he worked for the Hutt Valley Poultry Co Ltd of Upper Hutt, then the largest hatchery in New Zealand. Mr Doughty was probably the first New Zealander to qualify as a chick sexer.

In 1938, Mr K. Gibson of Mt Roskill, Auckland, stayed with the Evans' at Dundas, Sydney, while he was learning from Frank Evans. Frank remembers him as a very bright young man. He gained a first-class certificate NSW in 1938. He was only one chicken off gaining a special-class certificate.

Another New Zealander who learnt from Frank Evans was Mr Gordon Thomson, of Opoho, Dunedin. He also gained a first-class certificate from NSW in 1938.

The Japanese did not return to New Zealand after the war. All chick sexing was then done by New Zealanders.

The "machine" method gained some support during the 1950s and 60s. The New Zealand Department of Agriculture issued certificates to the candidates using the "machine" method.

Mr I. U. Laurie, of Fielding, sexed 200 chicks in 23 minutes with 100 per cent accuracy. Other successful candidates with the "machine" method included 200 chicks in 33 minutes with 100 per cent accuracy, 200 in 31 minutes with 99.5 per cent accuracy. Others with the "machine" obtained 98.5 and 97.5 per cent accuracy.

When the New Zealand Agriculture Department first introduced examinations using the "machine" method they stressed the importance of allowing the chicks to dry out for at least eight hours after hatching, otherwise injury could occur.

As well as the original Japanese Kizawa Chicktester, and two English versions, the 'Secura' chick-sexing machine and the Keeler company's 'Chixexer', there was also a version made by a New Zealander, Mr Hans Enzler, of Royal Oak, Auckland. His "machine" had a teaching version made especially for training students.[1]

Hans Enzler was probably the most successful "machine" chick sexer in New Zealand. He gained an International Chick-Sexing Diploma in Switzerland in 1953 with 100 per cent accuracy. He also obtained a NZ Government Certificate in 1958, again with 100 per cent accuracy.

Hans worked for four years in Europe before going to New Zealand in 1957 to work as a commercial chick sexer for Bromley Park Hatcheries. He retired from chick sexing in 1991.

Mr Enzler also taught the instrument method of chick sexing to the following students, all of Bromley Park Hatchery, all "machine" sexers: Christine Margaret Salmons, 100 per cent, 1992; Paula Cherie Salmons, 100 per cent, 1992; Queenie Oakes, 100 per cent, 1992; Naomi Hoete, 100 per cent, 1992; Susan Comer, 100 per cent, 1992; Karen Patricia Lopwood, 100 per cent, 1992; Marie Susan Robinson, 100 per cent, 1992; Ian Leslie Beazley, 100 per cent, 1992; Kevin Murphy, 98 per cent, 1992; Brenden Dobbs, 100 per cent, 1992.

Occasionally an Australian chick sexer is sent over to New Zealand to do several day's work for one of the large breeders.

Like Australia, New Zealand opportunities for new commercial chick sexers are few, and likely to remain so.

---

1 See the Section "Other Methods' of this study for photo of this instrument.

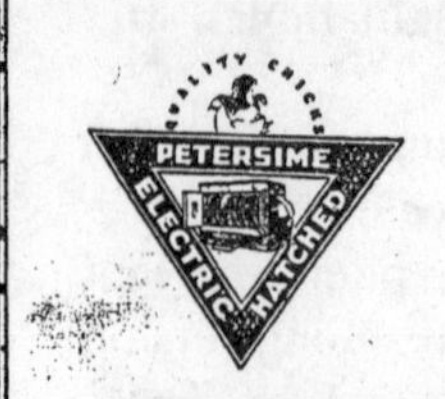

50,000

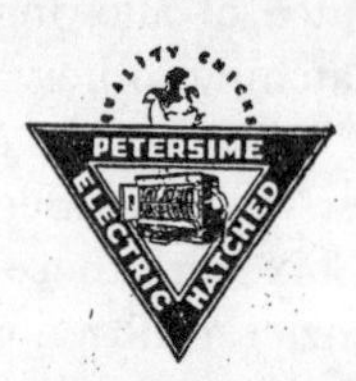

DAY OLD PULLETS

(90 PER CENT. GUARANTEED)

Have been disposed of in Melbourne since August 2, when Mr. Kataoka, the Japanese expert, arrived here. Approximately 100,000 chicks have been "sexed" by him, and several public demonstrations have been held, at each of which Mr. Kataoka has "sexed" about 100 chicks in from five to six minutes. The result of the "post-mortem" in each case has been

100 PER CENT. CORRECT.

That the value of CHICK SEXING is appreciated by poultry farmers in Australia, as in other countries of the world, is indicated by the demand for the services of the three Japanese Experts who were brought to Sydney, Brisbane and Melbourne through the enterprise of the manufacturers of the world-famous PETERSIME Electric Incubators.

Here in Melbourne innumerable hatcheries have applied for Mr. Kataoka's services, but he has been working overtime—Sundays included—since his arrival.

The demand for DAY-OLD PULLETS increases daily; orders should be placed at once for forward delivery with the following:—

W. GILLETT,
Centre Dandenong Road, CHELTENHAM, S.22.

E. A. LAWSON,
Hunter Road, EAST CAMBERWELL, E.6.
'Phone: W 4283.

W. McLISTER,
176 Hall Street, SPOTSWOOD, W.14.
'Phone: Williamstown 134.

SANDLAND'S Premier Poultry Farm
38 Cooper Street, PRESTON, N.18.
'Phone: JW 1371.

H. & A. WOODMAN,
4 Alice Street, COBURG, N.13.
'Phone: Brunswick 208.

S. T. J. HALL,
St. Hellier's Street, HEIDELBERG, N.23.
'Phone: Heidelberg 117.

SYDNEY N. LLOYD,
"Cranleigh," Cranbourne Road, FRANKSTON.
'Phone: Frankston 96.

H. H. LLOYD,
Box 10, FRANKSTON. 'Phone: Frankston 96.

H. OLIVE,
LARA.

M. WHITE,
Highton, GEELONG.

PETERSIME PULLETS ARE QUALITY PULLETS

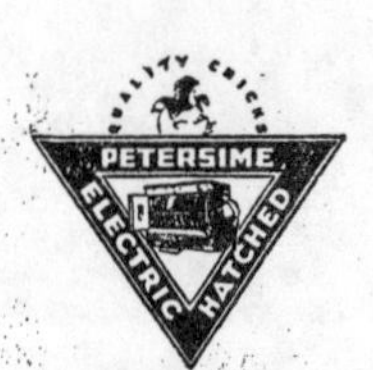

THE FARM & PASTORAL SUPPLIES PTY. LTD.

500 Bourke Street, Melbourne, C.1.

Central 8049.

Agents for Victoria and Tasmania for PETERSIME Electric Incubators and MANNGAMBLE Poultry Equipment.

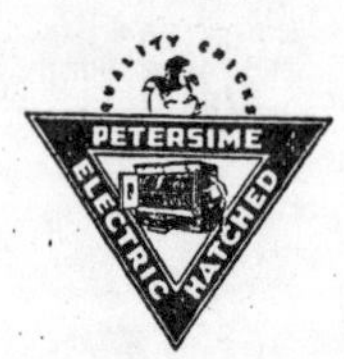

White Leghorn CHICKS and Started Chicks

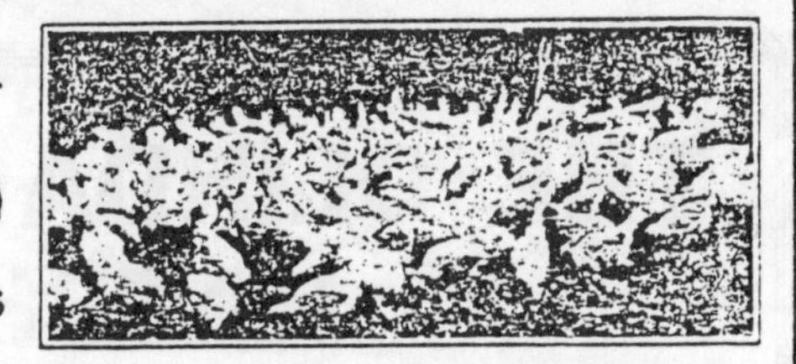

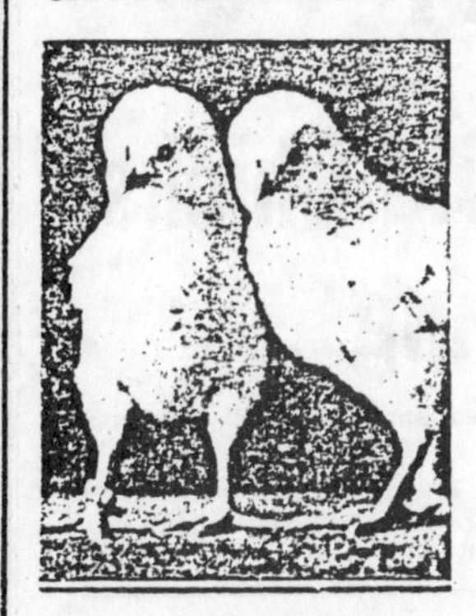

For the thirtieth season The Research Poultry Farm offers you their renowned White Leghorn chicks. During this time the farm has forged ahead and every purchaser of "Research" chicks has the satisfaction of knowing that thirty years of experience stands behind their purchase. Our continually increasing list of satisfied clients testify that the healthy, vigorous "Research" chicks are efficient money-makers.

Day Old White Leghorn Chicks, £3 per 100, £1/15/- per 50 (freight paid). Started Chicks (any age), prices on application. Pullets (eight weeks old), 3/- each. Sexed Day Old Pullets, £6/10/- per 100.

NOTE.—All sexing is done by Victoria's champion chick sexer, Mr. C. Bode, who has now made his services available to poultry farmers. Mr. Bode holds both the First and Special Class Chick Sexing Certificates with accuracy of 97 per cent. We welcome enquiries re chick sexing.

1936 Price Booklet now ready. Further particulars apply:

Research Poultry Farm

RESEARCH, VICTORIA.

'Phone: Research 4. Established 1906.

Day Old Pullets, Custom Hatching, Chick Sexing

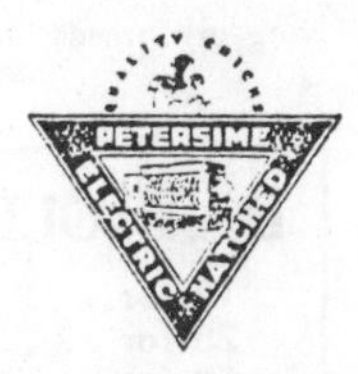

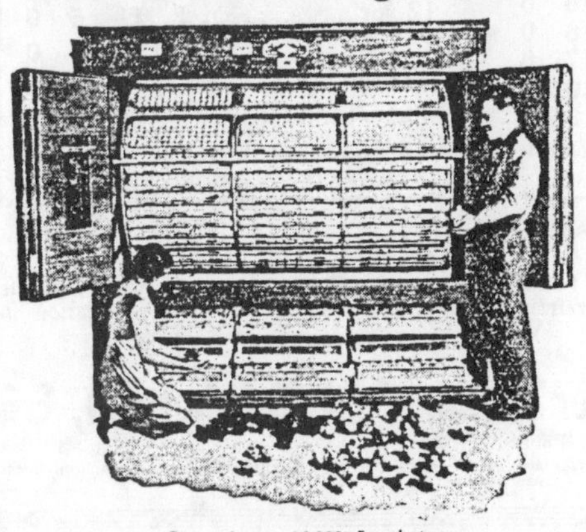

One of our 16,000 Incubators.

We now have two 16,000 Petersime Incubators, one for our day old chick business and the other for our custom hatching. Place your order with us.

We were the first to instal a 16,000 Petersime, and now we lead the way with chick sexing.

PRICES:

DAY OLD PULLETS, £6 per 100; £50 per 1,000

DAY OLD COCKERELS, 10/- per 100.

DAY OLD CHICKS, £3 per 100; £25 per 1,000. Sexing, 1d. per chick extra.

CUSTOM HATCHING, 12/6 per 100; £5 per 1,000. Sexing, 1½d. per chick extra.

S. T. J. HALL,

St. Helier's P.F., St. Helier's St., Heidelberg.
Charlesville P.F., Altona Street, Heidelberg.

'Phone: Heidelberg 117.

THE OLINDA HATCHERY

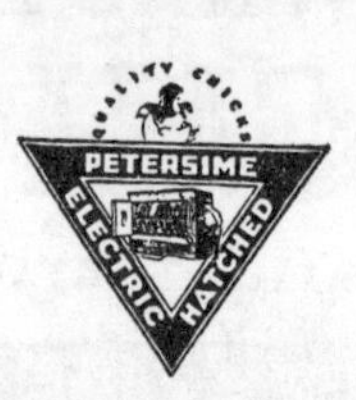

Day Old Pullets, Day Old Chicks, Custom Hatching

Owing to the big demand for Olinda Service, I have installed another 16,000 Petersime Electric Incubator, giving me capacity of over 30,000.

Wonderful results to date. The Japanese Expert has proved 100 per cent. correct in all selections. My brooder is full of pullets, the White Leghorn cockerels being killed off at day old, except what I reserve for stud.

Here is your opportunity to get new blood for next year. Specially Selected Day Old White Leghorn Cockerels, £1/1/- per hundred.

Note.—You don't buy these to kill. They will be at the head of your breeding pens next season. Introduce the Olinda Strain.

Remember, September is the best month to buy chickens. Buy Lawson's Day Old Pullets. Bred from Australia's Best. Bred to lay and always pay.

Note my breeds: WHITE LEGHORNS, RHODE ISLAND REDS and BLACK ORPS. I charge the same price for all my breeds.

PRICES:

DAY OLD CHICKENS:

12 for	£0	10	0
25 for	0	18	0
50 for	1	17	6
100 for	3	10	0
1000 for (White Leghorns only)	30	0	0

Previous orders for day-old chicks may now be converted to pullets.

DAY OLD PULLETS:

12 for	£1	5	0
25 for	2	5	0
50 for	4	4	0
100 for	8	0	0

With a guarantee of 90 per cent. correct, but invariably results prove 100 per cent.

CUSTOM HATCHING:

£1/2/6 per tray of approximately 155 hen eggs. Note.—Have your custom hatched chickens sexed at 1½d. per chick extra. I pay freight on all chickens to any railway station in Victoria.

E. A. LAWSON, Hunter Road, East Camberwell, E.6

'Phone: W 4283.

Take Wattle Park Electric Tram from Prince's Bridge and get off at the new stop, Middlesex Rd., and come down Lockhart Avenue.

Victoria's Leading Chick Hatchery

FIRST QUALITY ANY QUANTITY

SATISFACTION ASSURED

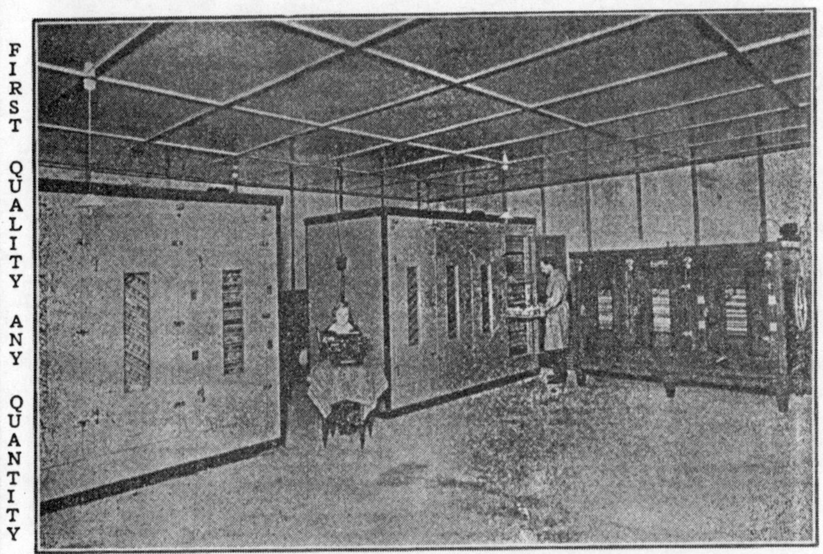

Every Machine filled to capacity and producing Chicks that please.

CUSTOM HATCHING

12/6 per 100; 6/6 for 50. 500 or more booked for the season, 10/- per 100.

Eggs remain in the same tray throughout the hatch, thus eliminating the possibility of eggs becoming mixed.

Eggs set every Monday and Thursday.

SEND FOR 1934 CATALOGUE

DAY OLD CHICKS

White Leghorns, £2/12/6 per 100; £25 per 1,000.
Black Orpingtons, £3/10/- per 100; £30 per 1,000.
Limited number of Langshan, Rhode Island Red, Brown Leghorn and Light Sussex at 15/- per doz; £5 per 100.

SEXED CHICKS.

White Leghorns only. Guaranteed 90 per cent. Pullets, £6/10/- per 100.
All Chicks sent out in new boxes.

Latest production. BABY MAMMOTH INCUBATOR, 1,200 to 1,350 Egg Capacity, £60. Mammoth construction and finish. This was the attraction at the Poultry Show. See it in operation.

H. E. Southwell

NEWPORT POULTRY FARM,
JOHNSTON STREET —— NEWPORT
'Phones: Williamstown 426, 354.
And at HANMER STREET, WILLIAMSTOWN.
Stock over 4,000 birds. Inspection invited. (Not Sundays.)

Rainbow, 16/7/34.

Mr. Southwell.

Herewith orders for 2,000 chicks this season. I hope that these dates will suit, and trust that we shall receive chicks of as good a type as last season, with which we were highly satisfied.—Yours,

F. F. K.

PART II

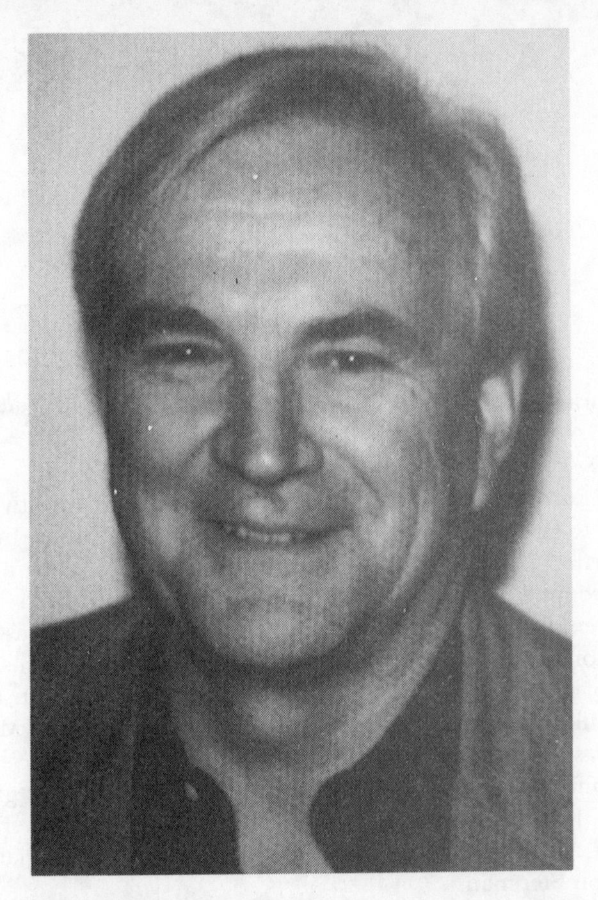

After an absence of 26 years from commercial chick sexing I have once again become involved with my former colleagues—I have met several of my boyhood heroes for the first time. I was brought up-to-date by a lifetime poultryman, Bill Stanhope, and by "my student", John Hammond.

In reflecting on my chick-sexing past, it seems almost impossible that I sexed just over 12 000 000 chicks during my twenty years as a commercial chick sexer; that I worked, as did many of my colleagues, seven days and seven nights a week, for the 12-week hatching season each year; that I managed to visit 17 farms and hatcheries each week, after spending three full days working at one large hatchery.

I claimed to sex chicks at the rate of 1000 chicks an hour (always working with a feeder and boxer), but it still took me 13 hours to sex 10 000 chicks.

Many of today's chick sexers can do their 10 000 chicks in eight hours, without a counter helping them, such are the improvements in hatchery technology and chick-sexing techniques.

A world view 1945–1994

After World War II there was a great demand for chick sexers worldwide.

EUROPE

All over Europe the breeding and laying flocks were greatly depleted and had to be built up during the spring hatching seasons. In England the interned Japanese chick sexers were released to teach and to sex chicks commercially. Many hatcheries in England and mainland Europe employed overseas chick sexers from America, Australia and Japan, working mainly through chick-sexing contractor firms.

One of the largest and oldest chick-sexing contractors in Europe is Hobo Chick Sexing of Waregem, Belgium. Its founder, Mr Junichi Hobo, was Belgium's first chick sexer.

He came from Japan to work in Belgium in 1935, after graduating from the Japan Chick Sexing School in Nagoya, with an average of 99 per cent accuracy. He was invited to Belgium by a Belgian farmer, Mr Gaston Stepman.

Junichi Hobo stayed on in Belgium and made it his home. He later married one of the daughters of Gaston Stepman, Marie-Louise.

When World War II broke out he was interned for three days, before being released by the Belgian Government to resume his occupation of chick sexing.

Since he first came to Belgium in 1935, Mr Hobo has seen the rapid growth of the poultry industry. Japanese chick sexers originally, came to Europe for only three months each year, when chicks were hatched in the spring, before technology made it possible to hatch all year round. They used to earn enough in those few months to last them the whole year when they went back to Japan.

In 1946 Mr Hobo, his wife and their three children moved from Anzegem to Waregem and set up the 'Hobo Chick Sexing' company. By this time hatcheries were getting bigger and bigger to cater for the cage egg farms, and as a result there was a growing need for more chick sexers. The Hobos built sleeping accommodation on their property for the growing number of visiting chick sexers from Japan.

Since 1981 his company has organised regular chick-sexing competitions in Belgium, the only such event outside Japan. Candidates from all over the world come to test their chick-sexing skills for accuracy and speed. A recent winner (1990) was from Brazil, Mr Antonio Taniguchi, 38. He was able to sex 100 chicks in 3 minutes 30 seconds with 100 per cent accuracy.

Hobo Chick Sexing is an agent for the whole of Europe. Their Japanese and Korean sexers have gone to Spain, France, Norway, Belgium, The Netherlands, and some of the nations which used to make up Yugoslavia.

The company is now run by Takashi Hobo, the son of the founder. In 1994 the firm sent 100 chick sexers to different hatcheries throughout Europe. It is interesting to note that all their chick sexers are either Japanese or Koreans.

ENGLAND

England has always had some chick-sexing contractors, as well as training schools for chick sexers. Even before the Japanese Chick Sexing Association sent their experts to England in 1935, there were classes held in 1934 by private individuals from Japan. At the outbreak of World War II there were many English chick sexers.

From the mid-1940s Australian, English and Japanese chick sexers worked in Belgium, The Netherlands, Denmark and France. There were also several chick sexing contractors set up in England, and Belgium (apart from Hobos), many of which taught as well as supplied chick sexers to the United Kingdom, Europe, South Africa, the Middle East and on one occasion to far away New Zealand.

The largest of the English companies was Chick Sexing Specialists (UK) Ltd, based in Maidstone, Kent. Apart from being agents for the Zen-Nippon Chick Sexing Association and Amchick of America, this firm also supplied English chick sexers to Europe, Zimbabwe, the Middle East and South Africa.

In the late 1940s to the early 1950s, through to the 1970s, there was a growing demand for the services of specialist chick sexers, so much so that in the early 1950s there was a world shortage of chick sexers. This was met, in part, by the development of an optical chick-sexing instrument by the Japanese in 1951. The "machine" age had arrived to the chick-sexing industry!

There were headings in the poultry Press such as: "Vent method chick sexing is on the way out", "Hatcherymen are beginning to use the Japanese 'machine' which assures a 100 per cent accuracy".[1] Another heading "Is hand sexing out-moded?"[2]

---

1 *Poultry Supply World*, April 1953 issue.

2 *The Australasian Poultry World*, July 1954.

This new, easier to learn method, and the possibility of a 100 per cent accuracy at examinations, seemed to be a threat to the livelihood of vent (hand) chick sexers. For a while, it did help overcome the shortage of chick sexers in some areas. In England it brought about a drop in chick-sexing fees. There is no doubt that the "machine" did discourage many students from seeing chick sexing as a secure and worthwhile career.

While the "machine" had some success in filling a gap in some areas, there is no doubt that its threat and then eventual failure as a commercial success in most countries did lead to another world shortage of chick sexers in the 1970s. This shortage was overcome by the development of feather and colour sexing in the industry. Also this world shortage was overcome by the arrival of the Koreans, and to a lesser degree, the Mexicans, on the international scene.

With the establishment of feather and colour sexing in Australia in the 1970s the demand for the specialist chick sexer was reduced to 30 per cent, compared to the peak years in the 1950s to 1960s. The drop in demand for specialist chick sexers was worldwide. A slightly higher number was needed in Europe and America because of their larger numbers of primary breeding stock, which still have to be sexed by vent sexers.

It is worthwhile spending a little time looking at why the "machine" method started off with such promise and in some countries had a remarkable success, yet by the 1980s this method was no longer taught anywhere and is now used by only a few sexers in New Zealand, Australia, Denmark and Russia.

In Australia in the 1950s there was an extreme shortage of chick sexers in Victoria. This situation brought about a rapid entry of "machine" sexers into the industry in that State, firstly sexing mainly broiler chicks and later layer replacement stock. Most of these "machine" method sexers were successful commercially; they were fast, up to 1200 plus chicks an hour, and in most cases were equal to their vent colleagues. Although some New South Wales vent sexers will dispute the latter claim, their accuracy was well within a satisfactory commercial range, particularly for broiler chicks. A couple of the slower "machine" sexers were proved to be close to 100 per cent accurate.

Some NSW breeders and hatcherymen were not impressed by the number of injuries of the chicks sexed by "machine". Many hatcherymen in NSW were also concerned about the possible effect of the instrument on the DNA pattern, which, it was argued, could affect the aims of the geneticist and cause a loss of breeding goals. There was also some debate about the spread of diseases.

Nevertheless in Australia and a few other places the "machine" method has survived for nearly forty years. No one has been taught this method in Japan since 1966. The last Australian to be taught this method was in 1978.

One hatchery in New Zealand had nine people taught the "machine" method in 1992 and another one, in 1994.

Onko Wallbrink, one of the world's most experienced "machine" sexers, said in an interview I had with him in November 1993, "the 'machine' is finished!"

It is pointless to argue whether this method harms the chick or not. The reality is that the cloacal (vent) method has proved over time throughout the world to be the more accurate and faster method. For sixty years, since its introduction, there has been a gradual improvement in the number of chicks an hour and a more consistent overall accuracy among commercial chick sexers in most countries.

JAPAN CHICK SEXING ASSOCIATION

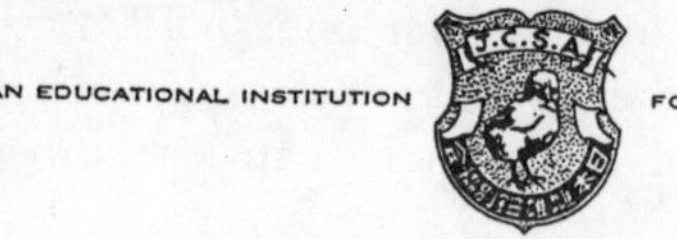

"AN EDUCATIONAL INSTITUTION FOR TRAINING CHICK SEXING EXPERTS"

DIPLOMA

This is to certify that Zyunichi Hobo, *First Class Chick Sexing Expert of* Gifuken, *Japan was successful in obtaining the following result at the Examination of Japan Chick Sexing Association.*

1st *100 chicks*........................ 98 *% Accuracy*

2nd *100 chicks*........................ 99 *% Accuracy*

3rd 100 chicks................100 % Accuracy

Average........................ 99 *% Accuracy*

Head examiner *Dr. Kiyoshi Masui*

Date November 1st, 1933. K. Masui

Dr. Ryoji Iwazumi

R. Iwazumi

President of Japan Chick Sexing Association.

CITY OFFICE, ROOM 208 NAGOYA, JAPAN.

Dr. R. Iwazumi — *Professor of Animal Husbandry, Imperial University of Tokyo*

Dr. K. Masui — *Professor of Veterinary Anatomy, Imperial University of Tokyo*

Diploma awarded to Zyunichi [Junichi] Hobo, November 1, 1933. (Courtesy of Takashi Hobo, Belgium)

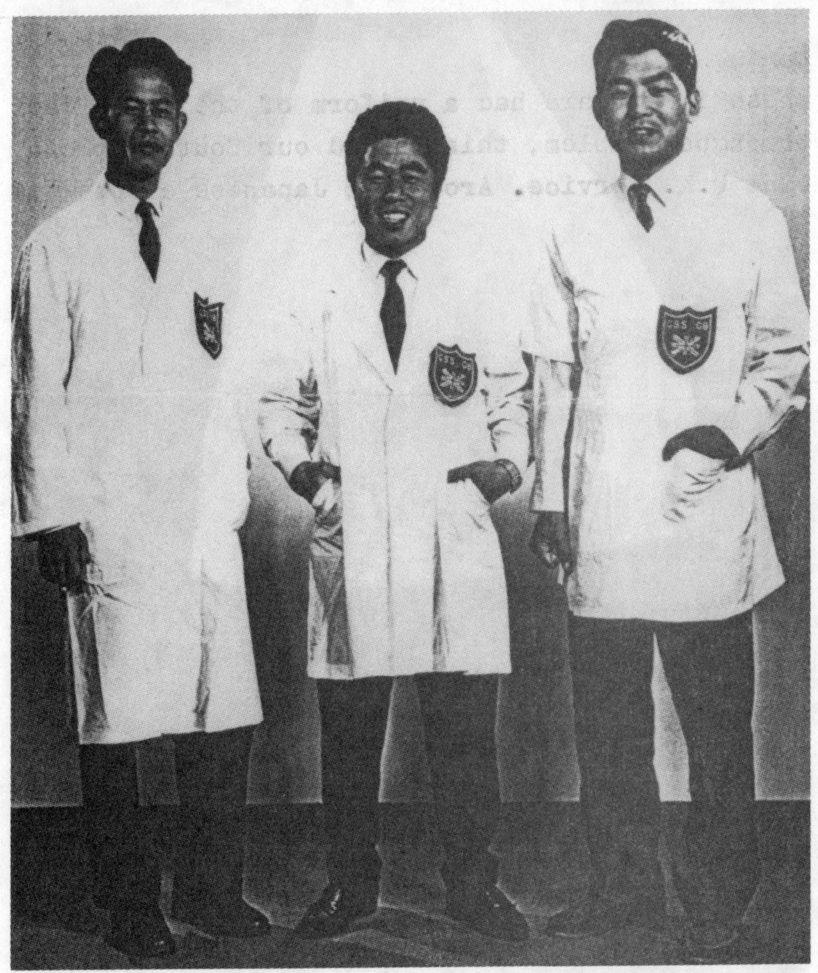

Three Japanese chick sexers working ''under the flag'' of Chick Sexing Specialists (G.B.). Later a springbok was added to the badge to signify this firm's South African connections. Apologies to the three experts for not being able to find their names. (Photo: C.S.S. (G.B.))

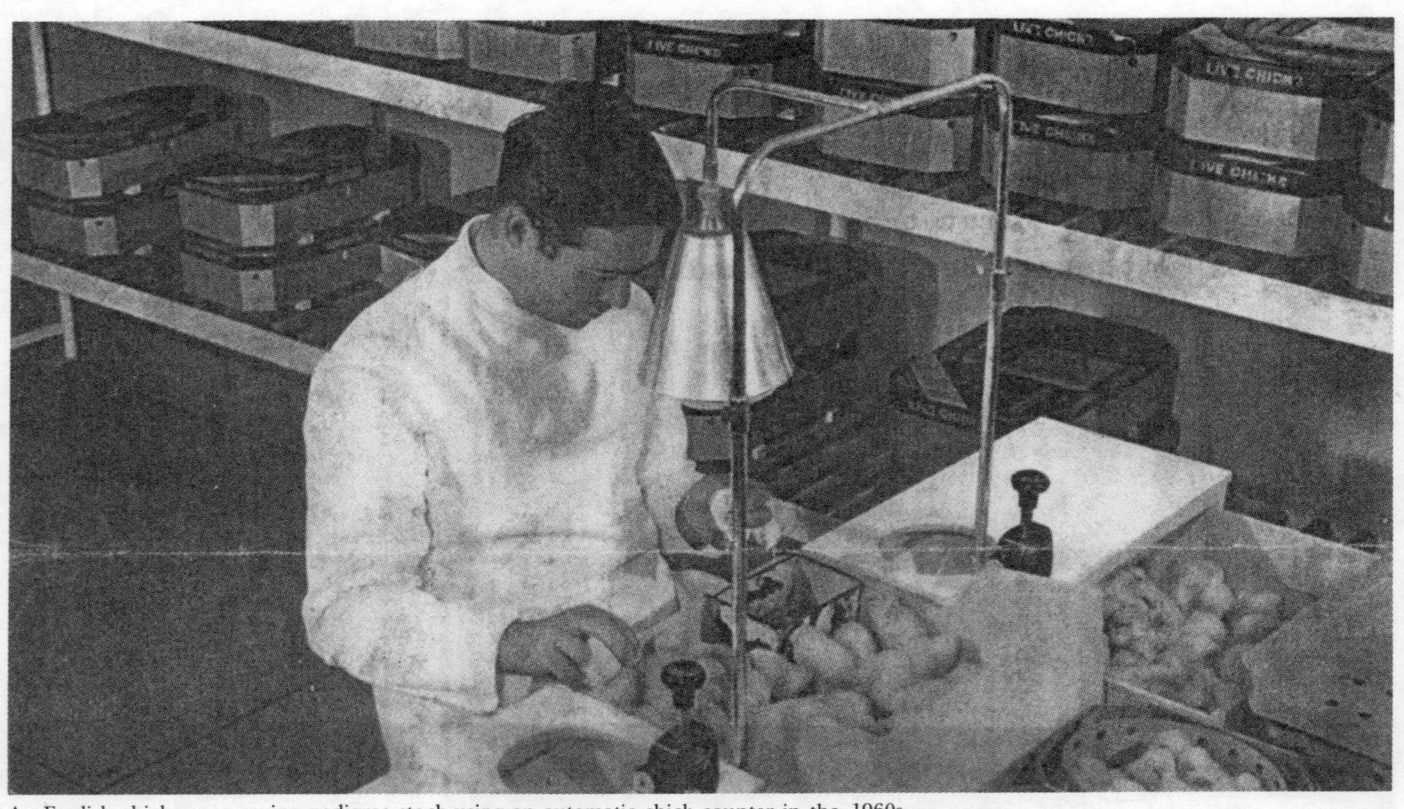

An English chick sexer, sexing pedigree stock using an automatic chick counter in the 1960s.

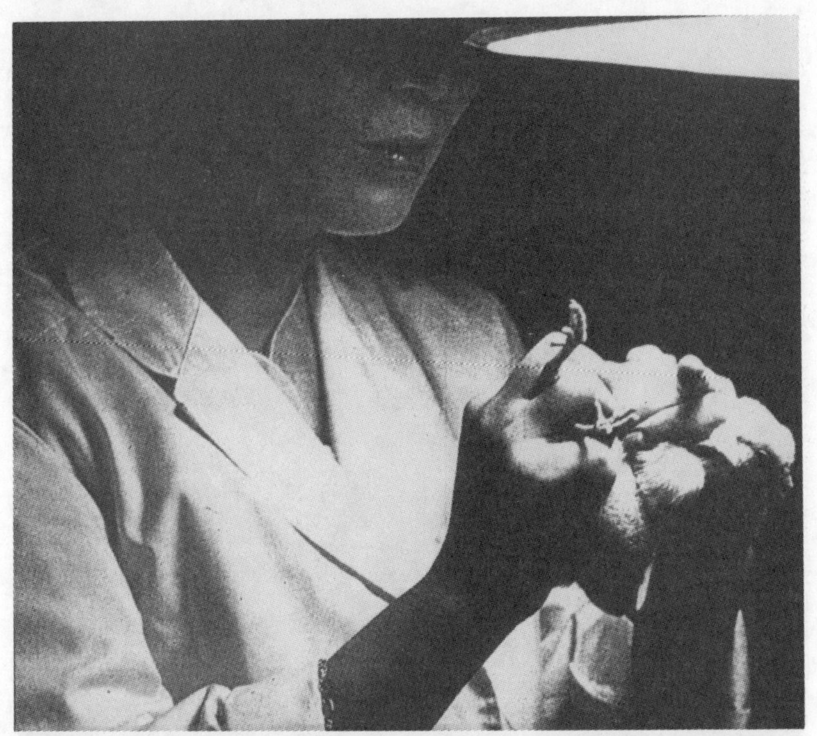

One of Japan's 22 women chick sexers at work. (5.7 per cent of all Japanese chick sexers).

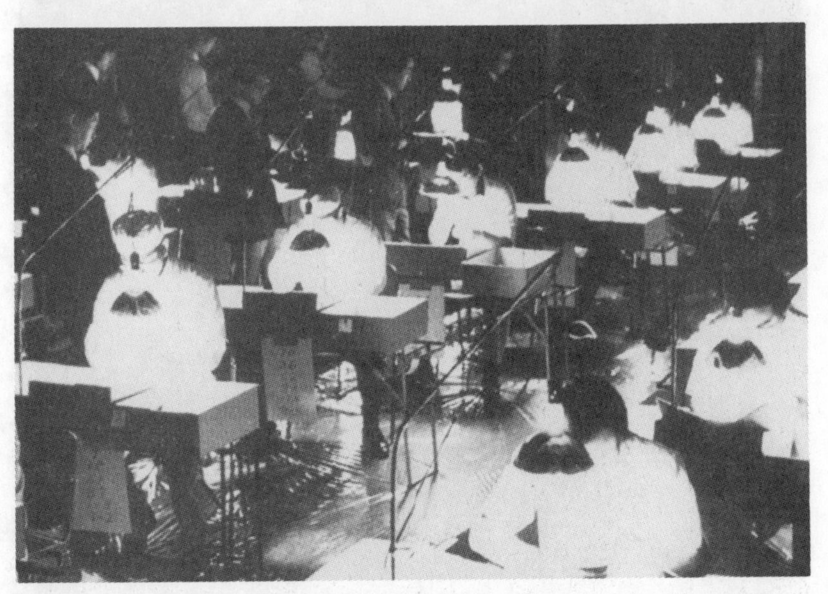

Japanese chick sexers competing at the annual chick sexing championships at Maronie Plaza, Utsunomiya City, Tuchiga-Ken, Japan. (Photo courtesy Zen-Nippon C.S.A.)

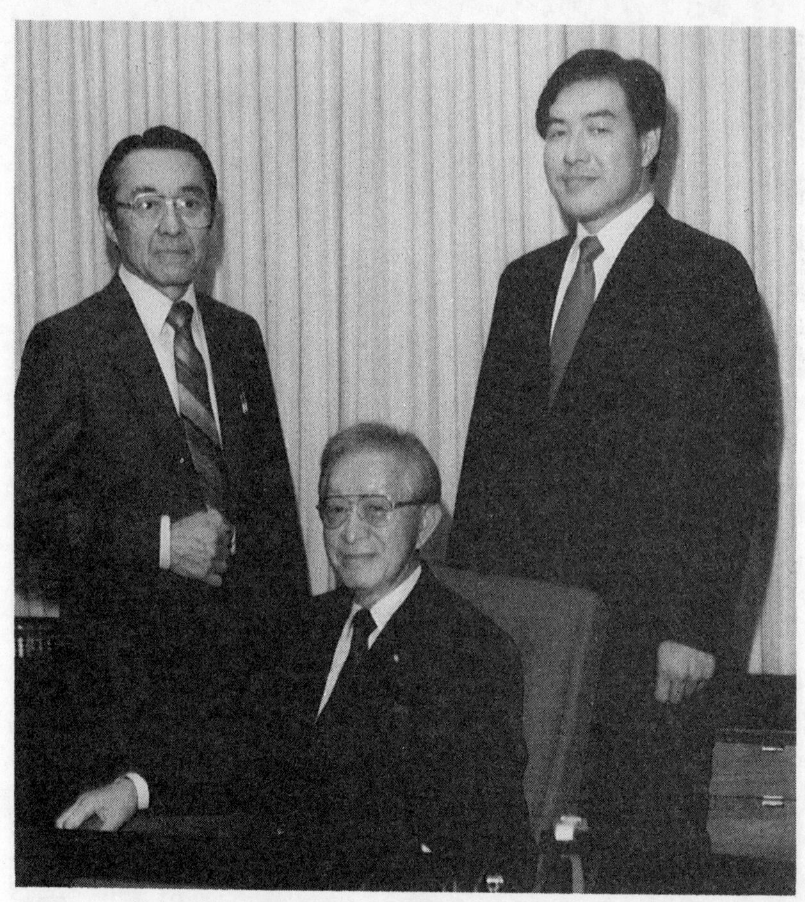

L to R: George Okazaki, S. John Nitta (seated), David Nitta of 'Amchick'.

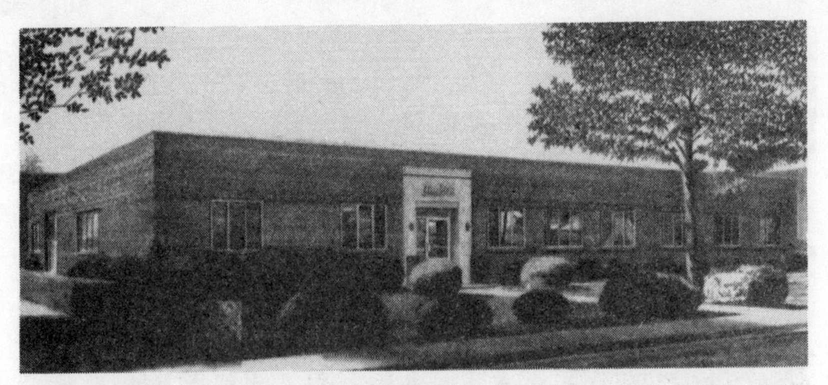

Amchick headquarters, located at Lansdale, Pennsylvania, 35 miles north of Philadelphia.

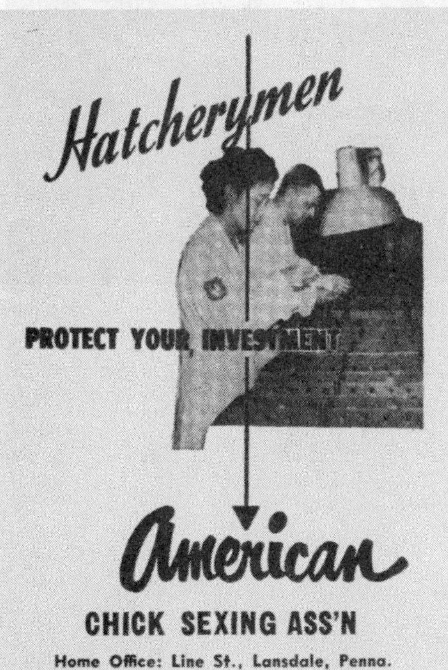

An advertisement of 'Amchick' from the 1950s then known as the American Chick Sexing Association.
(Permission to use these illustrations courtesy of Amchick.)

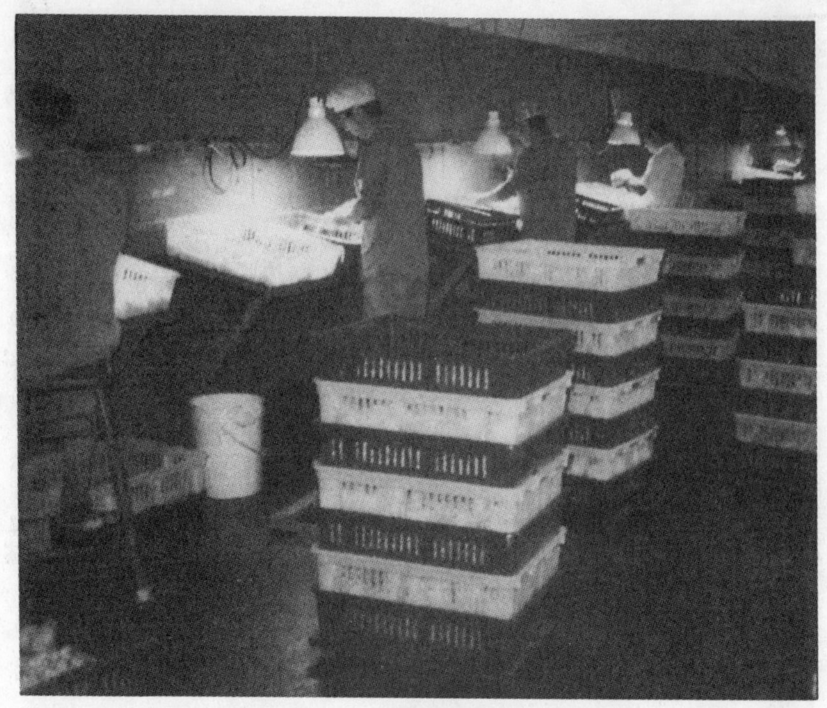

Japanese chick sexers working in an American hatchery. (Photo courtesy of Zen-Nippon C.S.A.)

As the poultry industry grew from the 1950s, more Japanese chick sexers started working in Europe and were later joined by the entry of Korean chick sexers into overseas service. Both the Japanese and the Koreans regularly worked in over 100 overseas countries by the 1980s. In 1993 there were, according to the Zen-Nippon Chick Sexing Association, 200 Korean chick sexers working in the United States and probably a similar number working in Europe.

KOREA

Most hatcherymen throughout the world are familiar with the literature from one or other of the Korean chick-sexing firms.

Korean Chick Sexers Services Association, through their Korean Chick Sexer Foreign Countries Employment Services Association of Seoul, estimate that there are about 2700 Korean chick sexers working overseas in over 100 different countries, and that this number is increasing. In their list of countries they include Australia. Up to 1994, there have never been any Korean chick sexers working commercially in Australia.

It is reasonable to assume that this figure of 2700 would include many people who have attended a chick-sexing class in Korea and then gone overseas, but not necessarily to work in the poultry industry. The Korean figures are difficult to verify as there are no over-all records kept.

The three Korean chick-sexing organisations I was able to contact supplied the following information, for which I thank them:

'Korean Chick Sexing Services Association/Korean Chick Sexer Foreign Countries Employment Services Association' and their chick-sexing school 'Korea Chick Sexer Institute' of Seoul, Korea supplied the following information and comments:

1) currently [June 1994] they have 50 registered chick sexers working in South Korea.
2) their training school the 'Korean Chick Sexer Institute' has a six-month training course for students of chick sexing.
3) their chick-sexing students must be able to sex 100 chicks in seven minutes with a 98 per cent accuracy (to pass the school test), so that they are able to sex commercially with this accuracy, and at the rate of 800 to 14,000 chicks per hour.
4) they estimate that there are about 2700 Korean chick sexers working overseas in over 100 countries.

The President of the above associations is Mr Jong-Ho Yoo.

Another Korean chick-sexing organisation 'Korchick International Services' is run by Mr Kyung Ho Kim of Pusan, South Korea. They have chick sexers working in Quebec and Edmonton in Canada, Italy, Chile,

Saudi Arabia and the United States. They supply feather-sexing services as well as vent sexers.

Another Korean chick-sexing service is a chick-sexing school and sexing service run by Mrs Kyong Mee Hah, of Pusan, with training centres in Seoul and Taegu, South Korea. Mrs Hah supplied the following information and comments:

1) she has been in the chick-sexing business since 1978.
2) the aim of her chick-sexing school is to turn out efficient chick sexers of good character and with an accuracy of 99 per cent, to work worldwide.
3) in 1986 a branch of the school was established in Taegu City, and in 1988 another school was started in Seoul.
4) the school aims to turn out students who can sex 1200 chicks an hour with a 99 per cent accuracy and, "with good human nature".
5) their graduates work in Korea, Europe, Asia, Africa and North and South America.

JAPAN

Zen-Nippon Chick Sexing Association

"Serving World Wide Since 1933"

The Zen-Nippon Chick Sexing Association of Japan still dominates the world's specialist chick-sexing scene, as it has since 1933. It has kept its dominance and reputation because it has always been professional in its dealings with its overseas clients, and has always maintained a high degree of accuracy through its permanent school in Nagoya and the annual chick-sexing competitions it conducts in Japan. The Japanese also have long-standing connections with ethnic Japanese experts in other countries particularly in the United States, Brazil and Europe.

The Zen-Nippon Association is always learning. It has always been generous in teaching others the skill and the latest developments, as well as supplying chick sexers to over 100 countries.

In 1994 there were 280 chick sexers in Japan, not all full time. There were nine students at the school in Nagoya.

The Zen-Nippon Chick Sexing Association has always had Japanese government and poultry-industry support in ensuring that there is only one chick-sexing body in Japan and that a high standard of professionalism as well as accuracy and speed is maintained on all who work in Japan and overseas.

The Zen-Nippon Association also has strong ties with Amchick of America and Hobo Chick Sexing in Belgium. In 1994 there were 180 Japanese chick sexers from Japan working in Europe, as well as those working in South America and in Asia.

The Zen-Nippon Association also conducts annual chick-sexing championships in Japan and has done so since 1934. The All-Japan chick-sexing championship contests are not only individual contests, but team contests between the different prefectures of Japan. Remarkable results in speed and accuracy have been achieved over the years.

These are the results for 1993 competitions. The team results have not been included.

The results of the Championships held at Maronie Plaza, Utsunomiya City, Tochigi-Ken, Japan on 30 October 1993
Individual event: 1 Tadashi Takamori, 100%, 3 min 18 sec (a little under 2000 chicks an hour); 2 Kimio Hatanio, 100%, 3min 29 sec.; 3 Takahiro Sasaki, 100%, 3 min 31 sec. (32 years old); 4 Katsutoshi Imaizumi, 100% 3 min 33 sec; 4 Hisayasu Watanabe, 100%, 3 min 33 sec; 6 Shiro Kato, 100%, 3 min 36 sec; 7 Hiroshi Shinmi, 100%, 3 min 43 sec; 8 Seiichi Saito, 100%, 3 min 44 sec; 9 Kiyoyuki Aizawa, 100%, 3 min 55 sec; 10 Mazazo Toyota, 100%, 3 min 58 sec (32 years old); 11 Kunimoto Fujita, 100%, 4 min 00 sec; 12 Shoei Furuyama, 100%, 4 min 04 sec; 13 Gusutabo Abe, 100%, 4 min 05 sec; 14 Takao Okuyama, 100%, 4 min 07 sec; 15 Hiroshi Iwase, 100%, 4 min 09 sec; 15 Toshinori Kanamori, 100%, 4 min 09 sec; 17 Masahiko Furubashi, 100%, 4 min 10 sec; 18 Emiko Hara, 100%, 4 min 11 sec (a little under 1500 chicks an hour), and Tadashi Akutsu, 100%, 4 min 11 sec; 20 Tomio Takasu, 100%, 4 min 15 sec; 21 Yoshikei Tanaka, 100%, 4 min 15 sec; 22 Tomoyuki Mutsuda, 100%, 4 min 22 sec; 23 Shonosuke Ima, 100%, 4 min 23 sec; 24 Tadaharu Kato, 100%, 4 min 26 sec; 25 Nen Ota, 100%, 4 min 27 sec; 26 Koichi Amikawa, 100%, 4 min 38 sec; 26 Yoshitaka Okada, 100%, 4 min 38 sec; 28 Kazuo Iwai, 100%, 4 min 41 sec; 29 Masaharu Yonezawa, 100%, 4 min 45 sec; 30 Katsuo Kawamata, 100%, 4 min 46 sec and Masako Tanitabe, 100%, 4 min 46 sec; 32 Toshiaki Todama, 100%, 4 min 47 sec; 33 Keiji Kushida, 100%, 4 min 49 sec; 34 Atsushi Nodera, 100%, 4 min 50 sec; 35 Tadashi Hara, 100%, 4 min 55 sec and 35 Hiromitsu Otiai, 100%, 4 min 55 sec; 37 Kiyoaki Takayama, 100%, 4 min 56 sec; 38 Yuzo Nariai, 100%, 5 min (1200 chicks an hour); 39 Yosao Mano, 100%, 5 min 01 sec; 40 Reiji Asai, 100%, 5 min 06 sec; 41 Akinoko Dtsubo, 100%, 5 min 29 sec; 42 Akimasa Koshino, 100%, 5 min 34 sec; 43 Toshio Ueda, 100%, 5 min 41 sec; 44 Toyoshi Hattori, 99%, 3 min 29 sec; 45 Hitoshi Miyata, 100%, 6 min (Executive Director: at the rate of 1000 chicks an hour); 46 Sadayasu Ishimaru, 100%, 6 min 03 sec; 47 Tatsuyoshi Takeuchi, 99%, 3 min 38 sec; 48 Mitsuru Fukui, 99%, 3 min 42 sec; 49 Toshio Usa, 99%, 3 min 43 sec; 50 Hideo Hirano, 99%, 3 min 46 sec; 51 Yasuji Takegami, 99%, 3 min 52 sec; 52 Yoshiko Baba, 99%, 4 min 02 sec; 53 Katsuhiko Kadowaki, 99%, 4 min 03 sec; 54 Junzo Mitani, 99%, 4 min 05 sec; 55 Yoshino Tanaka, 100%, 6 min 45 sec (73 years old; a fraction under 900 chicks an hour; one of the three women competitors); 56 Yoshio Kimura, 99%, 4 min 15

sec; 57 Hirofumi Hirata, 99%, 4 min 18 sec; 58 Mitsuyoshi Fudaki, 99%, 4 min 19 sec; 59 Eijiro Motohi, 99%, 4 min 23 sec; 60 Iwao Sakai, 99%, 4 min 24 sec; 61 Motohiro Nakamura, 99%, 4 min 24 sec; 62 Yoshihiko Kamitani, 99%, 4 min 35 sec and Hidekazu Takahashi, 99%, 4 min 35 sec; 64 Koichi Ogawa, 99%, 4 min 40 sec; 65 Hironori Hirano, 99%, 4 min 43 sec; 66 Yoichi Aida, 99%, 4 min 48 sec, Kazumi Suzuki, 99%, 4 min 48 sec and Shoji Suzuki, 99%, 4 min 48 sec; 69 Shuzo Takahashi, 99%, 5 min 10 sec; 70 Futoshi Suzuki, 99%, 5 min 20 sec; 71 Kazutada Onishi, 99%, 5 min 55 sec; 72 Chosuke Tanaka, 99%, 5 min 56 sec; 73 — Kusano[3], 98%, 3 min 27 sec; 74 Eizo Nishi, 98%, 3 min 36 sec; 75 Takashi Saiki, 98%, 3 min 44 sec; 76 Junichi Goto, 98%, 3 min 48 sec; 77 Fumio Urakawa, 98%, 4 min 17 sec; 78 Seizo Ishii, 98%, 4 min 36 sec; 79 Kazuti Osawa, 98%, 4 min 41 sec; 80 Hitoshi Sera, 98%, 4 min 45 sec; 81 Tsutomu Iwamoto, 98%, 4 min 47; 82 Iri Hirono, 98%, 4 min 51 sec; 83 Hirokazu Inagaki, 98%, 4 min 56 sec; 84 Ryo Ishizaki, 98%, 5 min 20 sec; 85 Kazuo Tamura, 98%, 5 min 24 sec; 86 Hidetada Okajima, 98%, 5 min 32 sec; 87 Seizo Murata, 98%, 5 min 53 sec; 88 Makoto Oka, 98%, 6 min 47 sec.

Unless otherwise stated, all competitors are over 40 years old. There were 107 participants: 46 obtained 100 per cent, 26 obtained 99 per cent, 16 obtained 98 per cent, and 19 were disqualified. There were also team events from the various prefectures of Japan.

BRAZIL

Brazil, with a population of 130 million, occupies fifth place in the world's egg production, behind China, the former USSR, USA and Japan.

Brazil's commercial chick-sexing is dominated by ethnic Japanese. American chick-sexing services and Zen-Nippon have sent chick sexers there, but now with less demand for specialist chick sexers most chick sexers are Brazilians.

Below is a list of Brazilian (B) and Japanese (J) chick sexers working in Brazil from 1927 to 1968, as listed in Koji Kato's Book *World of Chick Sexer* 1991 pp 34–35.

Shugo Tani 1927; Julio Hiroshi Terui 1928 B; Arnaldo Sasaki 1928 B; Keiichiro Minamoto 1928 J; Mioko Minamoto (Horie) 1930 J; Takashi Watanabe 1931 J; Shinichiro Maeda 1933 B; Masa Karube 1934 J; Joichi Yoshinaga 1935 B; Masakazu Tamura 1935 J; Hiroshi Sawaguchi 1935 B; Wataru Mifune 1936 B; Suekazu Honda 1936 J; Yoshio Toyoshima 1936 B; Hideki Sasaki 1937 B; Isamu Matuda 1937 B; Yujiro Taira 1939 J; Mario Kawahito 1941 B; Yoshie Terui 1941 B; Jorge Tsuneo Maruyama 1942 B; Mario Fujio Handa 1942 B; Hisako Tanaka 1942 J;

3 Regretfully, the given name could not be ascertained. The author apologises for this.

Shugoro Ito 1942 J; Shoji Usumoto 1942 J; Kiyoshi Sasajima 1943 B; Tadaomi Hara 1943 J; Noboru Nishimura 1944 J; Sanemasa Takaki 1945 J; Paulo Yoshiyuki Maruyama 1945 B; Tatsunobu Sakai 1946 J; Tacaaqui Mifune 1946 B; Claudio Irazuka — B; Yukinobu Yanaguizawa 1950 B; Mario Ogawa 1950 B; Marly Izuka 1951 B; Jorge Kusano 1951 B; Antonio Shizuo Taniguchi 1951 B; Natal Takashi Ami 1951 B: Coji Nakano 1952 B; Neusa Tomiko Tanaka 1953 B; Motoharu Kurosawa 1955 J; Gilson Massashi Toriumi 1958 B; Paulo Yatabe — B; Takeshi Sakai 1962 B; Marina Yoko Ide 1962 B; Midori Watanabe B; Auro Norio Yamakawa 1963 B; Jorge Utani 1963 B; Eduardo Norio Karube 1964 B; Lidia Aiko Kiguti 1964 B; Yasunori Ogura 1964 B; Mario Terauchi 1966 B; Paulo Koiti Ide 1966 B; Edson Takeski Nakamura 1966 B; Carlos Mutio Kon 1966 B; Minory Watanabe 1968 B; Americo Toshio Yamakawa; Nelsor Akira Fukai; Ana Naoka Nagashima; Paulo Maeda; Sandra Onishi; Masao Nishigori; and Tomoko Nishigori.

CHINA

There is no record of the number of chick sexers in China, but as China is the largest egg producer in the world there would be a need for many chick sexers if the pattern of other poultry-industry nations can be used as a guide.

According to Dr Hu Hisiang-Pih of the Chinese Academy of Agriculture in Beijing, there is widespread use of colour and feather sexing of day-old chicks in China. The cloacal (vent) sexing method is used for white chicks only.

All these (cloacal) chick sexers are Chinese. Some learnt the skill overseas and they in turn taught other chick sexers in China. There are no formal chick-sexing schools in China.

There are no chick sexers from China working overseas. This does not mean that there are no ethnic Chinese chick sexers living and working in other countries, for example one of Australia's top commercial chick sexers Norm Long (special-class certificate 1945). The Chinese have not entered the overseas service as the Japanese and Koreans have. The Chinese do not sex turkeys.

RUSSIA

The former Soviet Union was once the second largest egg producing nation of the world, marginally ahead of the USA and with about half the egg production of China.

The "machine" method of sexing day-old chicks is still widely used in Russia. No doubt genetic breeding of colour and feather sexing breeds have been introduced there, but there is no up-to-date reliable information on the chick-sexing industry in the former Soviet Union.

In Germany, as in most of Europe, cloacal (vent) sexing is used mainly for layers. All these specialist vent sexers are from overseas, presumably from Japan and Korea and occasionally from England.

Colour sexing is used mainly for brown-egg layers. Feather sexing is used for layers, broilers and broiler parent stock. In March 1994 Germany was testing an optical system to simplify colour sexing by video equipment, but it was not then used commercially.

In Europe, breeding work in poultry is continuing to further develop auto, colour and feather sexing stock.

The cloaca sexing of broiler PS and GPS is increasing in Europe, as is the demand for a feather sexable commercial broiler. The number of broiler PS is increasing worldwide.

In Europe almost all turkeys are sexed.

Comments from poultrymen about the poorer economic performance of feather-sexed layer replacement stock compared with stock that have to be vent sexed are not new.

When a poultry farmer in Japan was asked why there were so many specialist vent chick sexers working in Japan, his reply was that the farmers found that vent-sexed breeds were more economical than the feather-sexed stock. It should be noted that egg consumers in Japan prefer white-shelled eggs. In the past egg farmers in America have made similar comments when comparing results.

Feather, auto and colour sexing is not a new phenomenon. All were known and used long before vent sexing was developed. Even with the savings in sexing costs and not having to rear surplus cockerels, this type of stock was not used universally because of the far better performance of the white leghorn breeds or their crosses.

The Japanese claim that the development of feather sexing of layer replacement stock was brought about mainly through a world shortage of chick sexers at the time.

Worldwide, with some exceptions, there are about 70 per cent fewer specialist chick sexers than there were before the introduction of feather and colour sexing. The number of chick sexers working in Japan, while higher than most countries, is about 35 per cent of the number employed in the peak years. But as many work part-time or overseas it is difficult to arrive at an exact figure.

AMERICA

The oldest and largest chick-serving service in America is Amchick, now run by David K. Nitta, son of the founder S. John Nitta, who started the American Chick Sexing School in the mid-1930s. It is the only commercial licensed chick-sexing school in America. The American Chick Sexing Association has always had a close association with the Zen-Nippon Chick Sexing Association. Both associations have supplied chick sexers to South America and Europe.

There has been many other chick-sexing services in America, large and small, serving the industry at the height of demand for the specialist chick sexer. Among them were: Newton Chick Sexing Co., Pacific Chick Sexing Association, United Chick Sexing Association, International Chick Sexing Association, Sasamoto Chick Sexing Enterprises, Mid-West Chick Sexing and, of course the American Chick Sexing Association, now known as Amchick. All these names would be familiar to American hatcherymen.

The position in America is similar to the European practice, of vent sexing primary stock and most of the turkeys. However, in America there is still a great deal of vent sexing of white leghorn replacement stock and some heavy breeds, which still have to be vent sexed. As David Nitta of Amchick reflects: ''We'll always be around.''

There are chick sexers in America who still work at chick sexing in their sixties. Some are in their seventies. Many of these older chick sexers work on turkeys, which are easier to sex.

Most of the new vent chick sexers working in America are Koreans or Mexicans. None of the children of ethnic Japanese-American first- and second-generation chick sexers are interested in chick sexing as an occupation.

In 1994 there were 200 Korean chick sexers working in the USA, according to figures quoted by the Zen-Nippon Association.

Currently there are no chick-sexing schools in America.

A SUMMARY

Japan, China, Australia, Korea and possibly Russia are the only large poultry-industry nations in the world who do not employ any overseas chick sexers.

The proprietor of Chick Sexing Specialists (Great Britain) Ltd, Ian Bestwick, of Maidstone, Kent, formerly one of the largest services in Europe, had by the 1990s curtailed his business to a more compact organisation, but still supplies chick sexers to the United Kingdom, Africa and parts of Europe.

Hobo Chick Sexing of Belgium is now the largest chick-sexing service in Europe. It employs both Japanese and Korean sexers.

Ian Bestwick comments that ''Sexers must be up to 99 per cent accurate all day long to get by these days, as breeding stock is exported worldwide, including Japan.''

Ian Bestwick coordinates a successful chick-sexing school at Hadlow Agriculture College, Kent.

Chick Sexing Schools

In 1994 there are four chick-sexing schools, all teaching the cloacal method of sexing day-old chicks. At the beginning of these classes they had a combined total of approximately 68 students. The four classes were: one in Japan with nine students, two in Korea with about 36 students, and one in the United Kingdom with 23 students. In addition two students in Australia are being taught turkey sexing in Sydney.

UNITED KINGDOM (ENGLAND)

In England, at the Hadlow College, Kent, there were 30 students who began learning chick sexing in the 1993–94 class. The coordinator and chief instructor, Ian Bestwick, and his co-instructor, Mitsu Takasaki, are both expert chick sexers with a long experience in the industry.

A 1993 press statement said, "This project was brought about by Ian Bestwick and commenced in April 1993 using a European Social Fund Grant and managed by the National Council of Industry Training Organisation, whereby young people between the age of 18 years and 25 can learn the art of chick sexing.

"The course lasts up to a year, with a college diploma given to those students who attain an accuracy of 98 per cent with a working speed of 800 chicks an hour. Part of the course is used to provide general training in the work-a-day hatchery methods and teaching of guidance skills. The course is designed for 30 students.

"Mr Bestwick was encouraged by the Parliamentary Secretary and the Minister of State, along with the full support of Christopher Jackson, MP."

It is a part-time course. Successful graduates are offered a salary of £15 000 pounds (Aus $30 000) per annum. It is stated that an experienced chick sexer can earn up to £40 000 (Aus $80 000).

Skills in chick sexing in the United Kingdom and mainland Europe have been in decline. As a result, poultry breeders and hatcherymen have been engaging Japanese and Korean chick sexers. There would be very few countries in Europe who do not depend on overseas chick sexers. Until this course was started, there had been no training facilities in the UK for many years. It is claimed that at present there are more chick-sexing positions available than there are people in the UK to fill them.

The Hadlow project is managed by Tom McGuckin. The cost of the initial training scheme is put at over £300 000, with £100 000 coming from a European Social Fund grant. This class is open to young people up to the age of 25 who have been out of work for at least six months. Students come from many former occupations. The class had a roof tiler, a former bank worker, a newsagent manager, others who had worked on poultry farms, delivered milk and had many other varied city and rural occupations.

It is intended that Hadlow College will have a regular chick-sexing class of around 20 students each year.

According to documentation supplied by Ian Bestwick, Chick Sexing Specialists (United Kingdom) Ltd,[1] in association with its subsidiaries Chick Sexing Specialists (Rhodesia) Ltd and Chick Sexing Specialists (Ireland) Ltd was Europe's largest chick-sexing organisation. They were also agents for the Zen-Nippon and Amchick chick sexing associations. Eventually they were able to provide sufficient English chick sexers who were just as accurate at 98 per cent and able to sex 1200 chicks an hour.

As its former managing director, Ian Bestwick, states:

"Chick Sexing Specialists (UK) Ltd was, in its heyday, the largest world service outside Japan. Today, we are a compact outfit still trading overseas. We worked in Rhodesia throughout the War. Over the years we have trained more people than any other several times over, apart from the Japanese. [Not to mention Korea today, of course].[2]

Today sexers in the UK and mainland Europe work only with breeding stock and turkeys.

KOREA

It has been said that there is a "chick-sexing school on every corner in Korea". There has been a large entry of Korean chick sexers into the overseas chick-sexing service, a market formerly dominated by the Japanese. In Korea there are two chick-sexing schools, one with classes in Pusan, Seoul and Taegu City, and the other with classes in Seoul.

The Pusan Chicken Sexing School, run by Mrs Kyong Mee Hah, has its headquarters in Pusan and branches in Seoul and Taegu.

Mrs Hah is a chick sexer of 20 years' experience. Her school was started in July 1978. In December 1986 she opened a branch in Taegu City and another branch was opened in Seoul in January 1988. The

---

1 now contracted to: Chick Sexing Specialists (Great Britain)

2 documents: Ian Bestwick, 4 April 1994

courses consist of one year's training and one year of working in hatcheries. Successful students are issued with a certificate. The school's aim is to turn out chick sexers who can sex 1200 or more chicks an hour with 99 per cent accuracy.

A later innovation of this school is a training program to ensure that the successful students are graduates of good character with a high standard of professionalism.

The other school in Korea is Mr Jong-Ho Yoo's, Korea Chick Sexer Institute in Seoul. The school is part of Mr Yoo's Korean Chick Sexers Service Association and Korean Chick Sexers Foreign Countries Employment Services Association. This service has 500 chick sexers working in Korea.

The chick-sexing course at this school runs for six months. A student must be able to sex 100 chicks in 7 minutes with an accuracy of 98 per cent in order to graduate. They expect their students to be able to sex commercially at the rate of 800 to 1400 chicks an hour.

Both Korean schools supply chick sexers for Korea and overseas countries. There are no government subsidies for these schools and classes are open to everyone.

Other Korean chick sexers have learnt their skills from the Japanese, although the Zen-Nippon Chick Sexing School at Nagoya has not trained any Korean chick sexers since 1945.

JAPAN

Zen-Nippon Chick Sexing School Nagoya

In a cover story by Rosamond Green in the *Bulletin*, 2 May 1991 (English European Ed), on the Hobo Chick Sexing's founder, 73-year-old Junichi Hobo makes the claim that the Zen-Nippon Chick Sexing School is "the only official school in the world".

I would fully agree with this statement. The Nagoya school is without argument the only school that has had a permanent home since it was founded, in October 1934. It was the first chick-sexing school, where it all started. It has always insisted that its graduates must be expert chick sexers and also men and women of high ethical and professional standing, before being able to graduate or sent overseas by the Zen-Nippon Chick Sexing Association.

The school itself is a large two-storey building, with an entrance lounge, offices, a library and a large, hall-like classroom on the ground floor. Upstairs there is a large lecture and video room, with photos of some of the old masters and founders of the art. The school is a 20-minute taxi ride from the centre of Nagoya City.

Looking at the portraits of some of the past experts, the founders of the school and developers of the technique, the well-worn wooden chick boxes on the clean wooden floor, the battered light shades resting on the 200-watt sexing lights, all spotlessly clean and silent, you get that feeling . . . that many others have been there before you. A sacred shrine of professional chick sexers!

They came there in their mid-teens, listened to what they were told and practised. There were disappointments for some, success for others.

"They were sent to far-off lands, first by ship, later by plane, in their early twenties to demonstrate their new skills, and to teach others, whose language they could not understand. Later to return to Japan. To marry. To grow old. To see their successors pick up the 'baton' and go on improving the skills and techniques of the next generation of chick sexers."

When the school was first opened the students were taught throughout the year. The students were graded into three classes: primary, junior and senior. The first two classes lasted for one month and the last one for three months. An examination was held at the end of each term. A student had to pass an examination to move from one level to the next.

The requirements for advancement were:

To pass from primary to junior class, students had to sex 100 white leghorn chicks in 20 minutes with 86 per cent or higher accuracy. They then became a third-class expert.

To pass form junior to senior class, students had to sex 100 white leghorn chicks in 20 minutes with 90 per cent accuracy or higher. They then became second-class experts.

In the graduation examination a student had to sex 200 white leghorn chicks in 30 minutes, with 95 per cent accuracy or more. A first-class certificate was then issued.

As well as these examinations the Japan Chick Sexing Association held chick-sexing contests and a championship series to raise the skills of their experts.

These contests were held twice each year and the championships series once. They were held at the school in Nagoya.

Table I. Record of All-Japan Chick Sexing Championship Contest of 1934

June 21, 1934. At the Japan Chick Sexing Assn., Nagoya. 36 experts entered this year's Contest and 27 experts proved to be over 95% accuracy sexing 100 chicks.

Rank	*Name of participant*	*Time to sex 100 chicks*	*Errors in Male*	*Errors in Female*	*Accuracy*
1	T. Tanaka	6' 40"	0	0	100%
2	M. Takahashi	6' 55"	0	0	100

3	K. Takahata	9' 03"	0	0	100
4	K. Takahashi	6' 36"	1	0	99
5	I. Ikeda	6' 55"	1	0	99
6	H. Takahashi	7' 55"	0	1	99
7	K. Kato	8' 06"	0	1	99
8	S. Tanaka	8' 40"	0	1	99
9	M. Suzuki	8' 56"	0	1	99
10	Y. Masuda	9' 20"	1	0	99
11	T. Abe	11' 46"	0	1	99
12	N. Watanabe	7' 16"	2	0	98
13	Y. Sugiura	7' 48"	1	1	98
14	Y. Hoshi	8' 03"	0	2	98
15	I. Matsuoka	8' 09"	2	0	98
16	J. Hobo	9' 34"	1	1	98
17	J. Jo	11' 29"	2	0	98
18	T. Furuhashi	7' 05'	1	2	97
19	S. Hattori	8' 23"	2	1	97
20	I. Ninomiya	12' 27"	3	0	97
21	E. Kondo	14' 15"	3	0	97
22	Y. Yasuhara	11' 38"	4	0	96
23	H. Okuyama	11' 54"	3	1	96
24	Y. Imaizumi	14' 23"	3	1	96
25	G. Fukushima	9' 01"	5	0	95
26	S. Iyoda	11' 45"	4	1	95
27	Mrs S. Kazumori	12' 18"	1	4	95

Table II. Record of All-Japan Chick Sexing Spring Contest of 1935

April 30, 1935. At the Japan Chick Sexing Assn. Nagoya. 35 experts entered this Contest and 27 experts proved to be over 95% accuracy sexing 100 baby chicks.

Rank	*Name of participant*	*Time to sex 100 chicks*	*Errors in Male*	*Female*	*Accuracy*
1	T. Abe	7' 20"	0	0	100%
2	I. Matsuoka	9' 23"	0	0	100
3	G. Fukushima	9' 15"	0	1	99
4	K. Horii	9' 25"	1	0	99
5	M. Yokozaka	10' 52"	0	1	99
6	I. Ikeda	7' 05"	2	0	98
7	S. Uryu	7' 40"	2	0	98
8	K. Otani	8' 40"	1	1	98
9	K. Kato	9' 14"	1	1	98
10	T. Sato	10' 28"	1	1	98
11	T. Urabe	12' 00"	1	1	98
12	M. Yamada	7' 03"	1	2	97
13	S. Sagihara	9' 03"	0	0	97
14	T. Sakai	9' 47"	3	0	97
15	M. Suzuki	9' 48"	3	0	97

16	S. Tsuruta	12' 30'	2	1	97
17	F. Miyagawa	9' 26"	0	4	96
18	K. Hatanaka	10' 07"	2	2	96
19	S. Isa	10' 40"	0	4	96
20	Y. Machida	11' 05"	4	0	96
21	M. Kakiuchi	12' 00"	2	2	96
22	H. Kawaguchi	12' 02"	1	3	96
23	S. Obayashi	12' 15"	3	1	96
23	K. Fujiwara	12' 15"	2	2	96
25	N. Watanabe	9' 21"	0	5	95
26	K. Shiraishi	10' 34"	4	1	95
27	G. Adachi	12' 10"	3	2	95

Table III. Record of All-Japan Chick Sexing Championship Contest of 1935

July 15, 1935. At the Japan Chick Sexing Assn., Nagoya. 31 experts entered this year's Contest and 26 experts proved to be over 95% accuracy sexing 100 chicks within 10 minutes.

Rank	*Name of participant*	*Time to sex 100 chicks*	*Errors in* *Male*	*Female*	*Accuracy*
1934 Record	N. Tanaka	6' 40"	0	0	100%
1935					
1	H. Sato	6' 52"	0	0	100%
2	S. Tsuruta	8' 23"	0	0	100
3	I. Tsukiyama	8' 39"	0	0	100
4	A. Totoda	9' 18'	0	0	100
5	T. Abe	6' 21"	0	1	99
6	I. Ikeda	6' 43"	0	1	99
7	I. Ninomiya	7' 30"	1	0	99
8	Miss S. Okutomi	7' 55"	0	1	99
9	F. Miyagawa	8' 35"	0	1	99
10	T. Sakai	6' 55"	1	1	98
11	M. Suzuki	7' 25"	1	1	98
12	S. Uryu	7' 33"	1	1	98
13	F. Yakumaru	7' 39"	0	2	98
14	M. Kamiuchi	9' 25"	0	2	98
15	T. Ninomiya	7' 12"	3	0	97
16	S. Miyamoto	7' 18"	1	2	97
17	S. Kato	7' 40"	1	2	97
18	K. Horii	7' 52'	2	1	97
19	S. Niizuma	8' 39"	0	3	97
20	S. Isa	9' 30"	1	2	97
21	S. Aida	6' 28"	2	2	96
22	K. Goto	8' 27"	3	1	96

23	S. Iyoda	9' 23"	4	0	96
24	S. Inagaki	9' 30'	0	4	96
25	T. Kanada	6' 38"	0	5	95
26	G. Adachi	8' 34"	2	3	95

Table IV. Result of 500 Chick Sexing Examination

Name of Experts	*Group No.*	*Time spent*	*Errors in males*	*Errors in females*	*Accuracy*	*Points*
Nobuyishi Tanaka	I.	6' 45"	0	2	98%	95.513
	II.	6' 09"	0	0	100%	97.694
	III.	6' 27"	1	0	99%	96.605
	IV.	6' 44"	2	0	98%	95.526
	V.	6' 25"	0	0	100%	97.954
	Total	32 ' 31"		Average	99%	96.589
Tomeichi Furuhashi	I.	6' 16"	2	0	98%	95.697
	II.	5' 45"	0	0	100%	97.844
	III.	6' 50"	0	1	99%	96.463
	IV.	6' 25"	2	1	97%	94.666
	V.	6' 31"	1	0	99%	96.581
	Total	31' 47"		Average	98.6%	96.250
Hideo Kataoka	Total	34' 48"	0	6	98.8%	96.123
Koji Kato		37' 26"	5	2	98.6%	95.832
Isamu Ikeda		32' 27"	9	0	98.2%	95.813
Minoru Suzuki		37' 08"	10	0	98.0%	95.266
Shogo Uryu		40' 28"	3	6	98.2%	95.224
Isamu Ninomiya		43' 01"	4	5	98.2%	95.032
Masahiro Kakiuchi		42' 02"	3	8	97.8%	94.719
Tadashi Sakai		39' 30'	4	8	97.6%	94.710
Kunio Takashi		38' 57"	2	12	97.4%	94.559
Kiyomi Horii		41' 50"	7	5	97.6%	94.540
Shozo Yamamoto		42' 16"	7	8	97.0%	93.927

Records of All-Japan Chick Sexing Championships 1933–1934 courtesy of Zen-Nippon Chick Sexing Association, Tokyo

In 1933, before the establishment of this school, the Japan Chick Sexing Propagate Association had sent experts to Canada and America to demonstrate, teach and sex chicks commercially. After this successful trip the association was asked by many countries to send experts to them.

But by this time in Japan there were many small associations established, trying to imitate the work of the Japan Chick Sexing Propagate

Association. Several people from these smaller associations went overseas in 1933 and 1934, some to America, England and one to Australia and, in 1935 to 1939, New Zealand.

Many of the chick sexers working in Japan from these small associations were more interested in the "business ends" than the advancement of chick-sexing skills in Japan and overseas. As a result, executives of many of these small associations and other leaders from poultry organisations got together and amalgamated and established one new organisation on 28 October 1933. The association was called the "Japan Chick Sexing Association". This association established the Nagoya school in 1934 and set the standards set out above and also made sure that all its experts were of good character. The school has continued to set high standards of accuracy and develop better chick-sexing techniques, as well as maintaining its tradition of always setting a high ethical and professional standard for its graduates.

During my forty plus years as a chick sexer, company secretary, teacher, writer and researcher, I have never met, or heard of, a Japanese chick-sexing expert from the school who did not live up to this high ethical and professional standard. The most "daring" thing they ever did in Australia was reported by a Victorian hatcheryman, Mr Alf Woodman, of Coburg.

Mr Woodman got up early each hatching day to unload the chicks from the incubator, ready for the arrival of his Japanese chick sexer. On one occasion when he arrived at the hatchery at the usual early-morning time, he found a note on the door explaining that his Japanese sexer had arrived early, climbed through a window, unloaded the chicks from the incubator and sexed all the chicks, and left. He had done this, the note said, because he wanted to finish early so he could go to the horse-racing that day. I add here that all the Japanese chick sexers working in Australia had Australians drive them on their rounds and count and box the sexed chicks. Australians are great gamblers.

In April 1994 nine students began their chick sexing careers at the school. The eight young men and one young woman, all direct from high school, spent the first two weeks on theory and some video viewing, before starting their practical work on the day-old chicks.

The course at the school now lasts for three months. The students attend classes for six days a week. After completing the three months the students then work in hatcheries throughout Japan. It is usually two years before they graduate with a diploma. Most of them go overseas to work.

In 1994 a candidate has to demonstrate at an examination on 500 chicks, with a speed not below 100 chicks in eight minutes, with an average accuracy of 98 per cent, to be classed as an expert chick sexer.

To be a second-class chick sexer, who is considered a non-qualified sexers, a candidate must be able to sex 300 chicks with an average accuracy of 96 per cent, the speed being the same as an expert class, 100 chicks in eight minutes.

In 1994 there are 385 expert chick sexers and 30 second-class chick sexers in Japan. Of this total, 22 are women: 5.7 per cent of all chick sexers. There are no optical "machine" sexers in Japan.

A comparison in numbers from 1936

In a Melbourne daily newspaper *The Argus* 9 October 1936, the Japanese expert and managing director of the Japan Chick Sexing Association was reported as saying at an interview "that in Japan there were about 200 special-class (98 per cent) experts, and probably 800 holding the first-class (95 per cent) certificate. Practically all chicks in Japan were white leghorns. There were a few Rhode Island Reds and some similar Japanese breed".

Before 1933 most of the Japanese chick sexers of the first generation were self-taught: Dr Masui and his co-workers, Dr Hashimoto and Dr Ohno, had presented the theory and poultrymen Kojima and Sakakiyama had developed a practical way of distinguishing the male and female eminences in day-old chicks without weakening or killing the chick.

They had proved it could be done.

Who, then, did the experts of the 1920s learn from? They experimented with different ways of holding the chick and opening the vent. They taught themselves and each other.

As Hitoshi Miyata points out, in the foreword of this book, by 1929 there was an organisation aiming to market guaranteed sexed chicks, as well as training qualified chick sexers. It became well established in the Aichi Prefecture, in central Japan, which at that time was the centre of the poultry industry in Japan. As we have seen earlier, the City of Nagoya in the centre of this district had many large hatcheries.

It was natural that this district would become the birth place of commercial chick sexing in Japan, and eventually to the rest of the world.

The Zen-Nippon Chick Sexing School has had a long unbroken tradition in the development and teaching of chick sexing.

Mr Koji Kato, 77, of Nagoya is an early Japanese expert with links with the school since it was established. He is still a counsellor to the school and active in his own hatchery business a short distance from it. He has written a book, *World of Chick Sexer,* published in 1991 about his travels to many countries where Japanese chick sexers work, or have worked in the past.

Here is a transcript of an interview with him at Nagoya in March 1994.

PERSONAL HISTORY OF MR KOJI KATO

Date of birth: 7 February 1917

Record as chick sexer:

Dec 1930 first-class certificate 96 per cent (14 years old)

May 1935 NSW for three months, Victoria two months

May 1937 Brisbane for six months

1936, 1938, 1939: England

April 1948: Helped train Australian and New Zealand soldiers chick sexing in Kobe, at the request of the Allied Forces then occupying Japan.

Feb 1951 went to USA for six months

July 1958 went to India to teach chick sexing

July 1962 went to Sri Lanka to teach chick sexing

Record as an executive of Zen-Nippon

1959–1963: Director

1963–1973: Vice-President

Since 1973: Counsellor

1991: wrote *World of Chick Sexer*

Hatchery Business

Since 1950 Mr Kato has been running a hatchery, and is still active as President of Kato Yoken Co. Ltd.

Transcript of interview between Bob Martin and Koji Kato in Nagoya in March 1994:

BM: What made you take on chick sexing?

KK: I tell you that the chickens at the hatchery where I was employed at the age of 14, made me take on chick sexing. People at the hatchery tried to determine the sexes of chickens by opening the vent. I was the fastest of all to open the vent. So reputed was I to be the best of all, it motivated me to become a chick sexer.

BM: As an original chick sexer, how did you learn? Who did you learn from?

KK: Actually I taught myself to be a chick sexer. Given only a hint, while fingering around the vent of chicks, I happened to locate a process [eminence]. In due course, I succeeded in separating 30 cockerels out of 100 quite accurately. Consequently, I was much sought after by many poultry farms commercially.

BM: You and the other two chick sexers, Genbe Fukushima and Haich [Saichi] Hasegawa, have the reputation in Australia of being almost 100 per cent accurate. What was your "secret"? [1935]

KK: Dr Juro Hashimoto, one of the three discoverers of the theory of the chick-sexing method, published in 1930 a book called *The Development of the Phallus in the Chick* in Japanese. In this book, Dr Hashimoto clarified the presence of the two process-like folds [lambada folds] which enclose the phallus of the chick. The presence of this lambada-form folds paved the way to 100 per cent sexing. In the same year, 1930, a meeting to study how to attain 100 per cent accuracy was held with many chick sexers attending. Through this meeting, many sexers, including Fukushima, Hasegawa, etc., could improve their skills to be up to 100 per cent accurate.

BM: When you were sexing, did you ever depend on the folds to help you determine the sex of the chick? Explain.

KK: Not the appearance of the folds. I observed the above-mentioned lambada-form folds by opening the vent. I rather depended on the touch by so opening the vent, and then feeling when discharging excrements by squeezing the vent, etc.

BM: Do speed and accuracy go together?

KK: I think that accuracy comes first, then speed will follow through one's device and effort.

BM: What were some of your thoughts when you first came to Australia in 1935?

KK: Its vast land, and people living in a comfortable way. I felt envy of your people when compared with our people living frugally on a narrow land.

BM: In 1936 you went to Queensland. Were there many chickens to sex there?

KK: There were only a small number of chickens ready for the two sexers, one Australian and me. In this year of 1936, the number of the chickens I sexed in Queensland was only 150 000.

BM: Do you think intuition plays any part in being an outstanding chick sexer?

KK: I think so. Besides that, I think accumulation of repeated practice and long hours of concentration are indispensable to be an outstanding chick sexer.

BM: Would you like to tell us about some of your experiences when you were teaching Australians to sex chickens?

KK: I have taught chick sexing to many people of many lands in the same way, on the same conditions. Nothing special to mention about my experiences in your country.

BM: What age were you when you gave up chick sexing?

KK: I gave up chick sexing at 47 in 1964. My hatchery business advanced my retirement.

BM: Thank you, Mr Kato, for answering our questions and showing us over the school. We appreciate it very much.

UNITED STATES

In 1994 America has no formal chick-sexing school. The industry relies upon the current supply of American chick sexers and Korean chick sexers, of which there are 200 in America. Amchick, formerly called the American Chick Sexing Association, has been the main chick sexing school in America since 1937 but has not held any formal classes recently.

AUSTRALIA

Australia has lost its once dominant place in chick sexing. Australia does not have to rely on overseas chick sexers but no Australian chick sexers now work overseas and have not done so since 1955.

In the 1940s and 1950s Australian chick sexers worked in England, Ireland, Belgium, France and Denmark, often in hatcheries side by side with Japanese sexers. They also held classes in England and Belgium. One chick sexer from NSW also had a chick-sexing-contracting service in England which he sold when he returned to Australia permanently.

In the past, Australia had four chick-sexing schools. One in New South Wales was run by the NSW Chick Sexing Association, with Mr Frank Evans as teacher. This school ran for over ten years and was most successful in the number of accurate chick sexers it turned out to work in NSW and other States of Australia and New Zealand.

The other three schools were in Victoria and run by various chick sexers at their hatcheries. While they turned out some very accurate chick sexers, they never produced enough commercial chick sexers to meet the needs of the poultry industry in Victoria.

Nor was Victoria able to send any chick sexers from these classes overseas to work. Victoria and South Australia were the only two poultry States not to send chick sexers overseas after World War II.

Queensland, Western Australia and South Australia held classes or taught individual students as the occasion demanded.

I would argue that Australian chick sexers have adopted a defensive and inward-looking stance since the mid-1970s. They have been able to meet the greatly reduced demand for their services reasonably well, considering the current lack of opportunity for chick sexers in Australia. The most recent six chick sexers (all vent sexers) to be taught in Australia were taught by individual chick sexers, in some cases their kin. Some chick sexers in Australia have an understanding with their employers that before they retire they will train someone to take their place.

The average age of chick sexers in Australia is 50, the same as in Japan. The Japanese figure does not include their sexers working overseas. Australia does not have a reserve of young chick sexers working overseas. There are two students currently being taught to sex turkeys in NSW. Whether they will graduate to chickens remains to be seen.

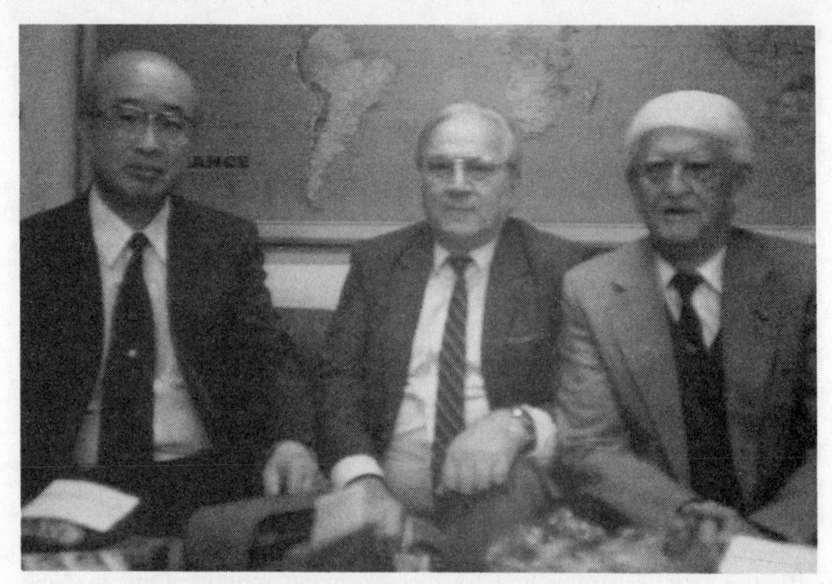

From left to right: Hitoshi Miyata, Executive Director, Zen-Nippon, Bob Martin and Hartley Hall. Tokyo 1994.

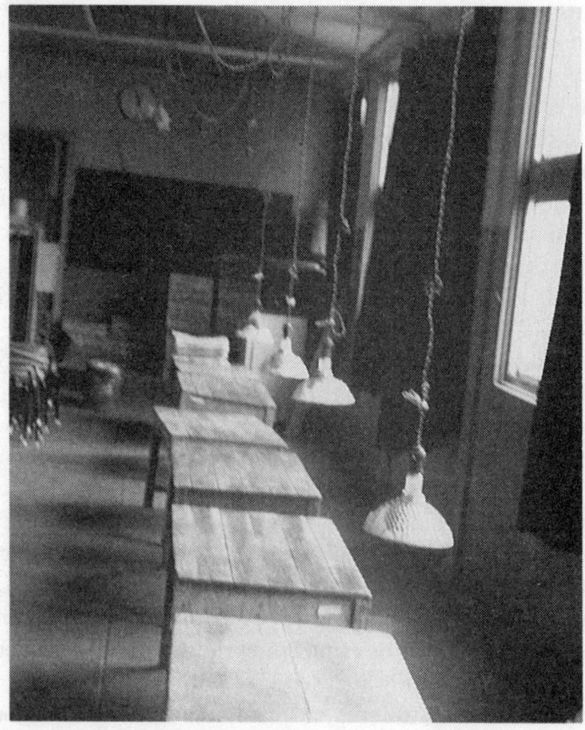

Chick-sexing school at Nagoya. March 1994

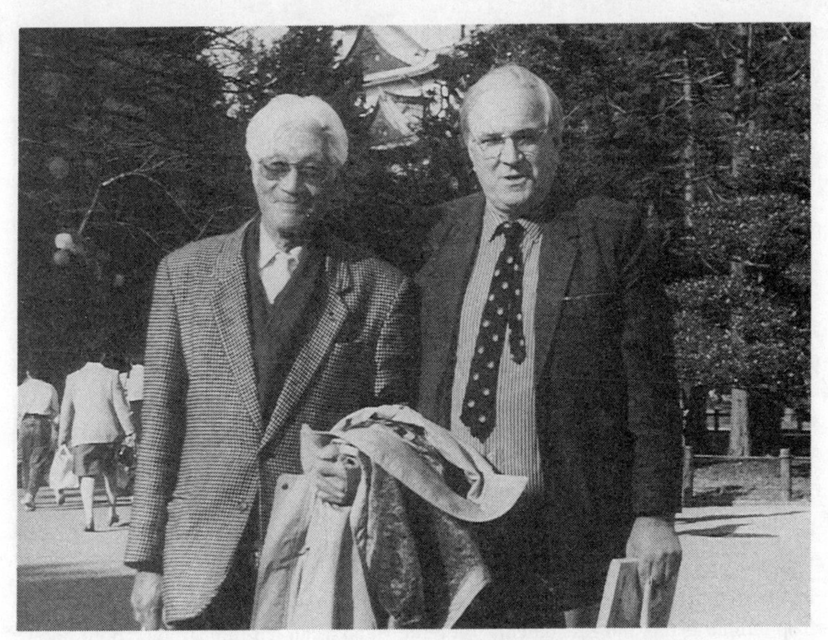

From left: Koji Kato and Bob Martin, two old-time chick sexers. March 1994.

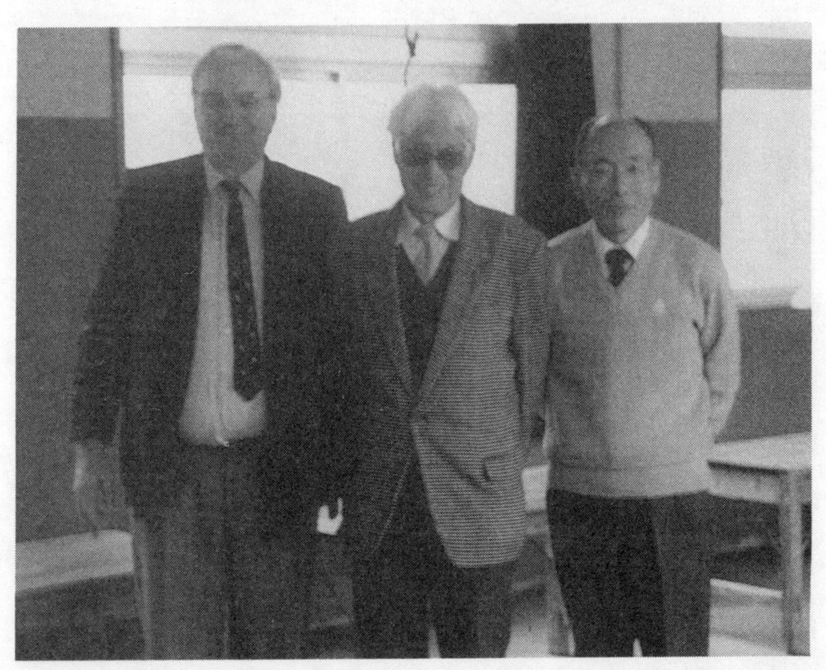

Bottom: From left, Bob Martin, Koji Kato and Yomio Mano at the chick sexing school in Nagoya.

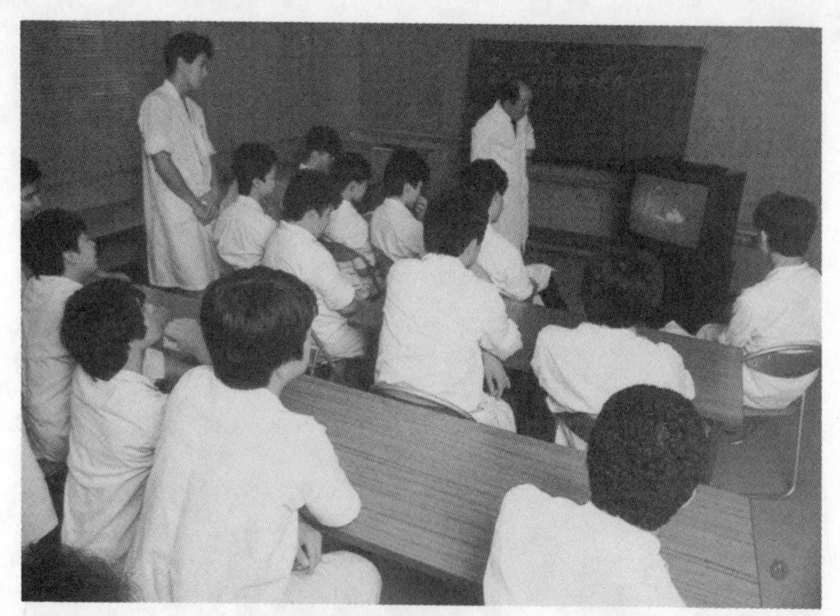

Top: Yomio Mano and his students using the video as an aid to learning. (Both photos courtesy of Zen-Nippon Chick Sexing Association)

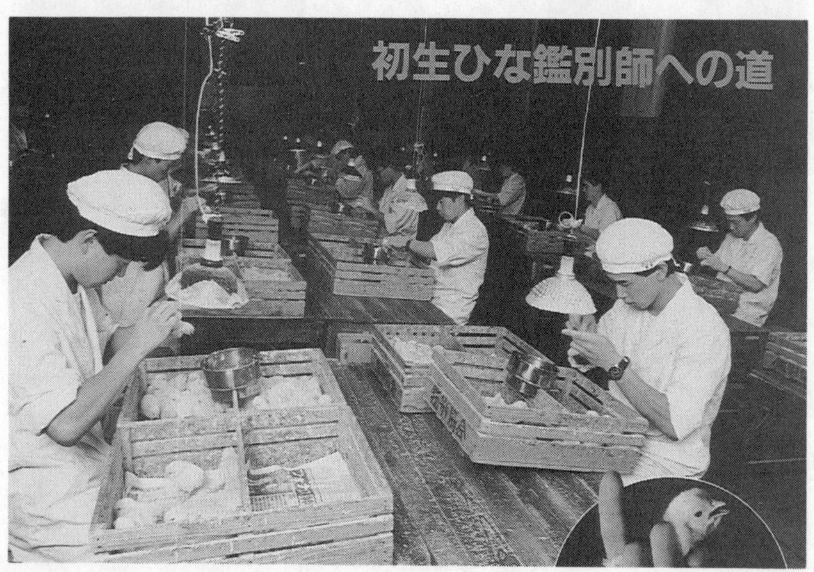

Chick-sexing students, mostly straight from high school, practising chick sexing, before being assigned to hatcheries.

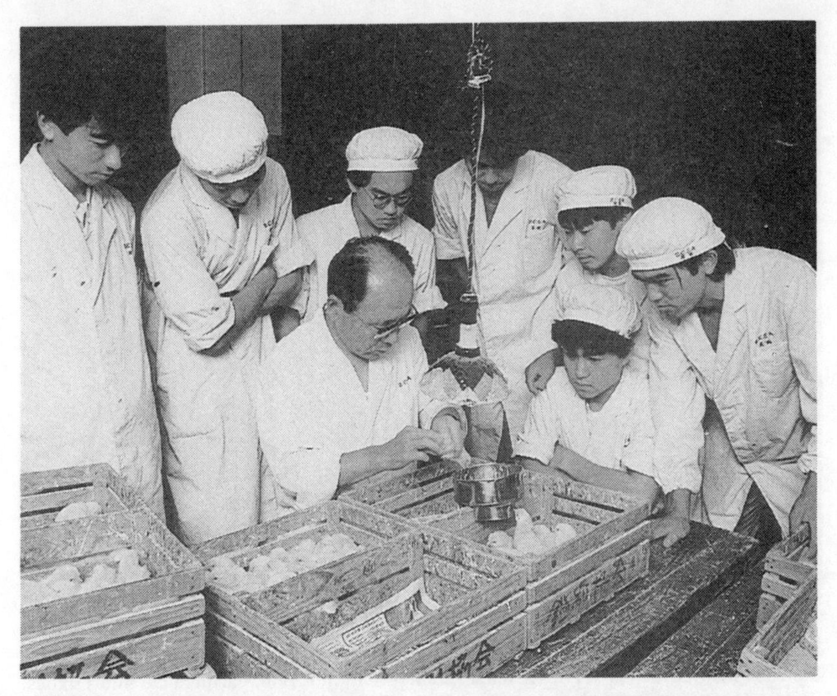

Zen-Nippon chick-sexing school, Nagoya. Yomio Mano demonstrating to his students. Below: The scrupulously clean classroom ready for the new students. March 1994.

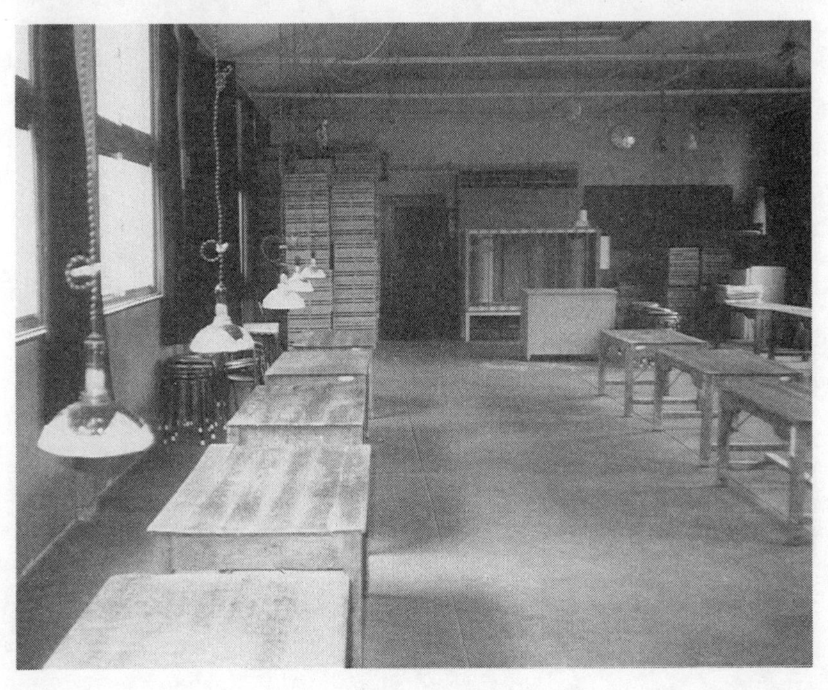

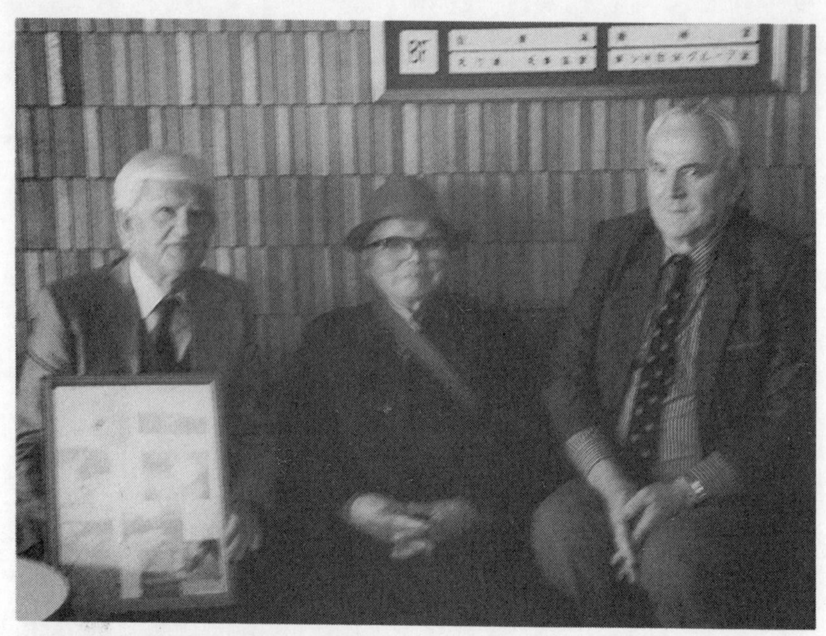

Hartley Hall (77) presenting to his teacher, Hideo Kataoka (83) a series of photos from the 1934 Melbourne classes of Mr Kataoka. On the right is Bob Martin, a lad in his sixties, a second-generation chick sexer. March 1994.

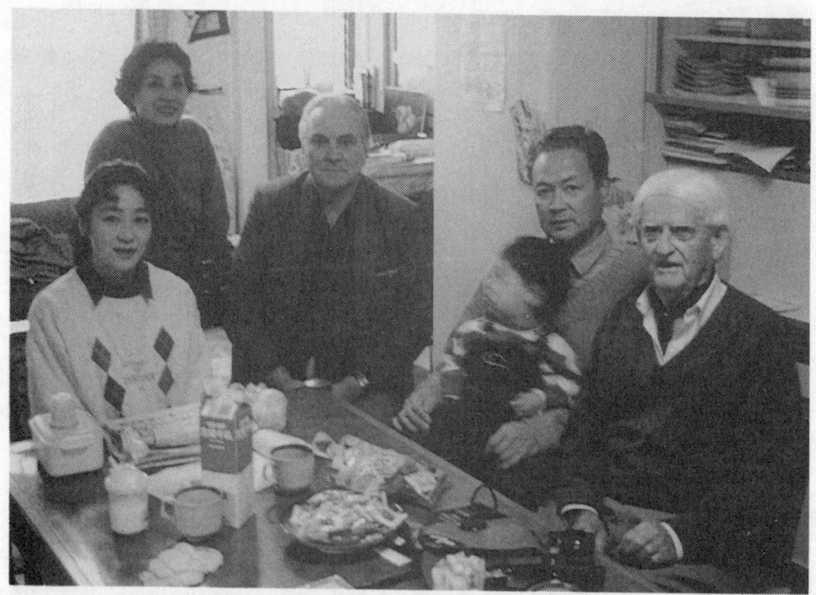

The Yamazaki Family of Sendai, hosts during Bob Martin's visit to Zen-Nippon Tokyo and Hartley Hall's reunion with his teacher of sixty years ago, Hideo Kataoka. March 1994. From left: Yumi Goto, Mayumi Yamazaki, Bob Martin, Yoshimi Yamazaki, Taiki Goto and Hartley Hall. March 1994.

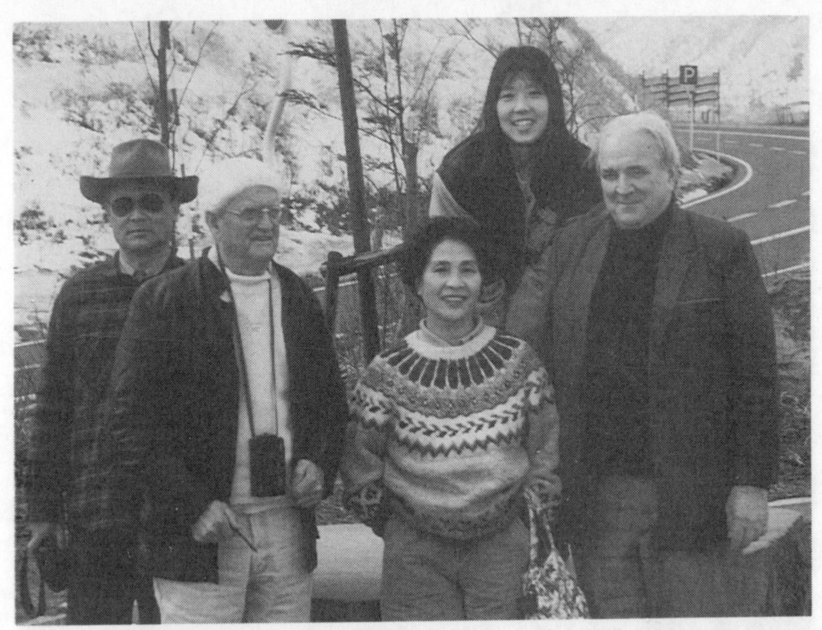

Hartley Hall, Bob Martin and the Yamazaki family on a snow trip to Mount Azuma, 150 kilometres from Sendai.

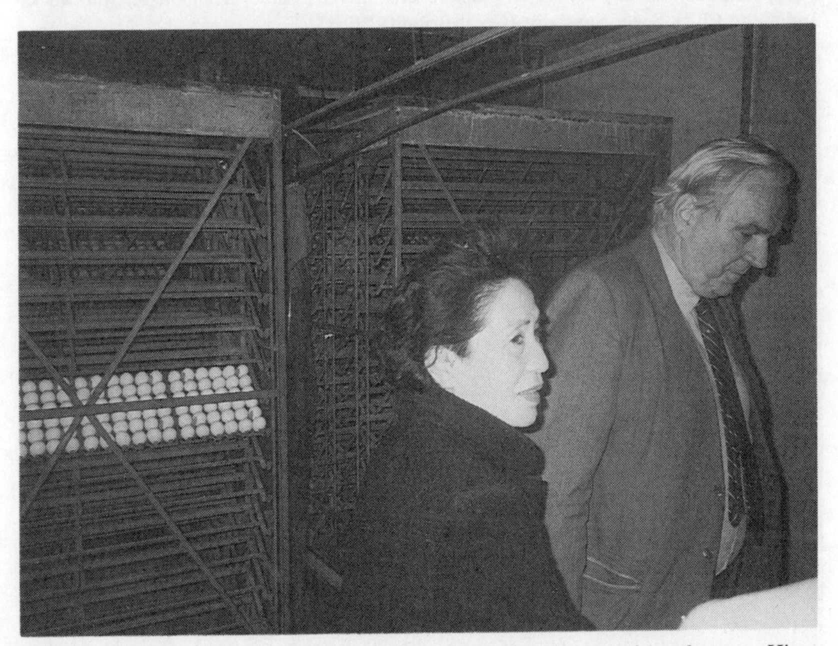

Mayumi Yamazaki and Bob Martin inside a forty-year-old 'Jamesway' incubator at Hisao Iwaya's hatchery in Sendai. Ryuichiro Iwaya, Hisao's father, the founder of the hatchery and poultry farm, was a chick sexer from 1929 till 1936. He did not sex chicks overseas.

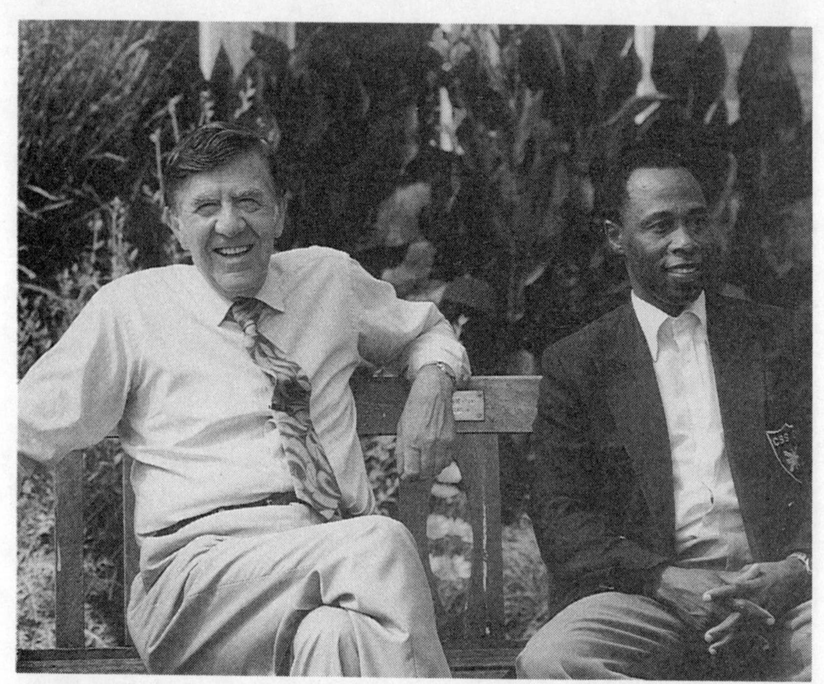

Above: Ian Bestwick and one of his chick sexers, Michael Cauley from Ghana, who works under the Chick Sexer Specialist (Great Britain) ''flag''.

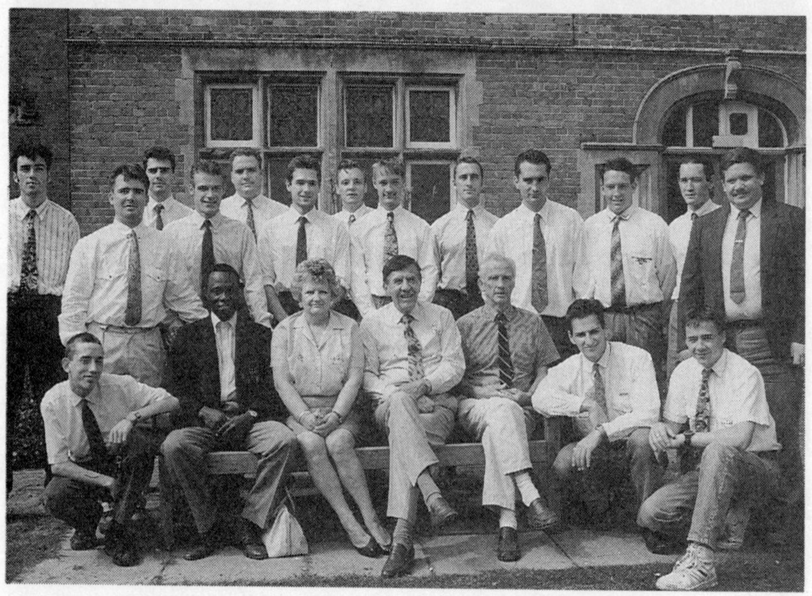

From front, left, seated: Michael Cauley (chick sexer), Theresa West (Instructor), Ian Bestwick (Coordinator) and Tom McGuckin (Manager) with their chick-sexing students from Hadlow College, Kent. (Photos courtesy Ian Bestwick)

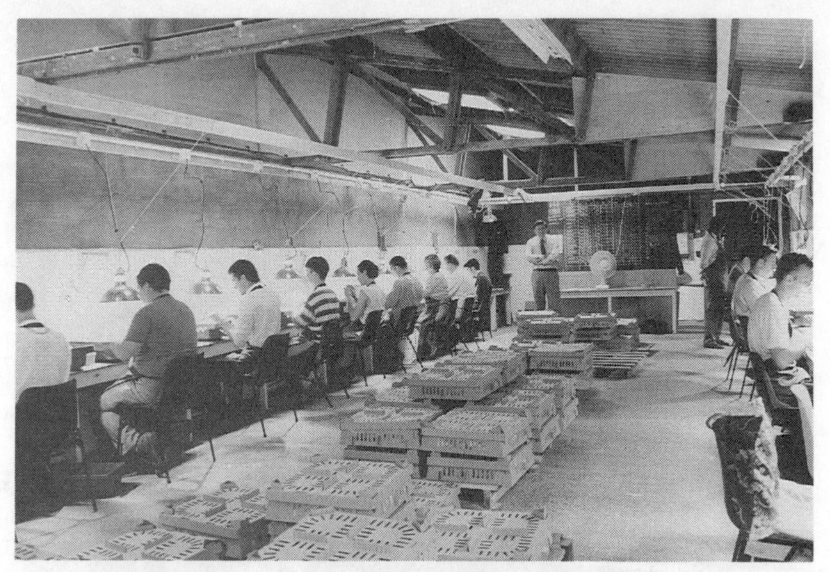

Ian Bestwick (background left) and his assistant teacher, Mitsu Takasaki, supervising the students at Hadlow College, Tonbridge, Kent.

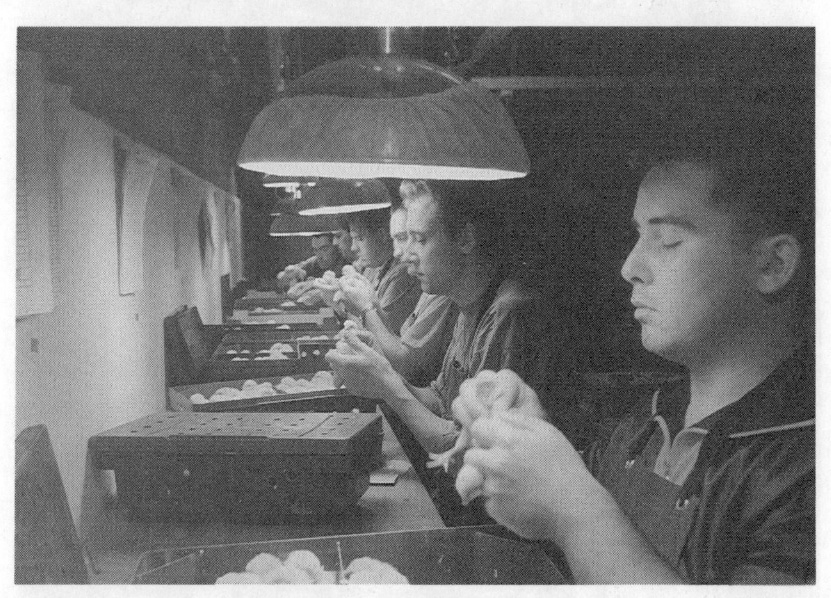

Chick-sexing students at Hadlow College. 1993–94.

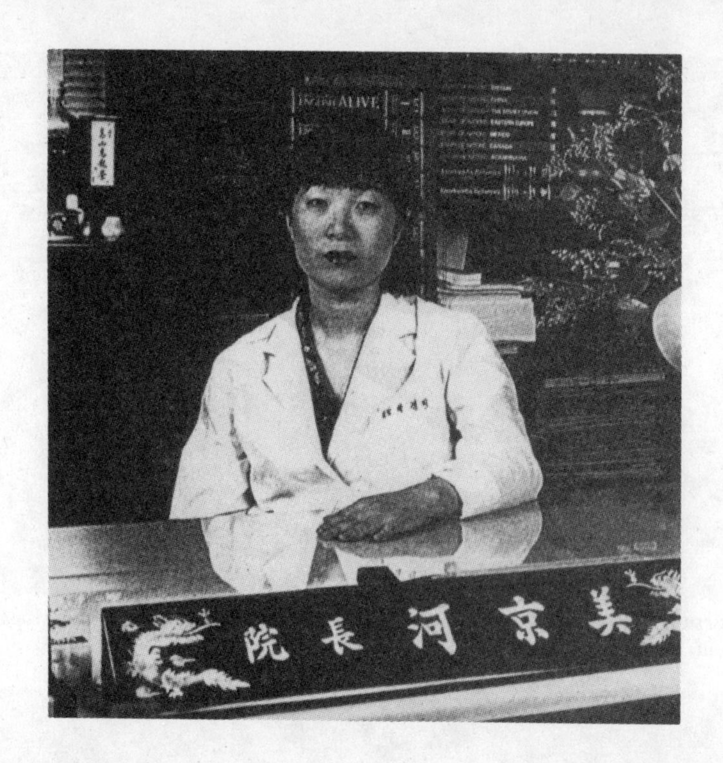

Mrs Kyong Mee Hah, President of Pusan Chicken Sexers School, Pusan, Taegu and Seoul, Korea.
Below: Students of Mrs Hah Pusan school at their practice. Korean chick sexers now work in Europe, Asia, Africa, North and South America.

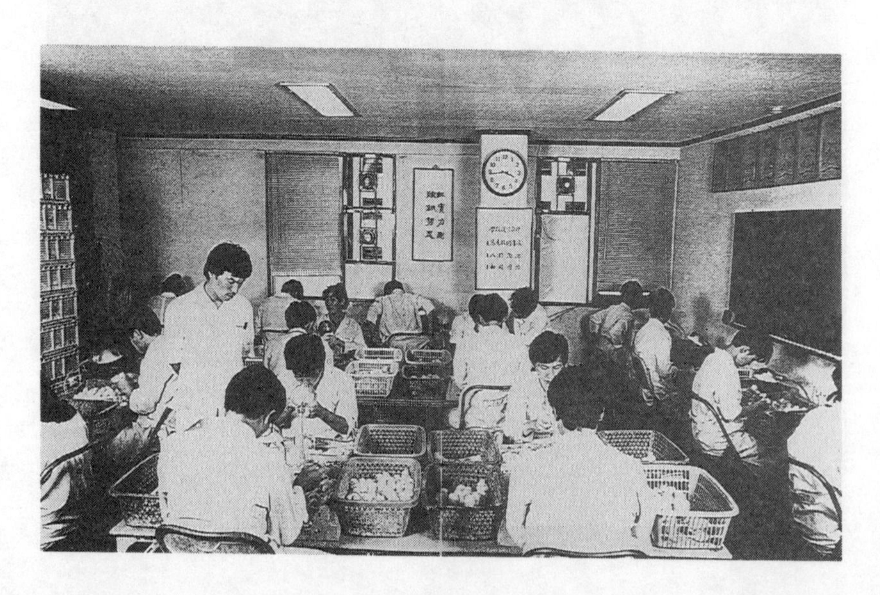

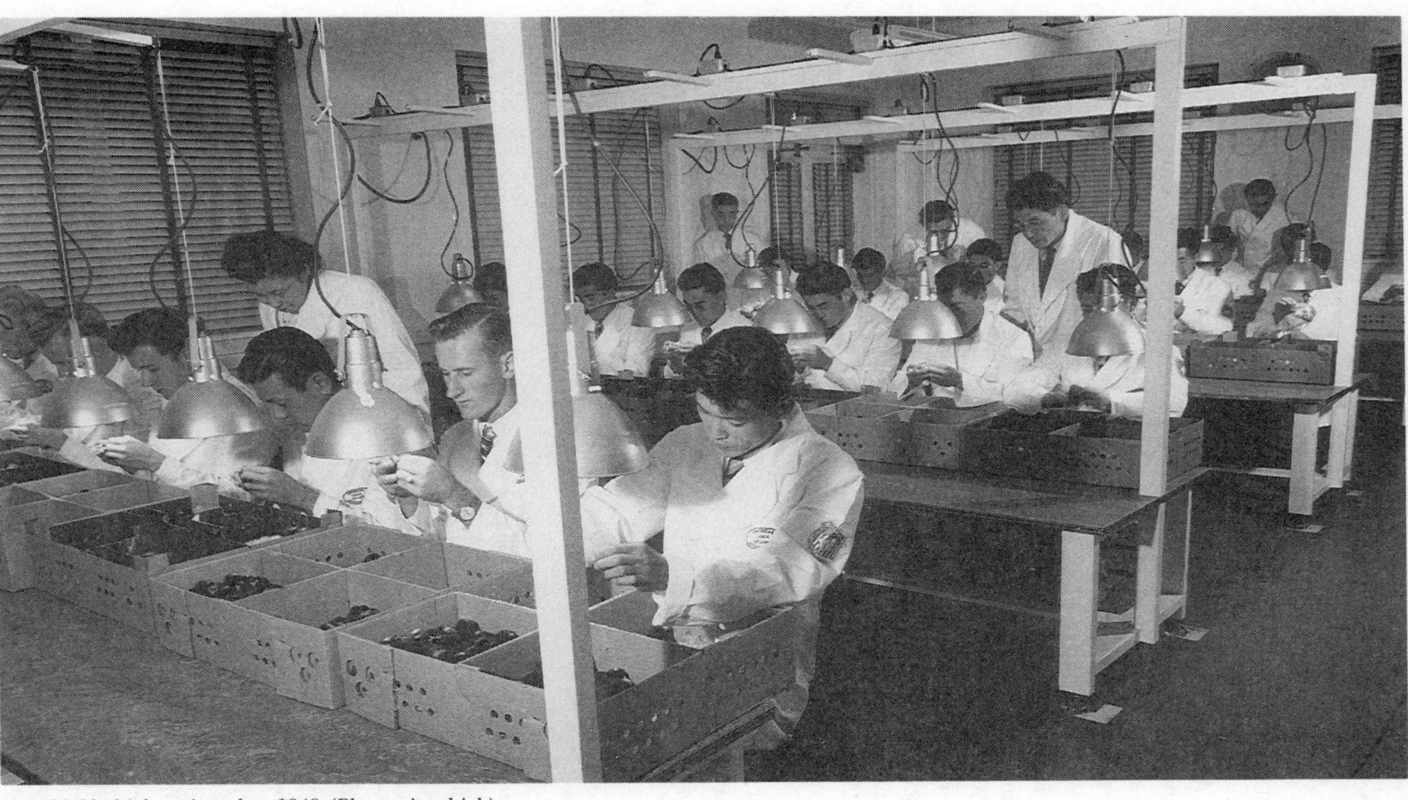

'Amchick' chick sexing class 1949 (Photo: Amchick)

I put forward the argument recently that Australia needed at least another four or five chick sexers to replace our ageing chick sexers and be ready for new work. The return argument was that there were plenty of chick sexers in Victoria at least who could fill any sudden demand for new sexers. One was recently on unemployment benefits. None of them were vent sexers.

At no time other than for the first generation of chick sexers does a newly graduated chick sexer have customers lined up for him or her. It is always a matter of replacing someone else, where and when the opportunity arrives. I leave the debate for others. Australia could again be an exporter of chick sexers.

If we look at the world's egg-production figures, we get some indication of the number of specialist chick sexers each country employs. Some countries, Japan and Korea, for example, have a much larger percentage of sexers to egg numbers than most other countries because their egg producers still use some vent-sexed strains, and of course many work overseas. In Japan many work only two or three days a week.

Australia, on the other hand, has fewer specialist chick sexers in relation to egg production because most hatcheries use overseas franchises for their primary breeder stock. However, turkey sexing is a big plus for many Australian sexers.

China is by far the world's largest egg producer, then the Soviet Union, closely followed by the USA, then Japan with about 60 per cent of the USA figure, then Brazil. All employ many chick sexers. In Russia, the "machine" method is still widely used, which suggests that there are not enough skilled vent sexers to meet the demand.

World Egg Production—1993 Rankings:

China, the world's leading egg producer is rapidly widening the gap between itself and the number two country, the USA. Japan now occupies third place, followed by Russia whose industry is still in decline.

Egg Production (million eggs)

China	180000	UK	10680	Argentina	6015
USA	71206	Spain	10400	Romania	6000
Japan	43100	Netherlands	10000	Colombia	5694
Russia	38000	Indonesia	9333	Canada	5560
India	27570	Korea Rep	8800	Philippines	5280
Brazil	26680	Thailand	8200	Pakistan	4934
Mexico	22445	Turkey	8200	Taiwan	4800
France	15352	Iran	7200	South Africa	4355
Germany	14700	Poland	7000	Hungary	4100
Ukraine	12000	Nigeria	6900	Saudi Arabia	3915
Italy	11780	Malaysia	6034	Morocco	3596

Kazakhstan	3304	Paraguay	732	Togo	126
Belarus	3300	Libya	700	Mauritania	122
Belgium/Lux.	3203	Croatia	670	Malta	117
Egypt	3200	Switzerland	631	Cyprus	112
Yugo. SFR	3000	Zambia	631	Gaza Strip	112
Czech. Rep	2980	Ireland	597	Oman	112
Korea DPR	2960	Sudan	567	Reunion	93
Australia	2842	Senegal	540	Burundi	92
Cuba	2550	Kyrgyzstan	536	Angola	89
Greece	2540	Georgia	535	Mauritius	89
Vietnam	2274	Nicaragua	510	Chad	84
Venezuela	2252	Jamaica	509	Kuwait	80
Peru	2200	Uruguay	475	Papua N. Guin	77
Chile	2021	Estonia	446	Haiti	72
Algeria	2800	Benin	416	Brunei	69
Ethiopia (former)	1990	Madagascar	405	Liberia	69
Israel	1900	Macedonia FY	390	Suriname	62
Sweden	1867	Burkina Faso	375	Bahrain	60
Austria	1700	Yemen	374	Rwanda	56
Portugal	1636	Costa Rica	367	Somalia	50
Bangladesh	1573	Uganda	364	Fiji	42
Uzbekistan	1571	Ivory Coast	358	Iceland	42
Guatemala	1555	Armenia	357	Cent Afr Rep.	39
Denmark	1495	Nepal	356	Namibia	38
Bulgaria	1429	Bosnia & Herz	340	Gabon	34
Syria	1400	Zimbabwe	340	Congo	33
Yugoslavia	1330	Puerto Rico	332	Barbados	32
Lebanon	1250	Latvia	330	FR Polynesia	32
Slovakia	1200	Cameroon	318	Hong Kong	32
Tanzania	1164	Guinea	318	Seychelles	30
Finland	1120	Tajikistan	286	Belize	29
Bolivia	1080	Ghana	286	Martinique	27
Tunisia	1074	Afghanistan	284	New Caledonia	27
El Salvador	1072	Mali	283	Mongolia	24
Ecuador	1065	Albania	280	Guadeloupe	19
Lithuania	982	Slovenia	270	Gambia	18
Iraq	950	Niger	269	Grenada	18
Kenya	933	Malawi	265	Lesotho	17
Norway	896	Turkmenistan	259	Comoros	16
Dominican Rep.	866	Cambodia	256	Guam	16
Azerbaijan	857	Singapore	252	Bahamas	15
Jordan	820	Zaire	249	Botswana	15
Moldova	804	Panama	243	Cape Verde	14
Laos	802	Mozambique	228	St Vincent	14
Sri Lanka	800	U.A. Emirates	218	Macau	13
Myanmar	793	Trinidad/Tob.	170	Guin Bissau	12
Honduras	790	Guyana	166	St Lucia	11
New Zealand	768	Sierre Leone	144	Bermuda	10

Neth. Antille	10	Eq Guinea	5	Virgin Is.	3
Bhutan	9	Fr Guiana	5	Antigua	2
St Kitts	8	Dominica	4	Cook Islands	2
Solomon Is	7	Pacific Is	4	Amer Somoa	1
Swaziland	7	Samoa	4	Montserrat	1
Tonga	7	Sao Tome	4	Nauru	1
Vanuatu	7	Kiribati	3	Wallis etc	1

This page courtesy of Watt Poultry Yearbook: International, Mount Morris, Illinois USA

Chick sexing theory

AN INTRODUCTION

Never lead a student where you have never been yourself.

Chick sexing is not something you learn from a book.

It can be argued, as Doctors Kiyoshi Masui and Juro Hashimoto did, "that the theory of chick sexing is rather too difficult for beginners to understand."[1] They advise the student to take some lessons first and read up the theory later. I do not agree with this. I believe a simple explanation of the theory is a help before the students begins the practical lessons.

Certainly a re-reading of the theory, once an accuracy of 85 per cent is reached, is a must if further progress is to be made. Looking at a text book of enlarged drawings and pictures showing the different types of eminences can be a help. But as Junichi Hobo observed at an interview once, when showing the journalist a book of diagrams used for teaching, "If only the chicks were this big in real life, it would be a lot easier."[2]

Many of the first Japanese experts were self-taught, but after reading the scientific findings behind the practice of chick sexing they still needed to compare with others what they saw, and to experiment with different ways of opening and holding the chick, and have much practice, a determination to be 100 per cent accurate, and be able to do the job quickly.

Almost without exception, the most skilled chick sexers I interviewed during the course of this study had sketches, photos and their own drawings of the various types of eminences as they saw and interpreted them during their early learning stage. They knew from reading the theory of Masui and Hashimoto why there was a small percentage of pullet eminences as well as cockerel eminences and while, at first, they

---

1 *Sexing Baby Chicks* by Kiyoshi Masui & Juro Hashimoto. Journal Printing Co. Vancouver. 1933.

2 *The Bulletin.* European Ed. 2 May 1991. "The profitable Art of Chick Sex Checking" by Rosamond Green.

seemed to be identical, there was a way of being able to tell the difference.

At first they learnt to group the different pullet and cockerel eminences. With more practice and experience, these groupings started to matter less and less. Soon accuracy and speed increased: it either had an eminence—it was a cockerel—or had no eminence—it was a pullet. At 800 to 1200 chicks an hour, it is there or it is not there. There is no time for observing different types of eminences or comparing the almost identical types of pullet and cockerel eminences. Yet they were able to achieve that 99 to 100 per cent accuracy, and with speed.

When they were learning, these groupings of cockerel's and pullet's eminences were an important part. Without being able to identify and group them, they would have never been able to get beyond an accuracy of 87–90 per cent.

If you have ever observed commercial chick sexers working for any length of time, you will notice occasionally they seem to slow a little and look at a chick before returning to their normal glance and throw. Sometimes, too, if they are not being observed, they will kill and postmortem a chick.

The aim here is to lead you through the transformation of a student in class analysing and observing the different groups of eminences to an expert 'glancing and throwing' at 1200 chick an hour.

The sex of a chick can be determined by examining the cloaca (vent), and by observing the absence of the genital eminence in a pullet, or the presence of the degenerate genital eminence in a cockerel. This absence of an eminence in pullets occurs in only about 85 per cent of them; in a further percentage the pullet eminence is so small it is easily distinguished from the male eminence.

As well as the genital eminences, there are also two roundish folds lying on either side and attached to it, the whole forming a raised area.

The eminence is usually in the central wall of the urogenital portion of the cloaca, just at the point where the second and third set of the above folds are. In the adult fowl the eminence is almost round in shape, white and measures about 3mm in diameter.

The genital eminence exists not only in the adult bird, but also at every stage of growth of the chick, even immediately after hatching. Therefore, sexing of chicks can be accomplished by reference to this sexual difference.

At this point it is important to explain what is meant by "genital eminence". The difference between the structure of the cloaca of the cockerel and the pullet chick is the presence, in the case of the cockerel, and absence in the case of the pullet, of a genital eminence.

The development of the genital eminence

The genital eminence and two round folds have been traced to the so-called phallus in the early embryonic stage of the chick's development. In this early stage of development in both cockerel and pullet chicks, the surrounding portion of the anal opening forms a ring-shaped swelling, the central part of which is a large tongue-shaped papilla. This tongue-shaped body is the origin of the genital eminence of the newly hatched chick, and is called the phallus. The size of the phallus, as well as its shape, is alike in both sexes until about the twelfth day of incubation. On about the twelfth day of incubation the shape of the phallus begins to change in both sexes. Depressions appear on each side of the tongue-shaped papilla. These depressions become more pronounced during further development. On the thirteenth day the phallus is distinctly divided into three portions, a cephalic and two basal portions. The difference in the phallus of the cockerel and the pullet begins to appear on the fourteenth day of incubation, and develops until it is quite distinct at the time of hatching.

In the cockerel, the cephalic portion of the phallus is seen as a sharp, round, raised body and the basal portion as two round folds at the end of incubation. In the pullet the cephalic portion diminishes. At hatching it remains, with some exceptions, only in the form of a flattened fold. In some pullet chicks the cephalic portion of the phallus, the genital eminence, exists even after hatching.

It is these "after hatching" pullet genital eminences that remain which is what chick sexing is about. Without these, the sexing of day-old chicks would be a fairly straightforward operation.

Masui and Hashimoto[3] go on to describe at length the various cockerel-type eminences and the importance of opening the cloaca (vent) correctly in order to be able to see and identify the cockerel and the pullet eminences. A student attending class, or being taught privately, will be shown diagrams or photos of some of these different types of eminences. I do not propose to go into any great detail here, except to include some drawings supplied at some of the chick-sexing classes in the past, and also some drawings that some of the most successful experts drew to help them identify the various types in their own early learning days.

Each student needs to see these types and be able to quickly identify them. Over time, with present-day genetic breeding, some of these genital eminence types will change. It is a matter of understanding why there are some pullet eminences still present at hatching time, and realising that there are differences which can be readily identified with practice, after some trial and error.

---

3 "Ibid", Masui and Hashimoto.

If a student could easily identify these cockerel and pullet eminences which are similar, sexing chicks would no longer be classed as a skilled occupation. One of the difficulties is to distinguish that small percentage of cockerel and pullet eminences that are almost identical.

Some of the methods used to help identify these difficult pullet eminences are listed here.

The genital eminence of the day-old pullet

1) the elasticity of the eminence: the pullet eminence is not as elastic as the cockerel eminence. If it is pressed with the finger tip it will be flattened and not come up quickly. Whereas the cockerel eminence is so elastic it is difficult to change its shape by pressing it or extending it with the finger.
2) The boundary and contour of the genital eminence: the pullet eminence has generally no distinct boundary or contour. This gives it an indistinct appearance, and this is important in gaining speed later.
3) The lustre and colour of the eminence: the pullet eminence generally has a transparent appearance, and its colour does not differ from the other part of the cloaca. The cockerel eminence has a distinctive lustre. This is one of the reasons the first look is the best, and again speed is possible. It is important to make a decision at first glance, because after manipulation an eminence will increase in size, and after too much manipulation a pullet eminence may enlarge so much that it will "unquestionably" be determined as a cockerel.
4) The difference in the position of the eminence: the pullet eminence is further inside than the cockerel. There are some exceptions, however, in which these differences are so indistinct that even experts are often unable to distinguish them.

Some of the cockerel and pullet eminences are the same small size, which makes it difficult to determine the sex of the chick. Some experts suggest that if you cannot distinguish these it is better to class them all as pullets. This way you will make fewer mistakes and will not be losing pullets among the cockerels. Some experts are able to distinguish these. Maybe here intuition comes into play. My own experience has been that I used to get these ones correct about half the time, but, at the cost of having to "look" rather than "glance and throw". Looking back now, I would have been better to have followed the suggestion of always classing these as pullets. But I was always aiming for that 100 per cent goal.

One of the early Japanese masters, Sakakiyama, gave this advice to his students: "Do not look at the eminence with your eyes, but with your fingers." He is quoted in Masui and Hashimoto, p 77.

The genital eminence of the day-old cockerel

The genital eminence of the cockerel varies in shape and size and can be divided into at least six different types, according to Masui and Hashimoto. However, most would agree there are far more types than these six, but classifying them, in my view, is not important, as most are unmistakably cockerels. But, occasionally, there are exceptions.

The (lateral) folds

I am unable to give a firm opinion about the importance of folds in helping to determine the sex. From my own experience I did not find the folds any help at all, but bear in mind that commercially I was a 97 percenter and 1000 chicks an hour, not great by today's standard.

When I asked the Japanese expert, Hitoshi Miyata, a 100 percenter, he answered that intuition was more important than the folds.

When I asked Koji Kato, one of the original sexers and to a degree self-taught, the same question about the folds he answered: "Not the appearance of the folds. I observed the lambada folds by opening the vent. I rather depended on the touch, by so opening the vent, and feeling when discharging excrements by squeezing the vent etc."

Yet Masui and Hashimoto when considering folds write (P.85 .4) "Two Round Folds. As has been stated before, in the adult fowl there are two round folds, situated symmetrically on both sides of the genital eminence. From the embryological study of the phallus (Hashimoto) it is seen that they are a part of the organ of copulation of the fowl.

"In baby chicks the round folds vary remarkably, according to individual chicks. They are very rarely found, as in the adult, to be regular in shape and situation symmetrically on either side of the genital eminence. On the contrary, in many cases these folds are irregular in shape, and remarkably variable in size. Sometimes only one fold is seen to exist, the other one remaining as a very small filament.

"With regard to the shape and size of the round folds, there is no distinct sexual difference. But from accurate observation it is seen that in the male chick they are more distinct than in the female. However, this difference is too slight to be of value in separating the sexes.

"It is to be remembered that although no sexual difference can be clearly seen in the size and shape of the two round folds, the boundary between the eminence and the folds is considered by some (Yogo e.g.) to be more distinct in the male than the female. This difference can practically be applied in sexing chicks."

In this extract of Masui's and Hashimoto's they quote Mr Yogo, a very accurate and fast commercial chick sexer, one of Japan's most experienced first-generation sexers. His observations are worth some thought.

One Australian sexer at least saw the folds as important aids to sexing. Hartley Hall, a first-generation expert, claimed that it was important to know something of these folds. He explains: "When the sexer is in doubt one of the main distinguishing features upon which he relies upon is the form and size of the folds, and for that reason these folds are important."

After explaining the appearance of the folds Hartley Hall continues. "Actually the folds in the pullets are less uniform in shape than the males.

"Sometimes folds are mistaken for the eminence, particularly when one fold is much smaller than the other. Very often it appears too small for a fold. Because of this, extreme care must be used by the sexer, otherwise he may mistake a female fold for a male eminence."

Hartley Hall was a very accurate chick sexer. His errors seldom exceeded 1 per cent in the days when 90 per cent of all chicks sexed were white leghorns. As a teenage student, I collected white leghorn cockerels from several of Hartley Hall's customers to practise on. Even after postmortems I never found more than one per cent of errors in the cockerels and among the pullets the errors were barely ½ a per cent.

One bonus in practising on Hall's cockerels was that he used a method of sexing which did not require evacuation of the excrement, so that I had practice at draining the excrement from chicks, even though they had already been sexed.

Hall, with the help of his father, Seth Hall, had developed a method of examining the vents without evacuating any excreta, a method he called "The Avoidance Method".

He used the Suzuki method of holding the chick (chick's legs away from the sexer). He achieved his "Avoidance Method" by compressing the chick's abdomen between the first finger and the thumb of the left hand, by giving it a sharp, jerky squeeze. The excreta was held back by pressing the first finger of the right hand on the intestinal duct immediately behind the cloaca in an upward and downward movement. This closed the walls of the intestine and blocked any excreta which may have been there. In the 1930s Hartley Hall was well known for this method. However, even though he held a chick-sexing class, no student was ever successful in learning this method. It was exclusively Hartley Hall's. In the 1930s, in Victoria, 4000 to 5000 chicks in a day was considered a big day's sexing. Hall sexed from 600 to 700 chicks in an hour. Whether his "Avoidance Method" slowed him down or not, I do not know, as he certainly sexed a large number of chicks both in Australia and England. That he was very accurate there was no argument. One can only go by what he has said and the results he obtained to assess the importance of the folds in his decisions.

Whether the folds are an important consideration is, in the end, up to the individual sexer.

Accuracy
The reason the Japan Chick Sexing Propagate Association in the 1930s originally set up a 92 per cent later and later a 95 per cent as the standard for a first-class sexer was because at that time these were the accuracies that could be achieved if a student could recognise the more easily identified pullet eminences.

It was found later that the student could soon get 95 per cent accuracy. This was the standard Australia followed, with 98 per cent for a higher or special-class certificate.

In Japan and elsewhere, as teaching methods improved, and more was learnt from practising chick sexers, many students were able to gain 98–100 per cent accuracy while learning.

In the sixty-plus years since commercial chick sexing began what was considered an outstanding performance both in accuracy and speed then is now the standard in the chick sexing world. Eight hundred, 1200, 1500 and occasionally 2000 chicks an hour are now possible, and it is expected that a chick sexer will sex all day long with an accuracy of near 98 per cent or more.

Chick sexing speeds
Gone are the days when a pimply eighteen-year-old Bob Martin arrives on his push bike, with light, jar and white coat balanced on the handle bars, to begin his first day as a chick sexer.

An 8 a.m. start, there are 4000 chicks to do. A counter/boxer helper is supplied, but still it takes till 7 p.m. to finish the 4000 chicks.

I am amazed that I have made in that one day more money than a man earns on the basic wage for a week's work. By the end of the twelve-week hatching season, I finish my 4000 chicks by 3 p.m. By the second season I have learnt to start at 5 a.m. (by myself until 8 a.m.) and finish the 4000 chicks by 10.30 and then go off to another hatchery to do another 4000 or 5000 in the afternoon and evening.

I always worked with a counter/boxer, usually the hatcheryman himself, who wanted to hear the news from the other hatcherymen I had been to that week, or sometimes to talk about an incubation problem.

With improved handling techniques, picking two chicks at a time, and more uniform hatching results with modern incubators, many chick sexers with over 40 years commercial experience have sometimes achieved speeds of up to 1800 chicks in an hour.

The oldest chick sexer in Japan, Yoshino Tanaka, a 73-year-old woman, was able to sex 100 chicks in 6 minutes 45 seconds with 100 per cent accuracy at the 34th Japanese Chick Sexing Competitions held in Utsunomiya City in 1993. Other competitors were able to sex the 100 chicks in 3 minutes 18 seconds. Of the 107 competitors, 46 were

100 per cent accurate and most of these were able to sex their 100 chicks in 3 minutes 30 seconds, 4 minutes 55 seconds and 6 minutes 3 seconds. All except two were over 40 years old.

A commercial speed of 800 to 1200 an hour with an accuracy of 98 per cent or more, all day long, would be expected by most hatcherymen who engage specialist chick sexers today.

Now, as always, an accurate chick sexer will always find work and attract premium payments.

A sexer who has chicks fed to him and taken away has an advantage, but few of today's chick sexers seem to work this way. My 51-year-old "student", John Hammond, who does 1200 chicks plus an hour and works by himself says of his "old teacher", "If you had worked by yourself and had not yapped so much while you were sexing, you would have got your 100 per cent accuracy."

My answer to this is, firstly, you didn't say that to me when I was teaching you. Secondly, if I did not talk occasionally, I would have been "madder" than I am. As well, the hatcheryman owner expected "intelligent conversation". It was partly what he was paying me for, part of my goodwill. Today's chick sexers are expected only to sex the chicks.

Nevertheless, what John Hammond is saying is correct. Laughing or fooling around is not the way to accurate and fast sexing. Sexers need to be left alone to work at their task.

The speed of sexing varies between sexers, of course. Once the most skilled experts worked at 600 to 800 and 1000 chicks an hour. It was once argued that if too much speed is obtained a lower degree of accuracy will result. The figure of 500 to 600 chicks an hour and 5000 chicks a day was quoted as the optimum.

I would agree that 5000 to 6000 chicks in a day is still a reasonable and a comfortable day's work. Many chick sexers will not agree with this figure, claiming that it is too low. Speeds per hour of 800 to 1400 chicks are probably a satisfactory rate for most sexers. Bear in mind that few of today's chick sexers work every day (they have rest days in between). This is a big plus when coupled with the all-year-round work which most sexers now have.

A ready reckoner of chick sexing speeds

Seconds per chick	*chicks per minute*	*chicks per hour*
10	6	360
8½	7	420
6½	9	540
6	10	600
5½	11	660
5	12	720
4.75	13	780

4½	14	840
4	15	900
3.75	16	960
3.6	17	1020
3.10	18	1080
3.3	19	1140
3	20	1200
2.85	21	1260
2.7	22	1320
2½	24	1440
2.4	25	1500
2.14	28	1680
2	30	1800
		2000

Making a decision

It is extremely important to make a decision at first glance because after manipulation an eminence will increase in size. After too much manipulation an easily identified pullet eminence can become "unquestionably determined" as a cockerel.

Pullet chick eminences tend to be placed towards the inside of the cloaca, unlike the cockerel eminence, which is on the outer ring.

To the experienced chick sexer the size of the eminence is possibly the chief determining factor. It is of no use to say that one is bigger than the other, or that the male is larger, because the difference to the beginner is so small as to be insignificant. Such decisions of course will come after practice and a wider knowledge.

There are times when a closer examination is necessary, but this is only with smaller types, which is not very often.

Perseverance and practice, and a quick decision is what is required. The first decision is almost without exception the correct one.

After a certain stage of accuracy and confidence is reached, speed and no hesitation in the decision making becomes automatic. Where intuition comes in, no-one can say, but at 1200 to 1700 chicks an hour or even 800 an hour there is not a great deal of time for analysis, and no time at all for hesitation.

How many times during Part I in this study have you read of a chick sexer say: "If it had an eminence I knew it was a cockerel, if nothing a pullet" . . . "It's either a cockerel or a pullet. It's that easy."

As a teacher of secondary-school English students and teaching reading comprehension, I always taught the students that your first decision is always the correct one. Once you begin having second thoughts you are in trouble. Whatever comes into your head first, that's it, put it down; providing you have read the article, of course.

Intuition

intuition: a) an understanding or perception arrived at without conscious reasoning.
b) the ability to perceive in this way.

—Heinemann *Australian Dictionary* 1976

intuition: Immediate apprehension by the mind without reasoning; immediate apprehension by sense; immediate insight, etc.

—The *Concise Oxford Dictionary of Current English* 1964

There have been several examples in this study of the role intuition plays in the skill of chick sexing at the commercial level.

Harry Pettigrove, a first-generation Australian chick sexer "I have sexed so many chickens I could do it with my eyes closed."

Ray Parkin, a New South Wales second-generation chick sexer, still sexing in his mid-sixties "There was nothing there, but I knew it was a cockerel."

Hitoshi Miyata, a 100 per center and executive director of Zen-Nippon Chick Sexing Association, saw intuition as extremely important.

Re-read what Frank Evans, Australia's dean of chick sexing, had to say about his record performance in 1936. Do you think he really looked at the various types of pullet eminences and compared their types with a small cockerel eminence!

Others in this study have also demonstrated, by what they have said, the role intuition plays in the cloacal method of sexing day-old chicks accurately, and at great speed.

It is essential that the student should learn the various shapes and sizes of the eminences and be able to grade them into the various types.

But the difference in sizes of some pullet and cockerel eminences are relative. There is no way of judging them, except intuitively.

Intuitiveness varies considerably with different people.

If you have the ability to determine the sex of chicks from the appearance of the eminence and in some cases the lateral folds, you have good judgment. With practice an accuracy of 90–92 per cent can be reached—an accuracy many earlier commercial chick sexers never got beyond.

To advance beyond this 90–92 per cent barrier is just a matter of perseverance, practice and a certain belief. Relax, and like my English-comprehension students, act on that first decision: throw, pick up the next chick. Never hesitate. If you believe in yourself it will come.

Attitude to success

As I interviewed and listened to the most successful of the "old-time chick sexers" what became apparent was that they all seemed to share six things in common.

1) They all thought it was easy. It's either a cockerel or a pullet.

2) They found personal satisfaction in being accurate at all times.
3) They acknowledged that some breeds and strains of chickens were difficult to sex.
4) They believed that without doubt 100 per cent accuracy is obtainable commercially.
5) They loved what they were doing.

And

6) They believed in themselves.

Cloacas of adult fowl
Top: male/cockerel
Bottom: female/pullet

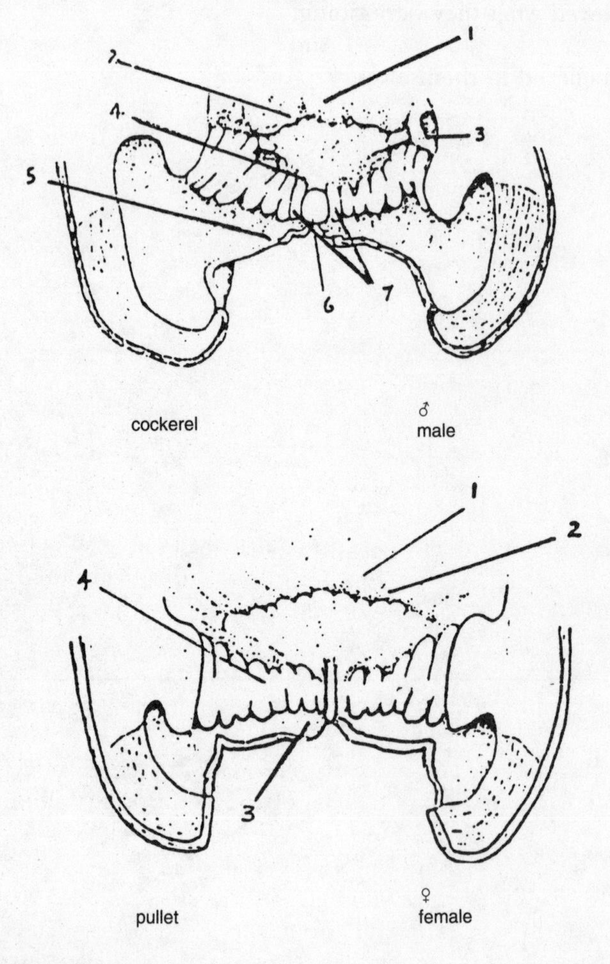

1) cloaca of the deferent duct
2) first set of folds
3) papillary process
4) second set of folds
5) third set of folds
6) organ of copulation
7) two round folds

From early instruction manual supplied by some of the early Japanese teachers in Australia.

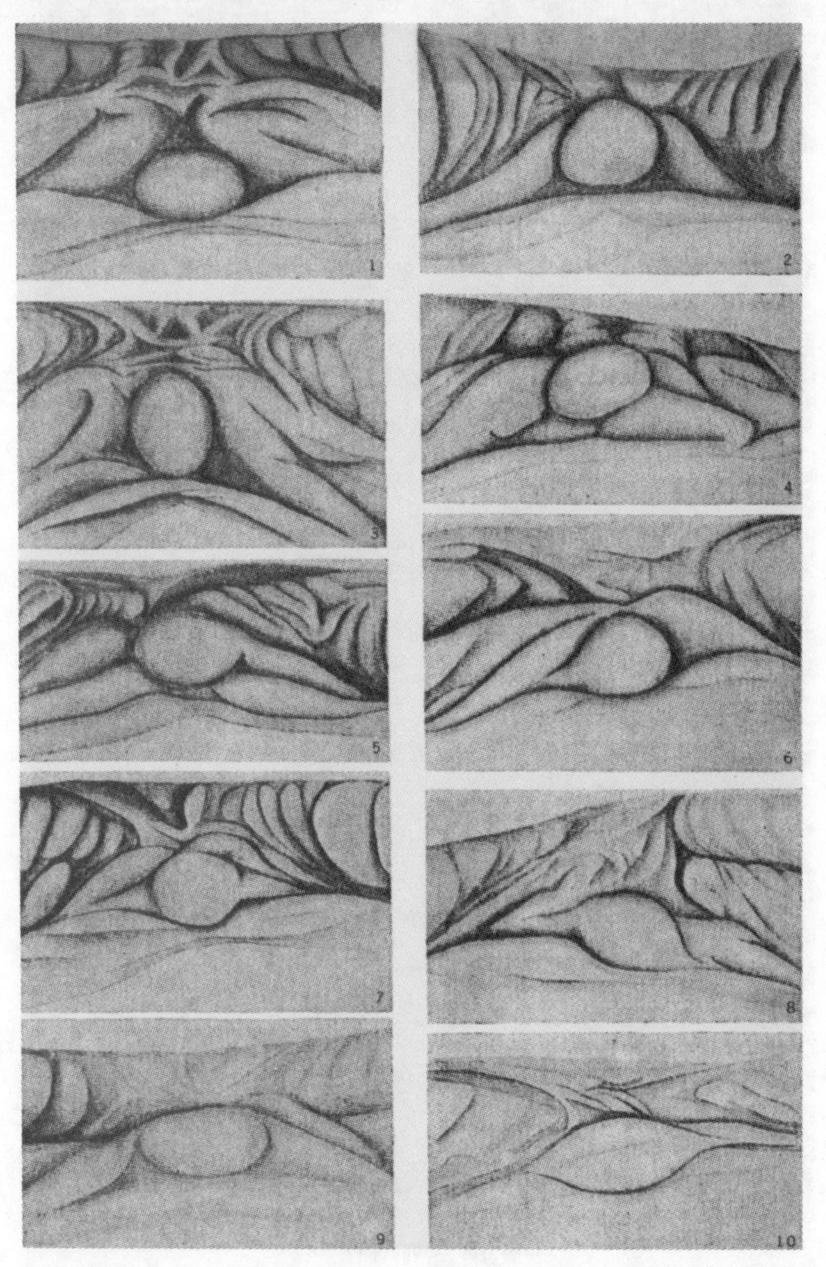

Male type A processes.

1–3. Typical processes are more than 0.6 mm long. 4. Folds are protruded markedly around the process, which is not so well projected. 5, 6. One side of the process is partly extended to form a fold. 7. Both sides of the process are extended to form folds, and the middle portion is spherical. 8. Both sides of the process are extended to form a fusiform structure. 9. The process is obscure, showing a low protrusion. 10. The process is a fusiform structure with a transverse groove, which divides the process into two protrusions.

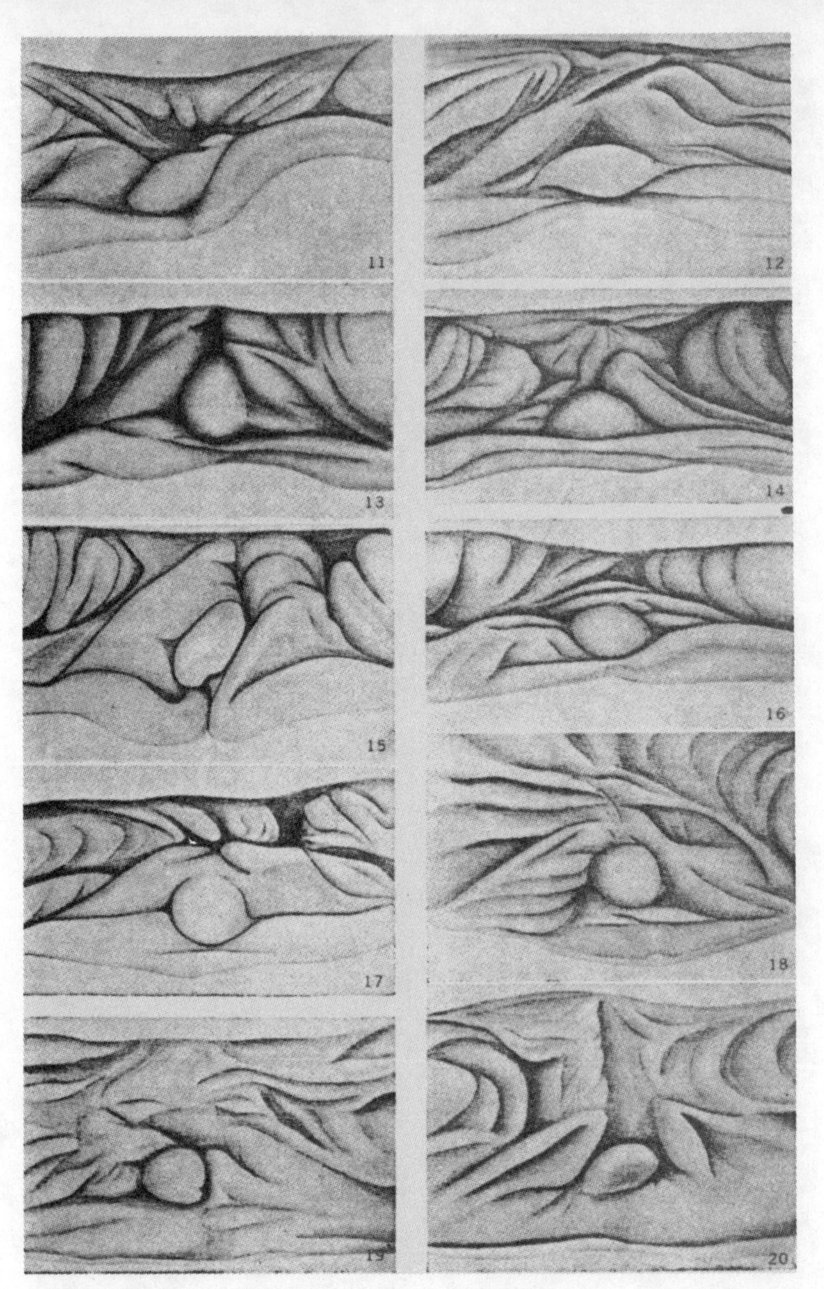

Small type A male processes.

11, 12. The process if fusiform. 13, 14. The tip of the process is directed toward the deep portion of the organ. Folds are well developed on both sides of the process. 15. Folds are particularly well developed on both sides of the process, which shows a low protrusion. 16. The process is a typical small male process. 17. Folds are particularly well developed on both sides of the process and join with each other anterior to it. 18. The process is spherical and a little smaller. 19, 20. The process is the smallest of the male type A processes.

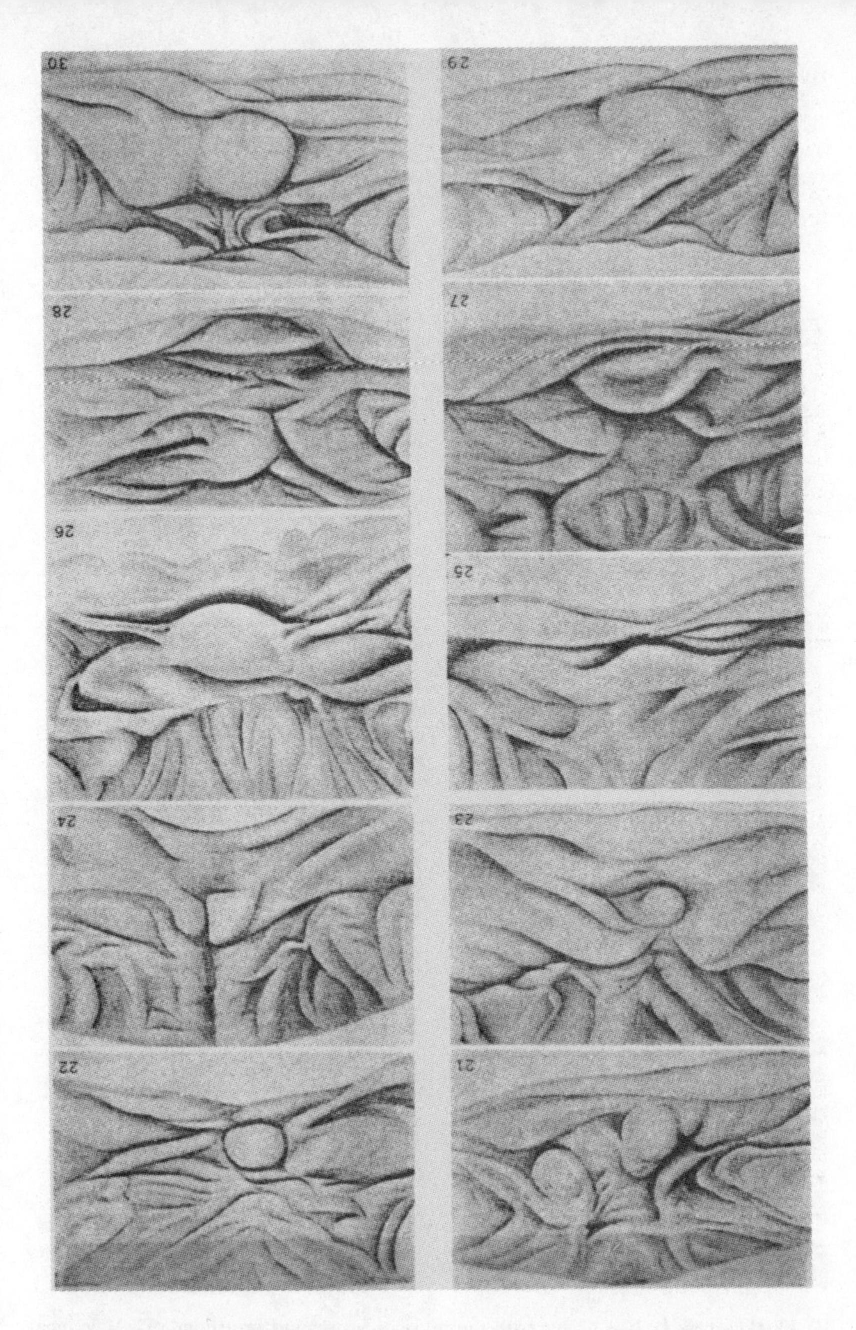

21, 22. The process is a large, male type B process. 23. The process is a small, male type B process, showing a low protrusion. 24. Male type B and irregular in shape, showing a low protrusion. 25, 26. Male type C and linguiform, protruding backward. 27. Male type C. Its tip is directed forward. 28. Male type C. It stands straight with a thin tip. 29. Male type D. It is united completely with folds which have developed on both sides of the process. 30. Male type D. The process is jointed with the right fold.

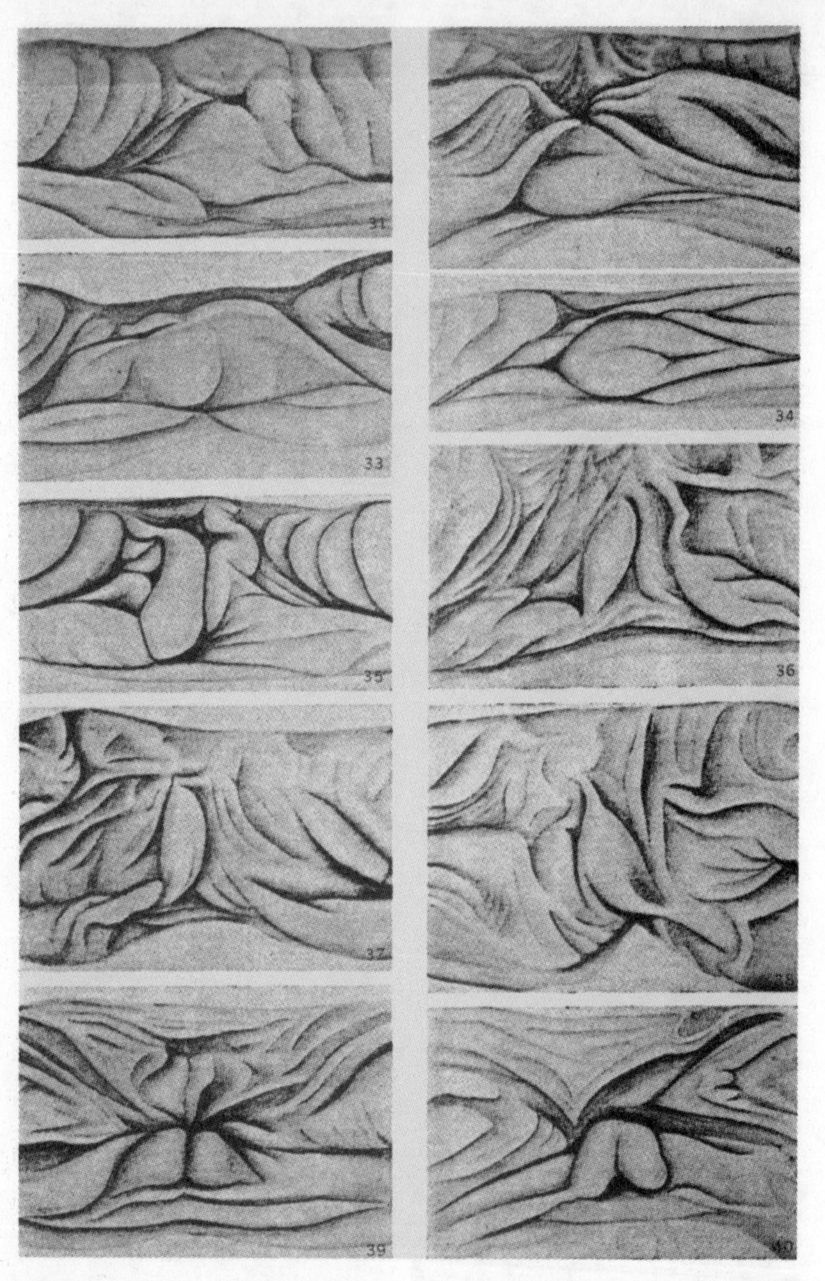

31, 32. Male type D. It is united with the folds anteriorly and protruded. 33. Male type D. It is joined with folds anteriorly. The folds may still be seen. 34. The process is joined with the right fold to form a large projected structure. 35. Male type E. Its back portion forms a spherical protrusion. 36–38. Male type E. It is fusiform and has no folds attached to either side of it. 39. Male type F. It is bilaterally divided by a groove. 40. Male type F. Its posterior is divided into two parts, but its anterior remains unseparated.

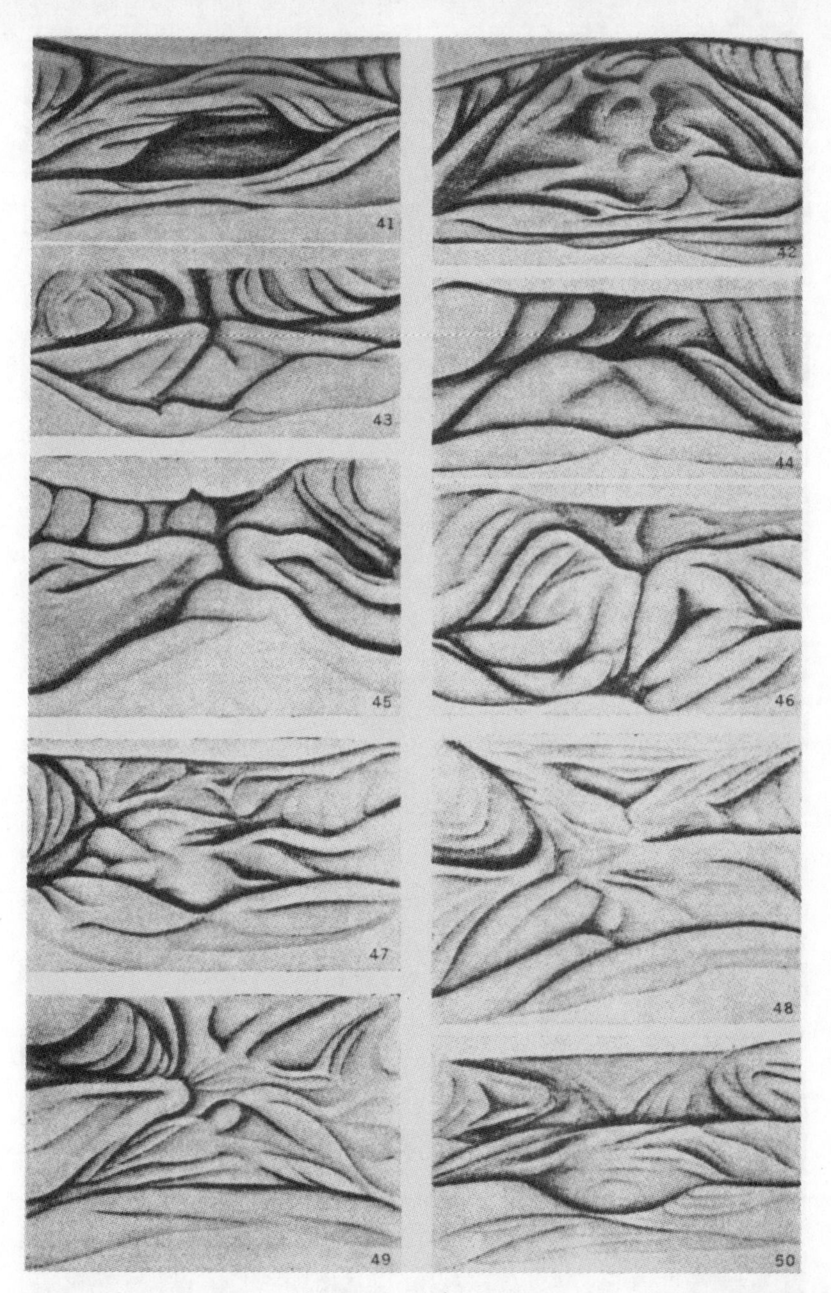

41, 42. Female type A. The process has thoroughly disappeared. No folds have developed on either side of the process site. 43, 44. Female type A. The process site forms a protuberance, and folds are developed on both sides of it. 45, 46. Female type A. The process has completely disappeared. Folds are particularly well developed on both sides of the process site. 47. Female type A. The process site forms a low protuberance. 48–50. Female type A. The process has almost completely disappeared. Only a minute rudimentary process remains.

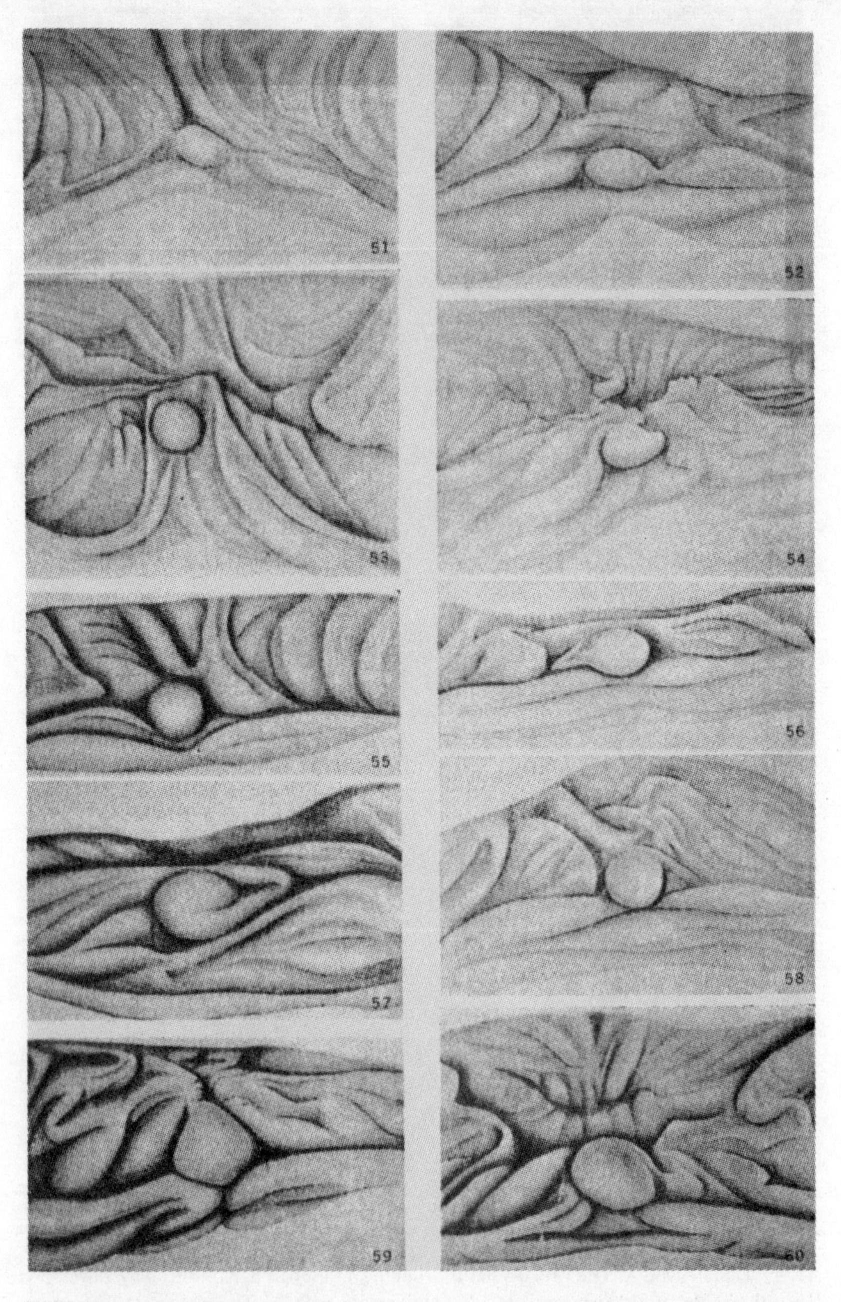

51, 52. Female type B. The process is small. 53, 54, 55, 56, 58. Female type B. The process is medium-sized. 57. Female type D. The process is joined to a fold developed on its right side and forms a large projected structure. 59, 60. Female type D. The process is well protruded, and both folds are well developed. The structure cannot be distinguished from the male type A process.

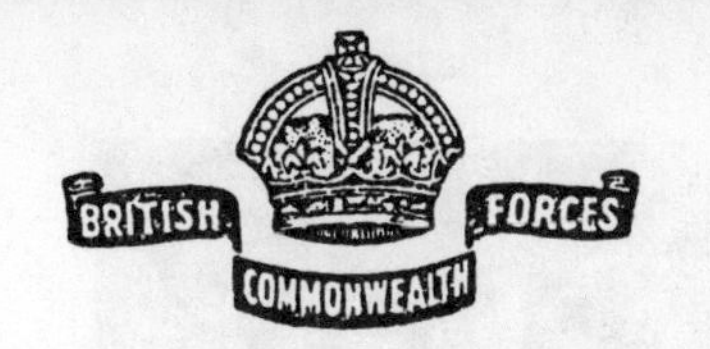

BRITISH COMMONWEALTH
OCCUPATION FORCE
JAPAN

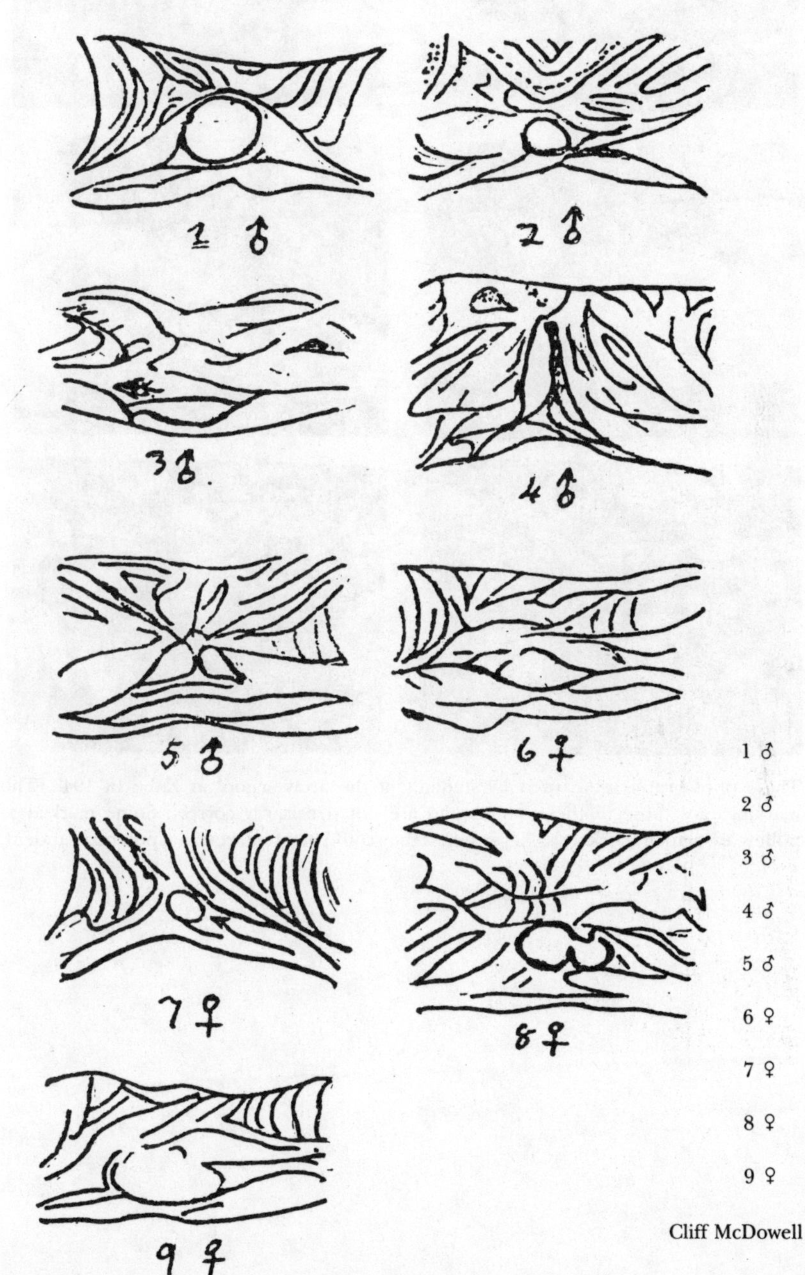

1 ♂
2 ♂
3 ♂
4 ♂
5 ♂
6 ♀
7 ♀
8 ♀
9 ♀

Cliff McDowell

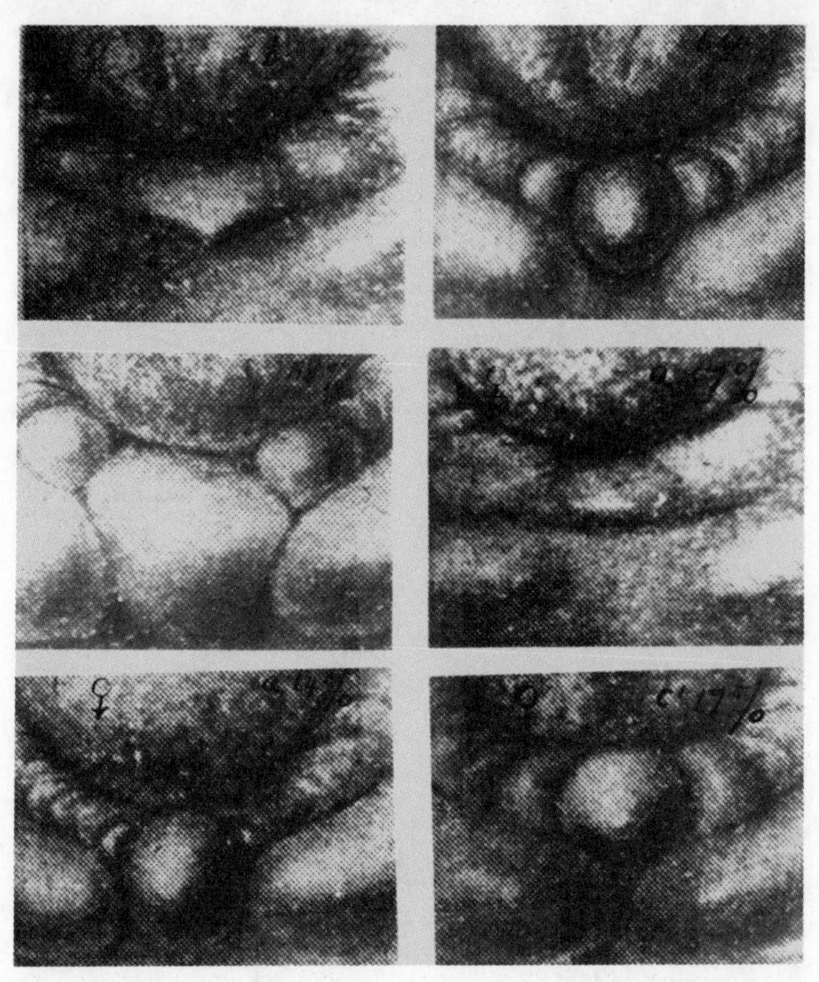

These photographs were used by students at the army school at Kobe in 1948. The markings are those of the students and are not necessarily correct. Some marked as pullets are actually cockerels. Nevertheless they could be of interest to a potential student.

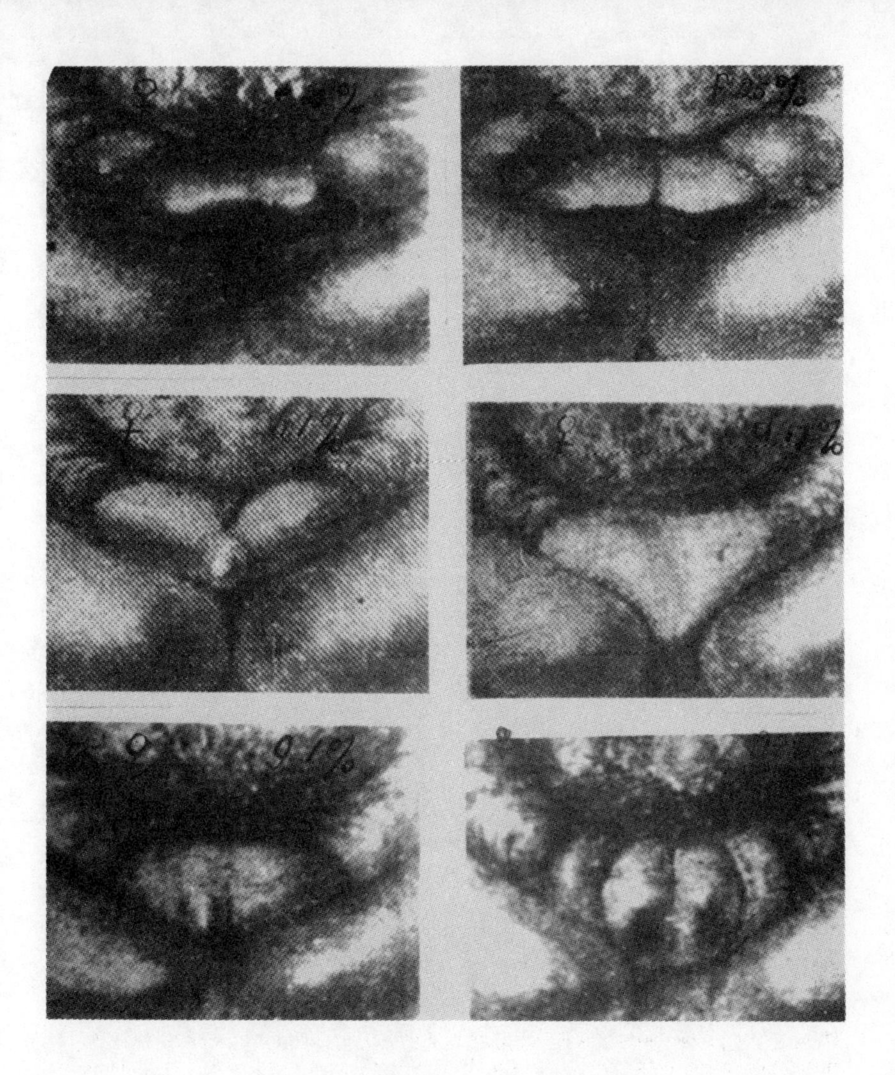

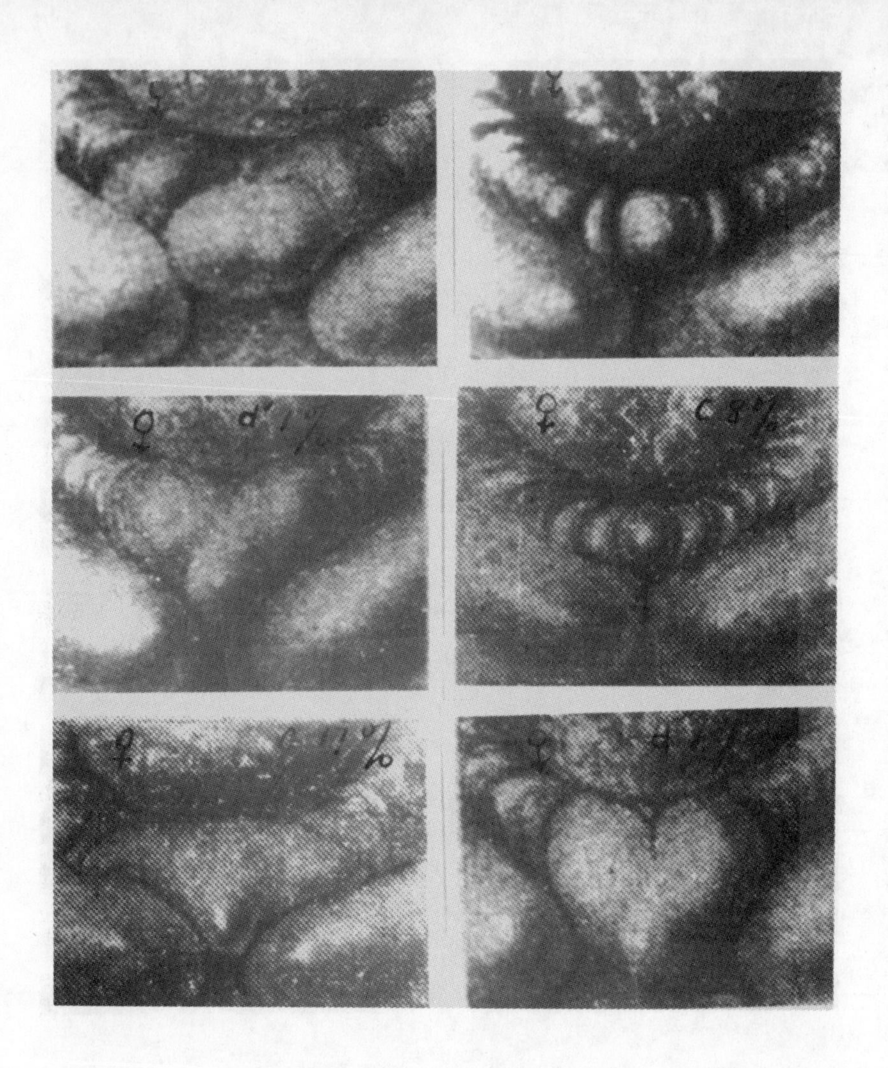

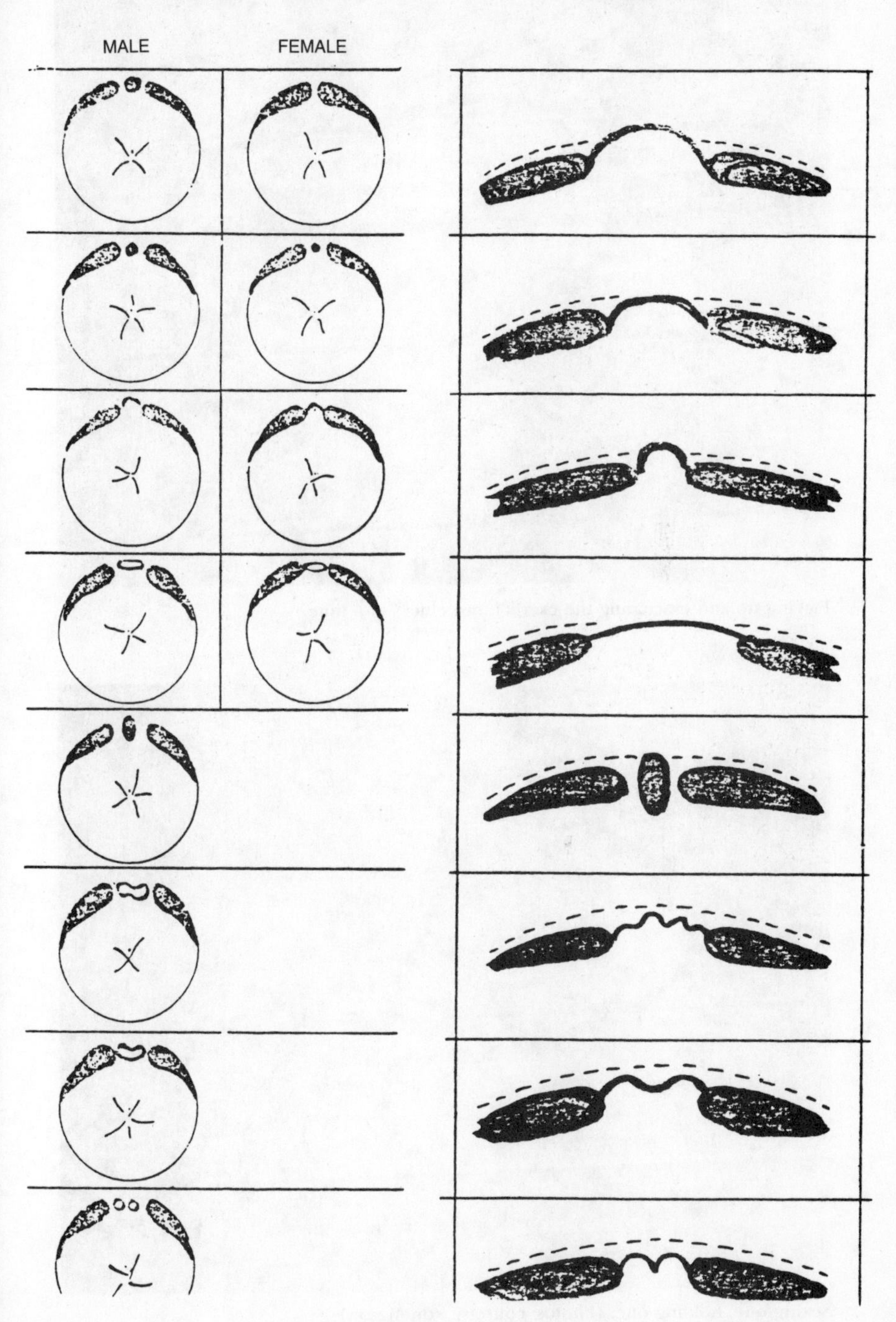

Hartley Hall

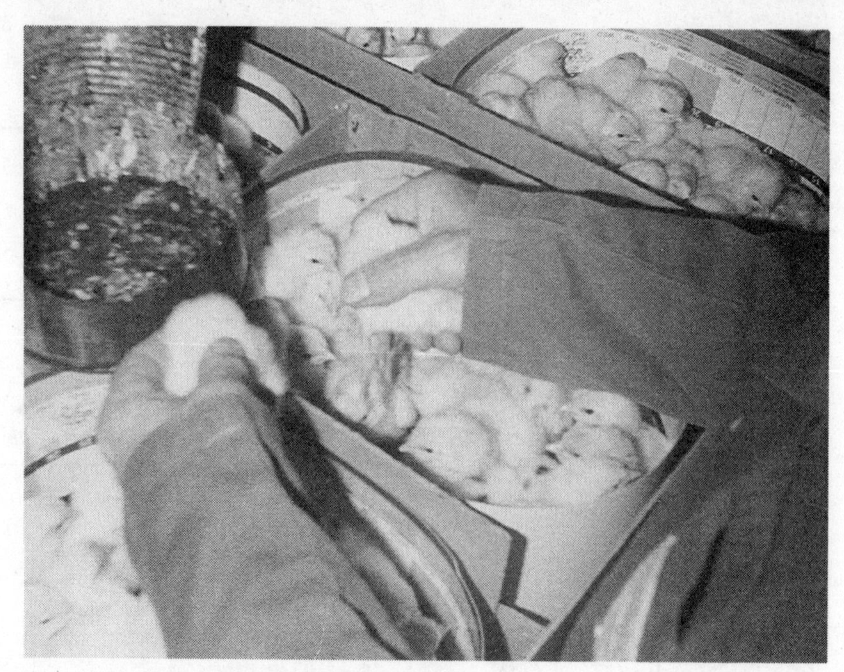

Picking up and evacuating the excreta, two chicks at a time.

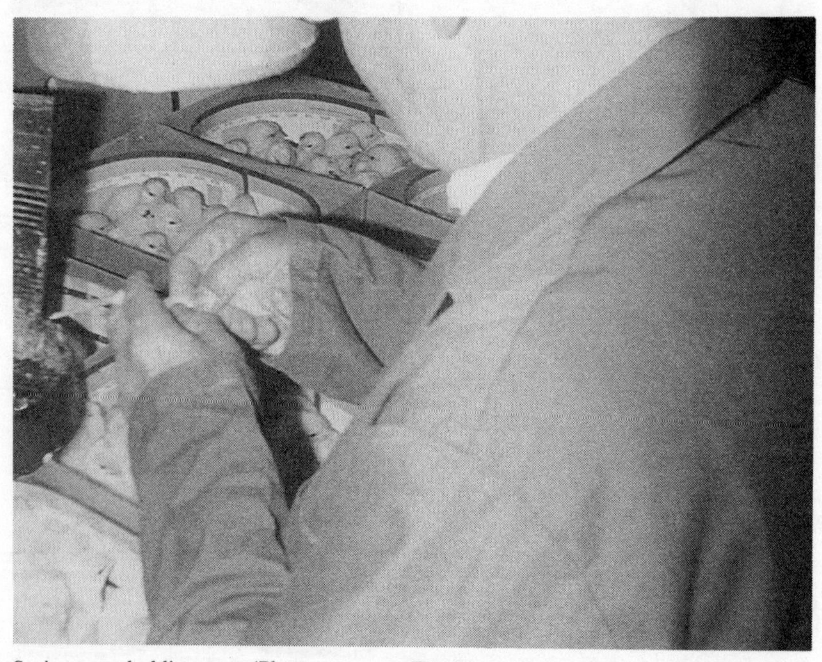

Sexing one, holding one. (Photos: courtesy Ron Mason)

Other methods of sexing day-old chicks

This study is about what I have termed the *Specialist Chick Sexer*, that is, the method of sexing day-old chicks by examination of the vent (cloaca) method. This method is also used for turkeys, guinea fowls, geese, ducklings and, with some variations, ostriches and emus. The other ways of separating the sexes of day-old chicks are:

Sex-linked crosses
The best known of these sex-linked crosses are the Rhode Island Red cockerel mate with a light Sussex hen. There are, however, many other combinations of crosses which produce different coloured day-old cockerels and day-old pullets, and are easily distinguished at hatching time.

Autosexing breeds
Autosexing is sex linkage applied within one pure breed. Unlike sex-linked crosses, autosexing does not require the development of two separate breeds of fowl. They were first developed in the 1930s. Since then many other autosexing breeds have been developed. The legbar was the most successful of these breeds, based mainly on the brown leghorn. Autosexing breeds never made any great impact on the world's poultry industry. Again, like the feather-sexing strains of the day, they were not competitive with other commercial laying stock.

Nevertheless, with the never-ending quest for greater efficiency in the production of commercial eggs and broilers, most of the world's brown-egg layers strains are now sexed by colour. So much so, that experiments are currently being conducted using an optical system to simplify colour sexing by using video equipment.

Feather sexing
Slow-feathering and rapid-feathering genes are used in breeding programs so that the sex of day-old chicks can easily be determined by hatchery staff after only a few hours' instruction.

Sometimes heavy breeds such as the Australian Australorp or the American Rhode Island Red, which tend to be slower feather breeds, are mated to the faster-feathering Mediterranean breeds, such as the leghorn. There are also fast-feathering strains of white leghorns bred with a slower feathering strain of white leghorn to achieve the same results.

Like auto-sexing and colour sexing, feather sexing is not new. It was known long before the development of vent sexing. But as these breeds were never competitive with other commercial laying breeds, most of the world's egg producers still reared unsexed chicks, with its greater costs, until the Japanese introduced vent sexing.

With the concentration of the breeding and hatchery industry throughout the world into the control of a few large breeding companies, who employ geneticists and technology, feather and colour sexing are now standard practices in most of the world's hatcheries.

While there has been a hint of some dissatisfaction with some of these laying strains when compared with breeds which have to be vent sexed, it is unlikely that there will be any rapid change to vent-sexed breeds, particularly in the broiler industry, except for primary breeders.

It is interesting to note that many specialist chick sexers can actually sex faster than the less skilled feather sorter sexers.

Feather sexing is used mainly for layers, broilers and some broiler parent stock.

Optical "machine" sexing

This method is usually referred to as the "machine" method, a misnomer as it is not a machine in any sense. It is an optical instrument with an illuminated glass tip which is inserted into the chick's bowel, enabling the operator to view the testicle of the cockerel or the ovary of the pullet.

A simple, direct decision; easier to learn than the vent method, resulting in chick-sexing changing from a highly skilled art to a semi-skilled occupation with big savings in sexing costs to the hatcheryman. At least, this was how the method was seen for the first decade of its use.

The reality was far different. While it is easier and therefore cheaper to learn, and requiring far fewer chicks for practice before entering the commercial chick-sexing market, it still depended on the skill of the operator.

This skill was not so much identification, judgment and intuition, but developing the knack of joining the chick and the instrument together gently and quickly. Concentration, reliability and the ability to work hour after hour after hour, day after day after day, was still needed. This is an ability not everyone has.

The arrival of the "machine age" into the chick-sexing business did solve the shortage of chick sexers in many countries. According to the

Japanese, this was the only reason it was introduced. Its introduction also resulted in a reduction in chick-sexing costs in some countries. The "machine" also discouraged many potential chick sexers from seeing chick sexing as a worthwhile occupation.

The original instrument, the "Kizawa Chicktester", was developed and introduced to the rest of the world by the Japanese in the 1950s. There have been several English versions of this first "machine", and one from New Zealand. Probably the best known after the Japanese Chicktester was the English version, the "Chixexer", put out by the Keeler Instrument Company of England.

Some observers believe the introduction of the machine made auto-sexing breeds less relevant, because of the reduction in chick-sexing costs, but I have found no evidence to support this view.

Most people in the industry are familiar with the arguments against the use of the "machine" method of sexing: it punctures the bowels of 5 per cent of the chicks; it is too slow and is not as accurate as the vent method; that the light from the machine affects the gonads (sex glands), causing a change in the DNA pattern which upsets the geneticist's breeding goals; that it is a cause of some respiratory complaints; and disease transmission is a greater problem with this method.

Most of these arguments are no longer relevant, as the cloaca method is now the method used almost universally by the industry when a specialist chick sexer is needed.

In Europe it was used from 1953 to about 1958. Denmark and Russia are the only countries who still use this method there. In New Zealand there is at least one hatchery which still uses this method.

Most of the chick sexers who are skilled in both methods tended to favour the vent method. The "machine" method is no longer used by specialist chick sexers entering the industry. Chick-sexing machines are no longer manufactured anywhere. The Tohzai Sangyo Boeki Co Ltd of Tokyo still have some instruments in stock. The five Australian chick sexers who use this method have their glass tips blown by an Australian glass blower.

I do not wish to enter further into the pros and cons of this method of sexing, except to observe that several Australian and New Zealand chick sexers have used this method for nearly forty years and have sexed millions of chicks with great speed and accuracy. I have no doubt that they will be successful chick sexers until they decide to retire.

Other applications for the "machine" method

Most poultry fanciers who hatch their own chicks would have little difficulty in teaching themselves how to use this instrument for small batches of chicks.

Below are a few hints which will help any poultry fanciers wanting to use the instrument to sex their own chicks. To sex large numbers of chicks commercially requires a different application, and it is unlikely that anyone would be able to teach themselves the special techniques which have been developed by others over 40 years.

Sex determination or control in the embryo stage

Just as my grandmother and others believed that the shape of the egg or holding a ring on a hair over an egg would determine the sex of the future chick, most agriculture departments have had devices for determining the sex of eggs or chicks submitted to them over the years. Some of these devices for determining the sex of future chickens in the egg that caused much excitement in the poultry world of Victoria (Australia) in the mid 1920s were known under various names such as: Sex Detector, Sex Indicator, Egg Indicator, Genderometer and so on. It was claimed that thousands of these instruments had been sold throughout the world.[1]

Many authorities have carried out tests on these "detectors" during the pre-chick sexing days—needless to say the results were not in accordance with the claims made for them.

As a 19-year-old chick sexer I can remember reading in a poultry magazine the heading "New Method of Controlling Sex of Baby Chicks in USA". It went on, "It controls chick sex with an application of hormone solution to the fertile egg . . . as cited in the patent show that 98 to 100 per cent of the eggs treated can be hatched in the desired sex."[2]

In 1994 I read a small piece in *Poultry International* about a project under way at Jerusalem College of Technology under the supervision of Professor Natan Avivi, where the sex of chicks can be identified when they are three hours old. Quote: "With state-of-the-art technology, it is possible to produce digitised video images of the chicks.

"Algorithms are then made on the picture, which differentiate between males and females. The project has achieved an accuracy of 85 per cent after seven months of development. The project goal is to cut costs of sexing in half.[3]

Nothing is new, nothing ever changes!

1 *Journal of Agriculture*, Victoria, from an article by H. F. Clinton, poultry expert, 1 March 1946.
2 *Poultry* NSW (from a US corrrespondent) July 1949.
3 *Poultry International*, 'Three-Hour Embryo Sexing' p 49. February 1994.

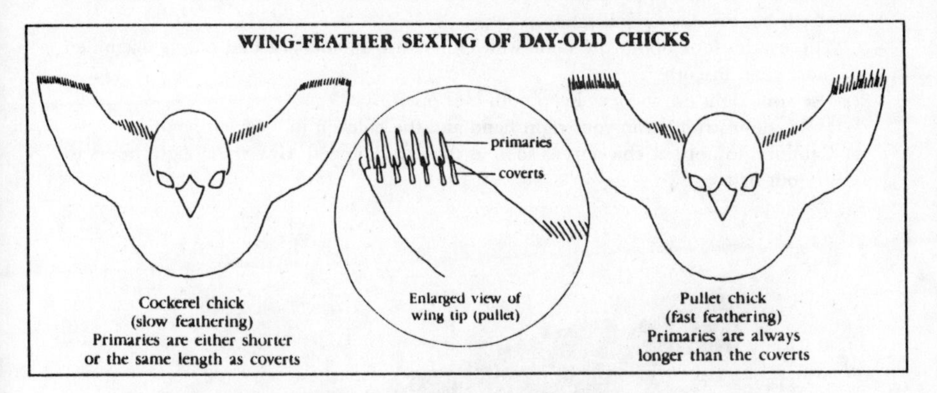

Sexing day-old chicks by differences in the formation of wing feathers.

Above: The method of feather sexing by crossing a fast-feathering with a slow-feathering parent stock, producing offspring that can be sexed by the feathers as shown above. Occasionally this system breaks down.
Below: One example of autosexing: the pullet is one colour; the cockerel another. A simple straight-forward operation, which no doubt will soon be able to be done without human contact at all.

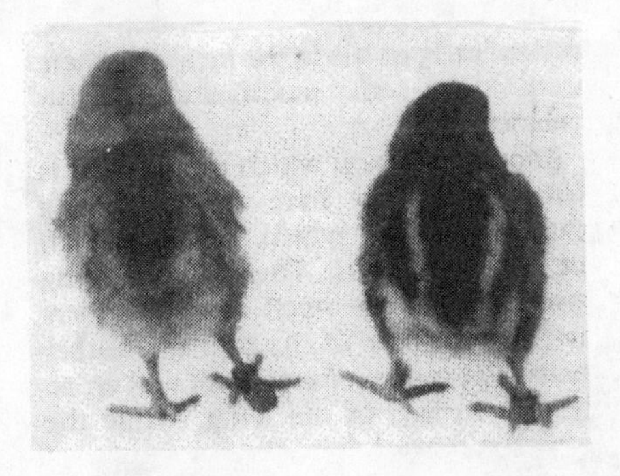

Legbars are an autosexing breed. The male chick is on the left and the female on the right. Ministry of Agriculture, Fisheries and Food, U.K.

Illustrations and photo courtesy of *Australasian Poultry* Vol 2 No 5 Dec 1991–Jan 1992. Vol 2 No 6 Feb–March 1992

"KEELER CHIXEXER"

Instructions: For sexing day-old chicks by either this "machine" or the Japanese "Chicktester machine".

1) to sex a few hobby chicks, it is fairly straight forward. The testicle shows up like a grain of rice on the Japanese machine, or as illustrated on the English "Chixexer", which has greater magnification.
   The ovaries look about the same with either instrument, just that one is magnified more than the other.
2) Use your right eye to view. Keep both eyes open.
3) Hold the instrument in your right hand and the chicken in your left hand.
4) Caution: do not sex chickens as soon as they are hatched. Give them eight hours to dry out first.

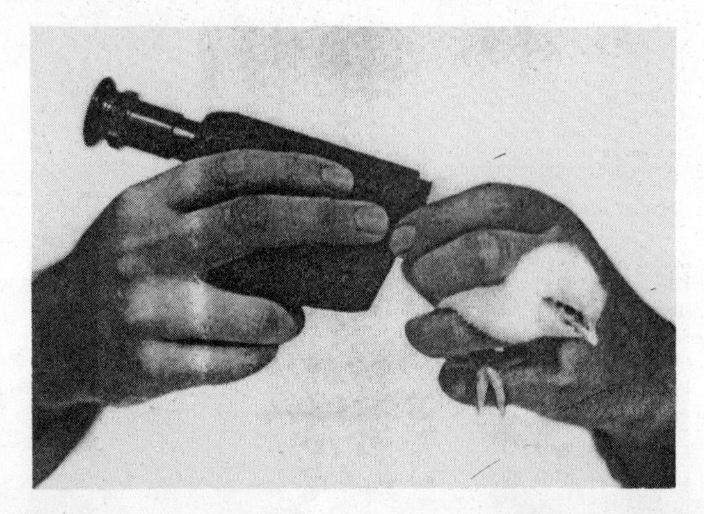

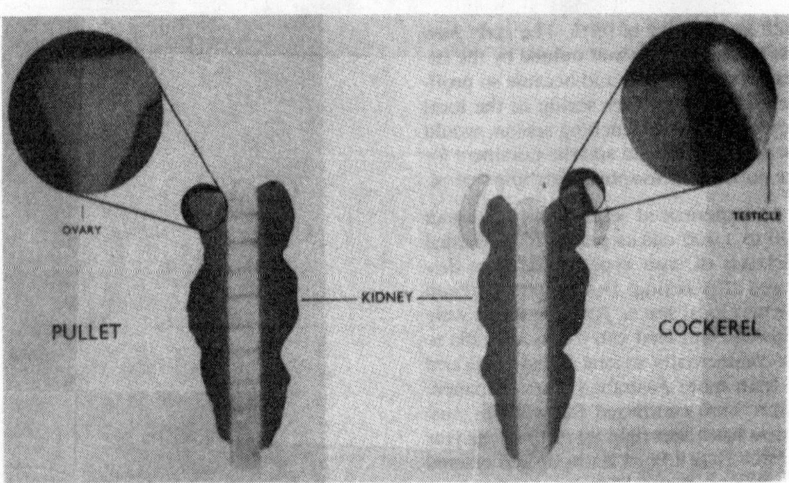

The position of the sex organs relative to the backbone and kidneys. The inserts show the field of vision and represent the magnified image of parts, of an ovary and a testicle.

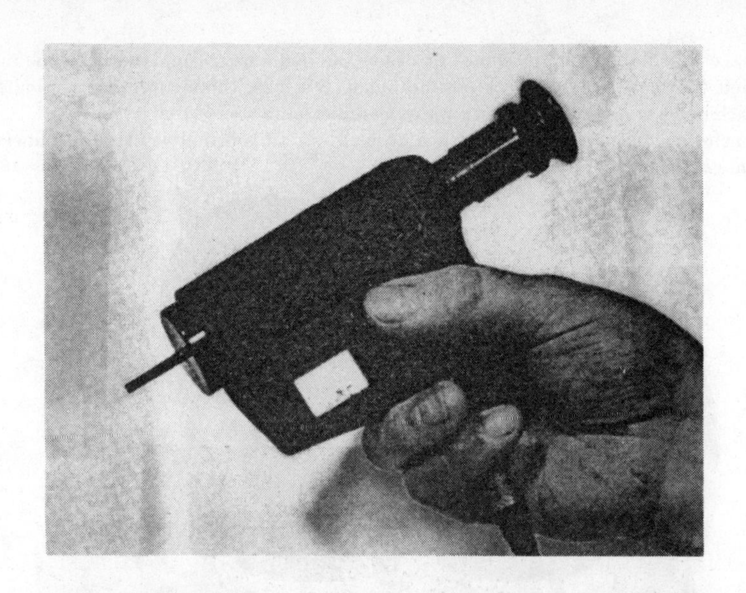

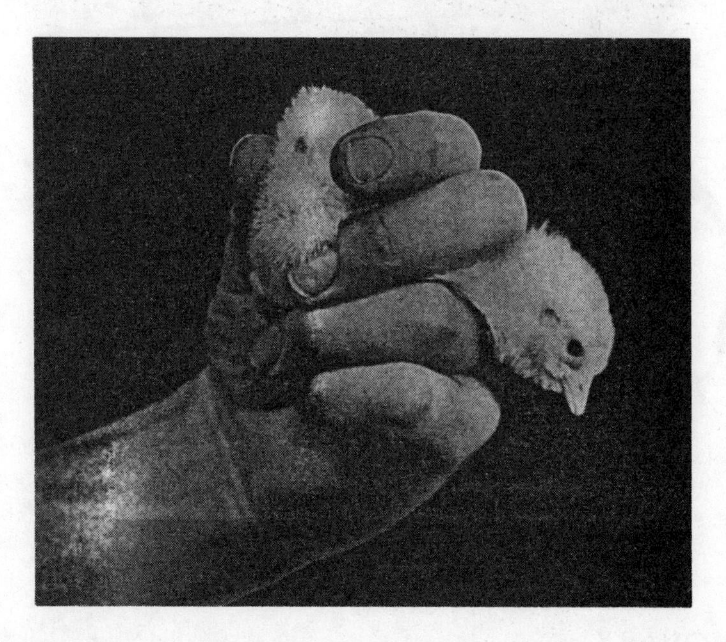

5) On the right is the testicle—easily identified usually a white-yellow colour, sometimes with a bit of black.
6) If there is no testicle on the right, move the instrument to the left and locate the left (normal) ovary. The right ovary is diminished and unclear. The left ovary is yellowish, shaped like Tasmania; a triangular shape with the point towards the bottom of what you see. The ovary on the right is similar but much narrower and paler than the right (normal) ovary. The reason for looking at the left's if it is not recognised as a cockerel on the right.

It was claimed when the "machine" first came out that a sexer could use either the right or left (normal) ovary to recognise the pullet. But most commercial sexers using the "machine" use the left ovary for positive identification.
*Puncturing the bowel is not usually a problem . . . if you find you start to puncture them give it away.

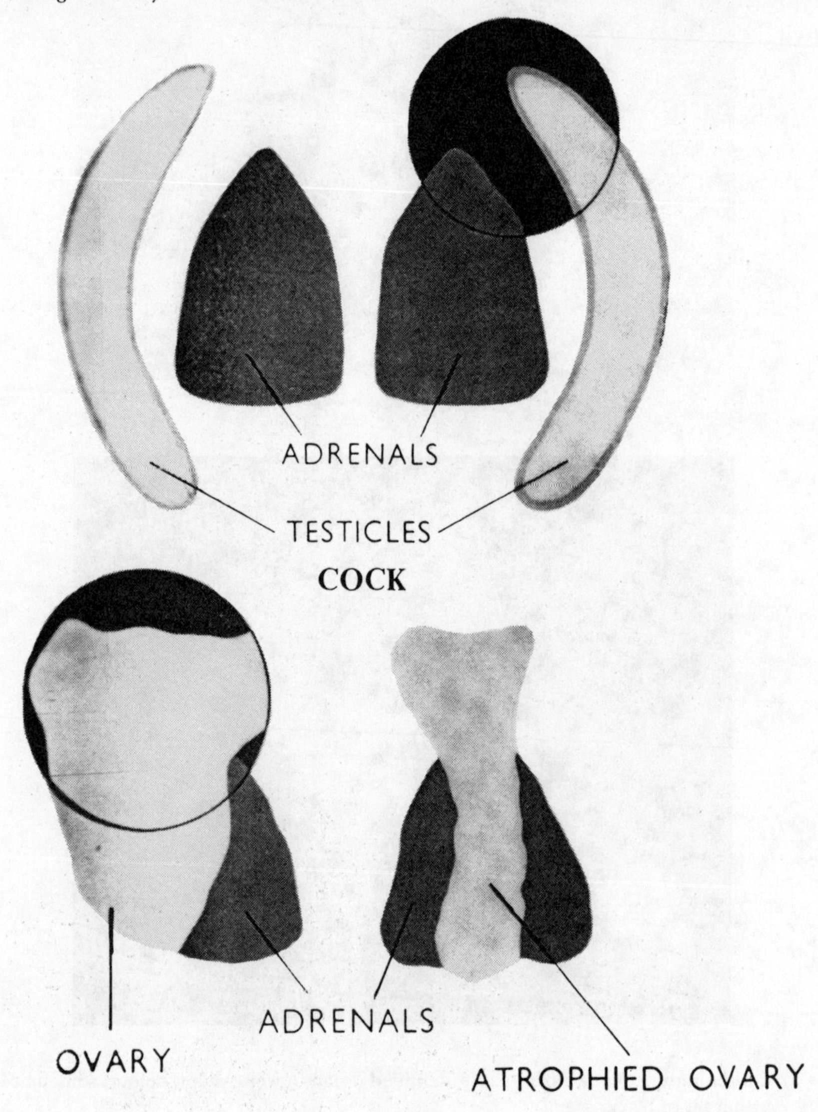

PULLET

It is not difficult to teach yourself to do small numbers of chicks. To sex large numbers it is necessary to be taught a "few extra tricks", and this method of sexing chicks commercially is no longer taught.

This instrument does not magnify as much as the English "Chixexer" instrument, but the ovaries and testicles are clearly visible. It is a matter of which "machine" is available. The results are the same.

What you see:

To determine the sex of the chick, insert the glass tip into the vent of the chick and look for the testicle on the right. If it is there then it is a cockerel.
If there is nothing visible, a slight movement of the tip to the left will reveal the ovary. (Learn to recognise the ovary. Do not mistake the adrenal glands for ovaries as both cockerels and pullets have adrenal glands.)

A simple quick recognition is all that is required. It is as simple as that.

*It is not necessary to drain the excrement from the chick before inserting the glass tip.

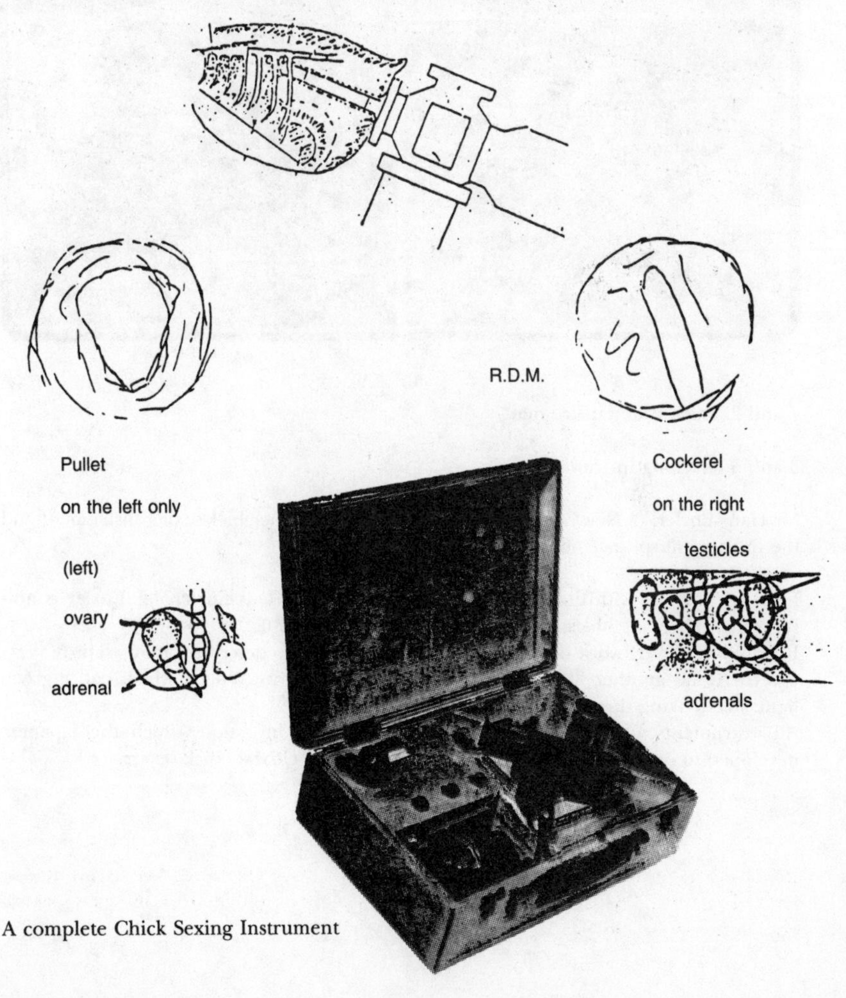

A complete Chick Sexing Instrument

ENZLER CHICK SEXING INSTRUMENT

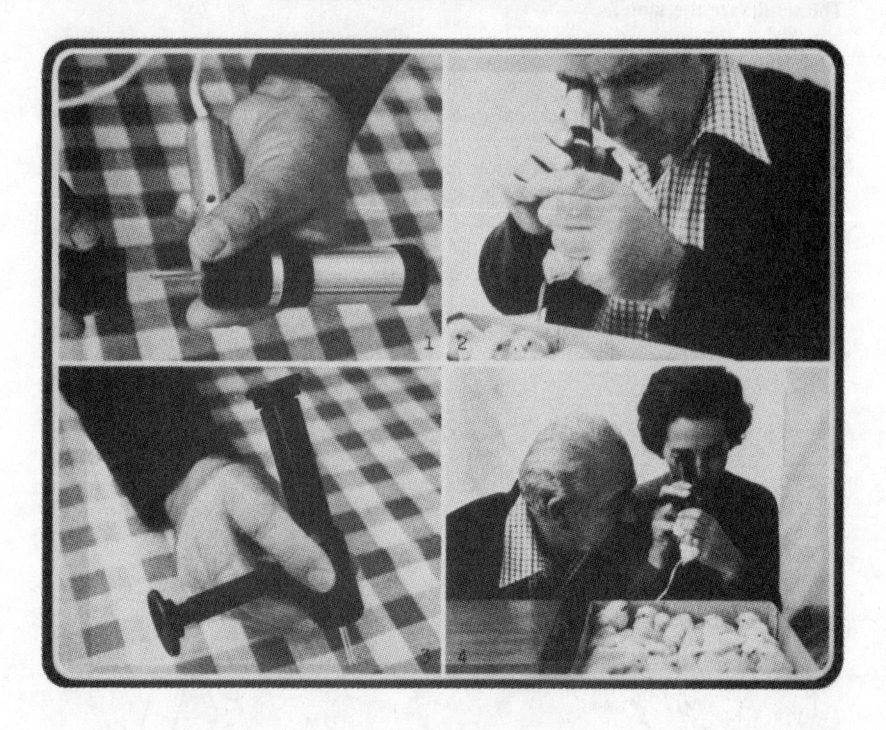

1 and 2: chick-sexing instrument

3 and 4: teaching instrument

Mr Hans Enzler, of New Zealand, demonstrating his unique chick-sexing instrument and the instrument specially made for teaching.

I am not familiar with the New Zealand "machine" of Hans Enzler. Mr Enzler is now retired and lives at: 30 Vagus Place, Royal Oak, Auckland 6.
It would, however, work on the same principle as I have described above. Thirty years ago there was another European version of this sexing instrument, which had a green light: like looking through a green fish bowl.
All instruments are versions of the original Japanese invention, which the Japanese developed to overcome a temporary world shortage of cloacal chick sexers.

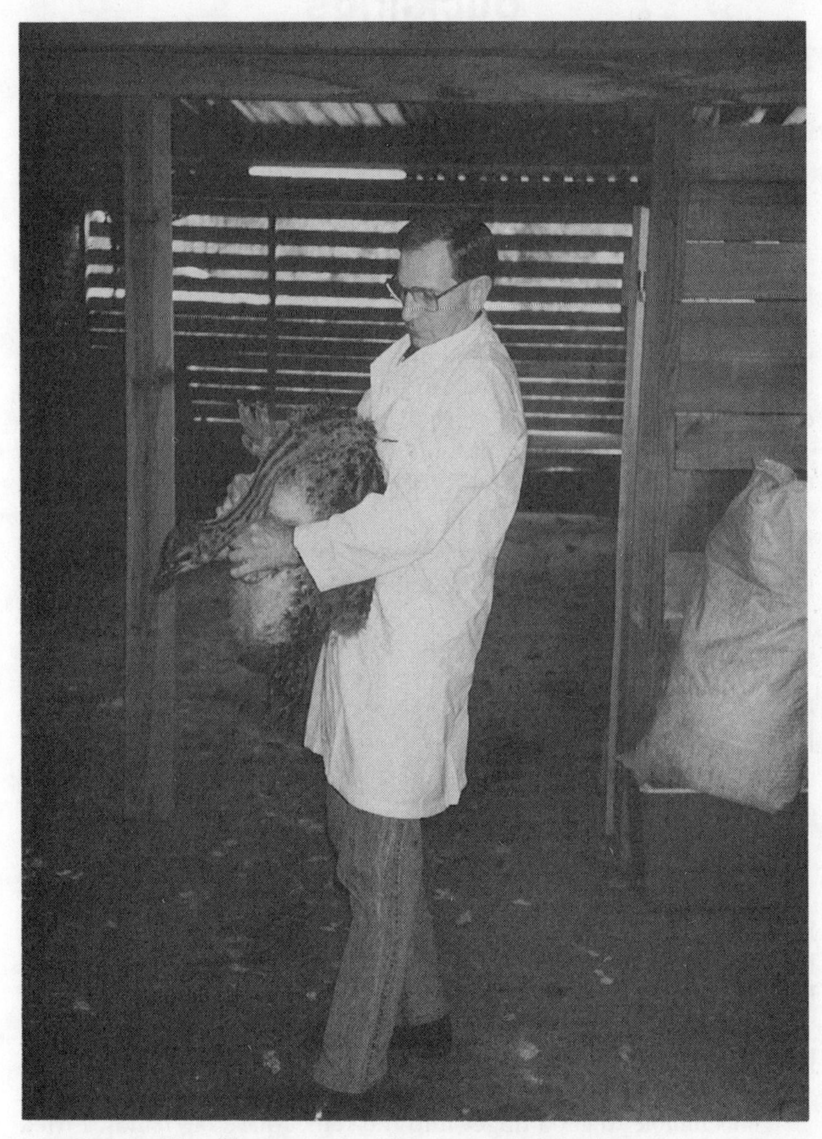

John Hammond handling a young ostrich before determining its sex.

Sexing ostriches, emus and ducklings

(With some thoughts on the cloaca sexing of parrots)

OSTRICHES

With some practice, ostriches can be sexed accurately at about six weeks of age by vent manipulation. It is not recommended on older birds because of the difficulty handling them. At older ages, the sex can be determined by the feather colour.

In a discussion with my colleague John Hammond he describes the two vent methods he has used to determine the sex of ostriches at six weeks.

BM: Can you describe how you sex ostriches?

JH: There are two ways: one is to invert the clitoris or penis . . . you insert a finger into the cloaca and flick the penis or clitoris out of the body of the ostriches . . . they are almost identical, a very subtle difference.

BM: What is the difference then? Can you tell?

JH: You can tell the difference, but it is very hard to do. The other way is to insert the finger into the cloaca, and press the genital against the *sternal* bone inside. The degree of thickness of the genital against the sternal bone inside: the degree of thickening or thickness will tell an experienced person whether you have a male or female.

BM: What age can you do each of these methods?

JH: Six weeks.

BM: It is claimed in a book[1] I was reading that you can sex emus the same way.

JH: I don't know. All I am saying is it said on the emu tape[2] to wait until they are 16 months of age. I tried emus at six weeks but I was unable to get a finger into the vent. I have big hands. I tried them again at six months but I was just unable to tell, but I am not practised. Given a bit of time, I may have had more success.

---

1 *Sexing all Fowl—Baby Chicks, Game Birds, caged Birds* by Loyl Stromberg. 1977.

2 *21st Century Video Productions* Script: David Marshall. Emu Tech Pty. Ltd.

EMUS

In America some emu breeders use *laparotomy*, or testing of DNA samples to determine the sex of young emus. This method requires the services of veterinary surgeons, but is 100 per cent accurate. Because some emus in America are valued at thousands of dollars this sexing via surgery can be justified.

For emu farmers in Australia this expense is not justified or necessary, as most specialist chick sexers, with a little initiation, could determine the sex of an emu during the first six days, by examining the cloaca. The manipulation of the vent is the same as that used for sexing day-old chicks.

After the first week, it is not possible to tell the sex of an emu by examining the vent because of the growth in the cloaca area, making it impossible to open the vent far enough to see the genital eminence. It is not until the emu is over 12 months of age that the sex can again be identified by examining the cloaca by the method described by John Hammond above, and repeated, with illustrations, below.

Sexing emus is a much slower process for the chick sexer and the numbers are small as most commercial chick sexers would not find the task worthwhile.

Chick sexing is not a skill which can be self-taught from a book, nor is sexing newly hatched emus.

The first Japanese experts in the 1920s did actually teach themselves to open the vent (by trial and error) after they knew the theory, but they were not practising on birds that were valued at $260 at day old.

It is possible that some emu farmers could learn to sex their own birds within the first few days of hatching, if they were shown how to open the vent by a person skilled in this operation. Because of the day-old value of emus, a farmer would need to be shown the vent-opening procedure on day-old cockerel chicks first, before attempting to try the same procedure on newly hatched emus. The operator needs to be very skilled at opening the vent of newly hatched emus. I have set out the procedure here.

Give the newly hatched emu eight or ten hours to dry out after hatching, or they can be left for two or three days. They need to be examined before they are seven days old, because the genital eminence is further inside the cloaca after this time.

As with chick sexing, a 150–200-watt shaded light is recommended.

The main purpose in opening the vent (cloaca) is not just to expose the genital eminence or clitoris, but to bring it into such a position that it may be easily seen by the sexer, and to make sure the eminence is always in the same position in relation to the sexer. This is how speed is obtained.

There are several ways of opening the vent. Whichever method is used, the important thing is that the vent should be properly and quickly opened. Opening the vent is the easiest part of emu sexing to learn, and is the most important part. Everything else depends on this correct, rapid and gentle opening of the cloaca. Once thoroughly mastered, it can be done automatically without giving it any thought at all. Here I describe one method of opening the vent. The other method is equally effective. What you see is the same except the eminence is at the bottom of the opening rather than the top, as described here.

Holding the emu chick—see illustrations

1) Method one. Get someone to place the chick on its back and hold it for you, with the vent towards you and its head away from you.
2) Method two. Lay the emu chick on its back on a table or preferably a raised support stand.

Place the emu's right leg between your left ring finger and little finger.

The left leg of the chick is placed between your right ring finger and little finger. Sometimes this is not necessary and the right hand can be left free to open the vent without restriction of movement. People with smaller hands could hold the chick only by the right leg.

Opening of the vent

The main purpose of opening the vent is to expose the eminence so that it can be easily seen.

To do this, it is necessary to press both sides of the vent furthest away from you with your thumbs and at the same time pull the fold back towards the chick's legs. At the same time use your right forefinger to get under the ridge of the vent and under the genital eminence and press upwards, so exposing the genital eminence, or in the case of some female emu chicks, nothing between the folds.

It is this opening of the cloaca which is important. It must be opened quickly and gently.

What you see

In the male emu chick there will be a small (usually round) genital eminence. It can vary in shape and size, and is usually light or clear in colour.

The female emu chick's clitoris is generally much smaller and has a more reddish colour and sometimes has a small tip on it. Some females will have virtually no visible clitoris at all.

The female sex organ, unlike that of the male, does not grow or change much from birth to maturity.

A lot more caution is necessary when sexing very young chicks.

Unless the birds are being sold and it is necessary to sex them it would be better to wait until they are older.

PARROTS

(Some thoughts on the cloaca/vent method of sexing parrots)

It seems that with some species of parrots the only sure way to determine their sex is by surgery.

This study does not attempt to cover the various methods of determining the sex of many breeds of parrots, as most breeders would be familiar with them. The question here is, can those parrots which have to be sexed by surgery be sexed by the cloaca chick-sexing method with any degree of accuracy?

One of my former chick-sexing colleagues, Charlie Bode, attempted to vent sex parrots several years ago, but the birds bit him and he soon lost interest. However, since then, Charlie and I have discussed making a cone shaped holder which we could drop the bird into to prevent it biting while its vent is being examined.

The difficulty with parrot sexing is the value of the birds. There is no opportunity to hold postmortems on them as there is when learning to sex day-old chicks.

In Australia the hatching season was several weeks after the deadline for this manuscript and therefore we were not able to include any results of our proposed examination.

Even with my limited knowledge of parrots I see no reason why they could not be vent sexed when they reach the size of a day-old chicken.

The publishers or I would be happy to hear from anyone who has had success in this area, or has some thoughts on sexing parrots by examination of the cloaca and the eminence.

* * *

The only effective way to learn to sex quickly and accurately any bird by the cloaca/vent method, is with a lot of practice, on many birds, of different ages. Some check on the results is essential.

SEXING NEWLY HATCHED EMU CHICKS

It is sometimes difficult to differentiate between some of the male organs and the small female clitoris of these very young emu chicks. It would be better to leave these ones and re-sex them when they are older.

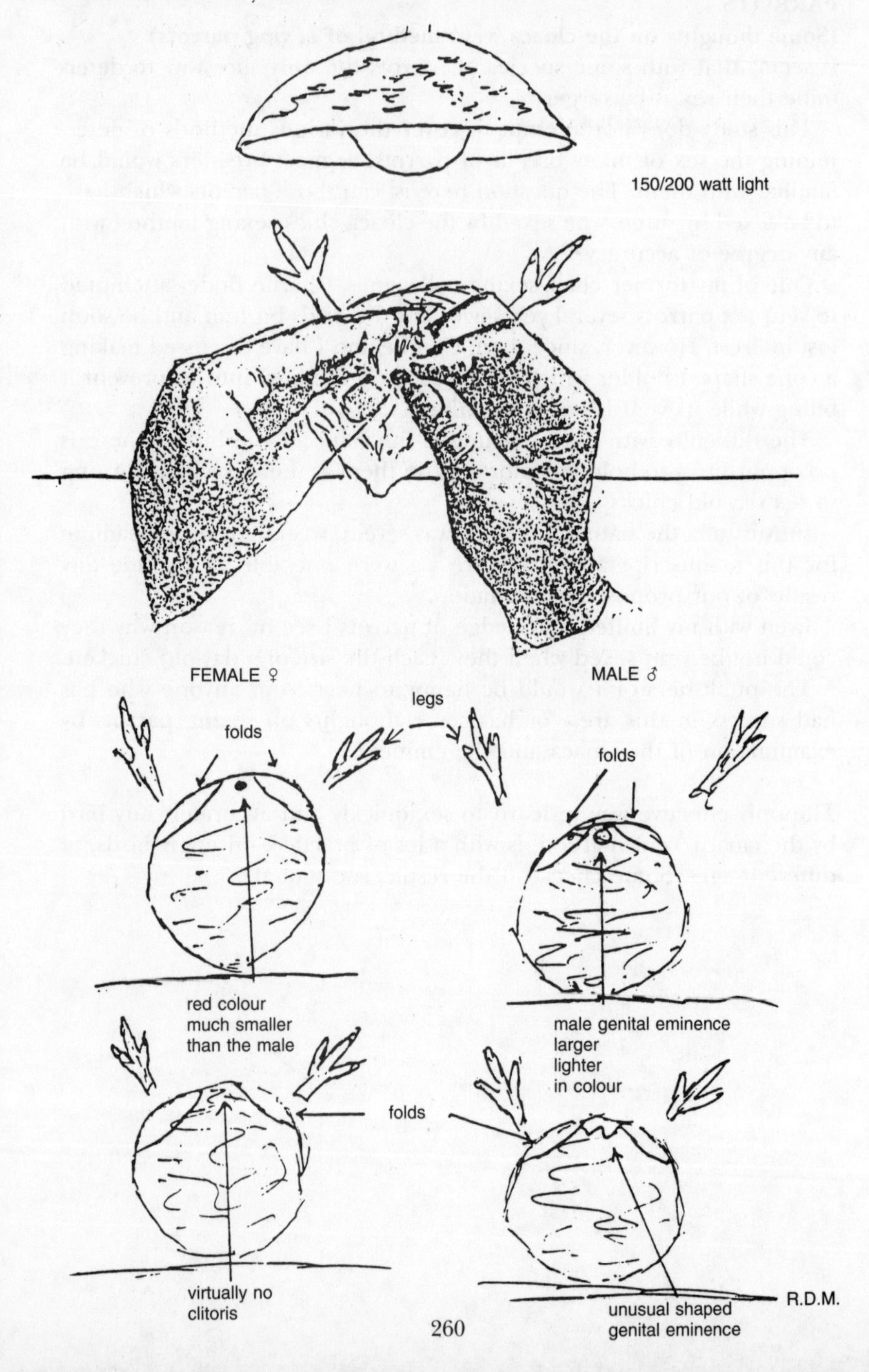

EMUS: SEXING THE ADULT BIRD

At 16 months of age an emu can be sexed as described by John Hammond. With one hand around the chest while standing behind it, leaving the other hand free to manually sex the bird. Using a latex glove, either the thumb or forefinger is placed inside the cloaca/vent while the bird is standing up. In a male emu the phallus is 35mm long and at this stage is most often erect and is easily identified. The female emu's clitoris is about half the size of a phallus and feels soft compared with the male's organ. It is exactly in the same position as the phallus is in the male bird. It can vary in size from about 20mm long to virtually nothing. It is rarely thicker than 10mm.

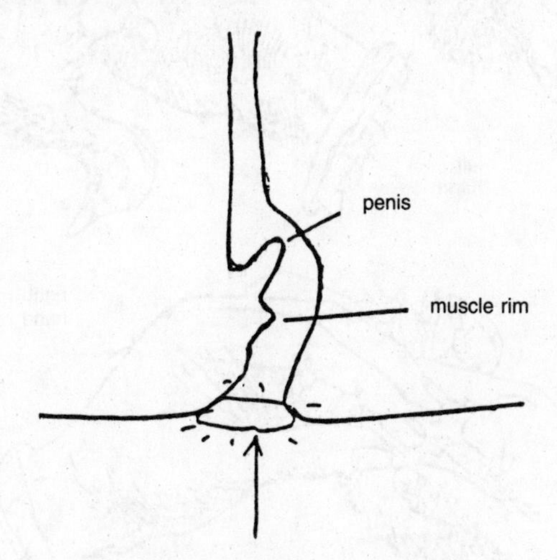

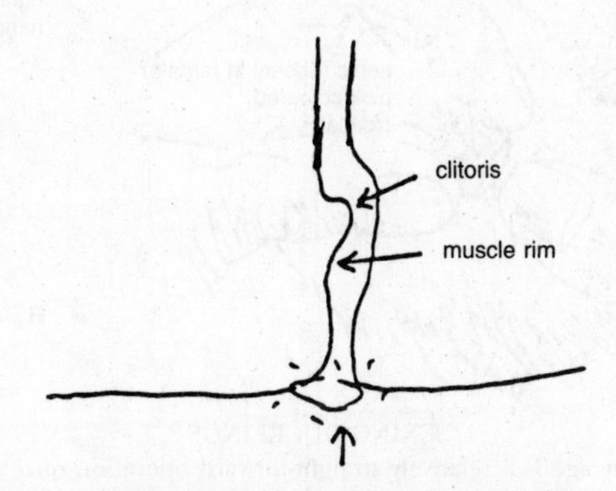

DUCKLINGS

The sexing of ducklings is a relatively simple, straightforward operation as the illustrations below show:

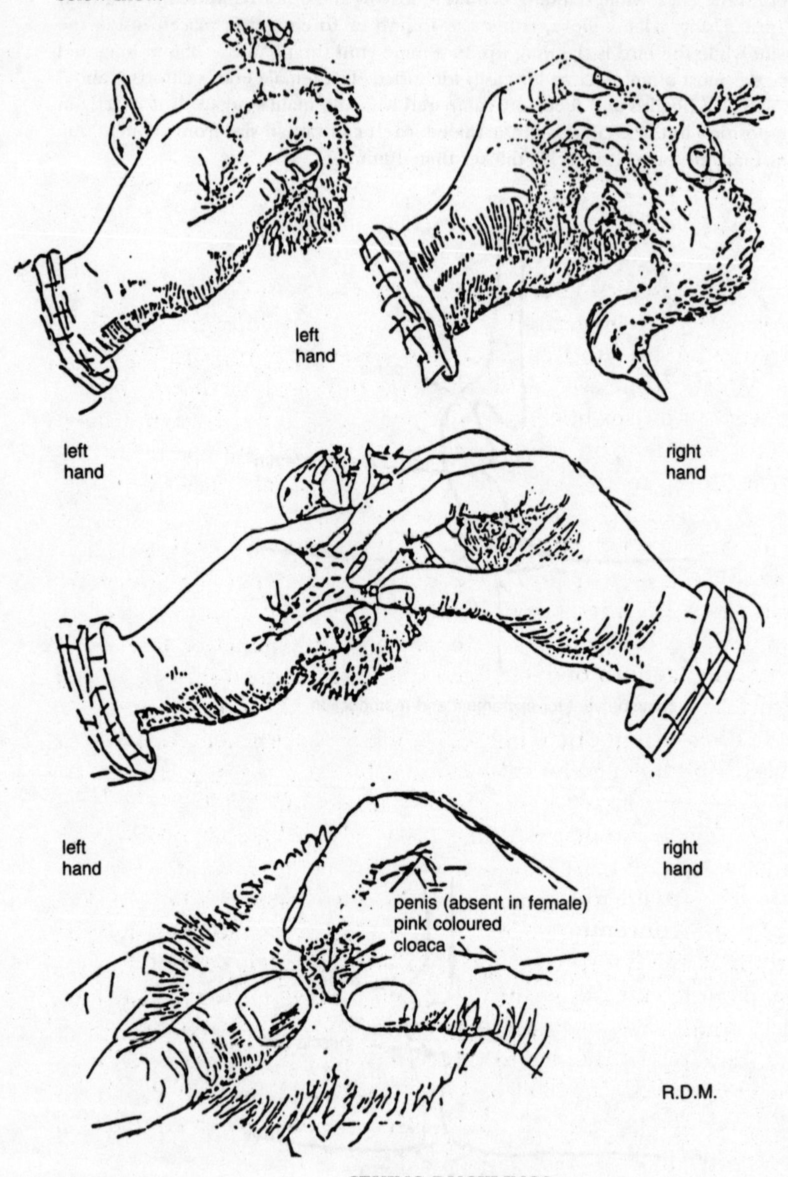

SEXING DUCKLINGS

Sexing ducks at any age is a relatively straight-forward operation once the technique of manipulating the vent, as illustrated above, is mastered. The male (drake) has a clear easily distinguished penis about the size of a pencil point, the female (duck) has nothing. It is as simple as that. No artificial lighting is needed unless large numbers are being sexed indoors.

Future prospects

Bill Stanhope, assistant editor of *Australasian Poultry* and former Principal Poultry Officer with the Victorian Agriculture Ministry, described the position in the Australian poultry industry during the last two decades, and what he sees as future world trends in the industry.

His article is on sex-linked crosses, auto sexing and feather sexing, with some comment on the effect the "machine" method of sexing had on breeding tends at the time. Below is a brief extract from the article:

"In Australia today, sexing of crossbred layer chicks by wing feather examination is now standard practice in most commercial hatcheries. Overseas, most brown-egg layer stock are sexed by colour, using the dominant silver (S) and the recessive gold (s) genes. Some international white leghorn breeders have utilised sex-linked slow and rapid feathering genes (K,k) within different lines of white leghorns to permit feather sexing of commercial white leghorn strain crosses.

"Both feather sexing and colour sexing have been applied in broiler breeding. The sex-linked gene for slow feathering has been inserted into some female broiler breeding lines. This allows day-old feather sexing and separate rearing of the sexes if necessary.

"This rapid trend to the use of sex-linked crosses has been accentuated by the concentration of the breeding and hatching industry around the Western world into the control of relatively few large breeding companies. This has justified the employment of highly qualified geneticists and other technical staff to undertake research and development work. So, by the end of this century, these geneticists will have largely superseded the skilled vent and 'machine' sexers in the never-ending quest for greater efficiency in the production of commercial eggs and broilers."[1]

This forecast on future trends in relation to chick sexing is shared by many, both in Australia and elsewhere in the poultry industry. It does reflect the present situation in most advanced poultry-industry countries of the world.

---

1 *Australasian Poultry*, Vol. 2 No. 6 Feb/March 1992 "Sexing Day Old Chicks" Part II

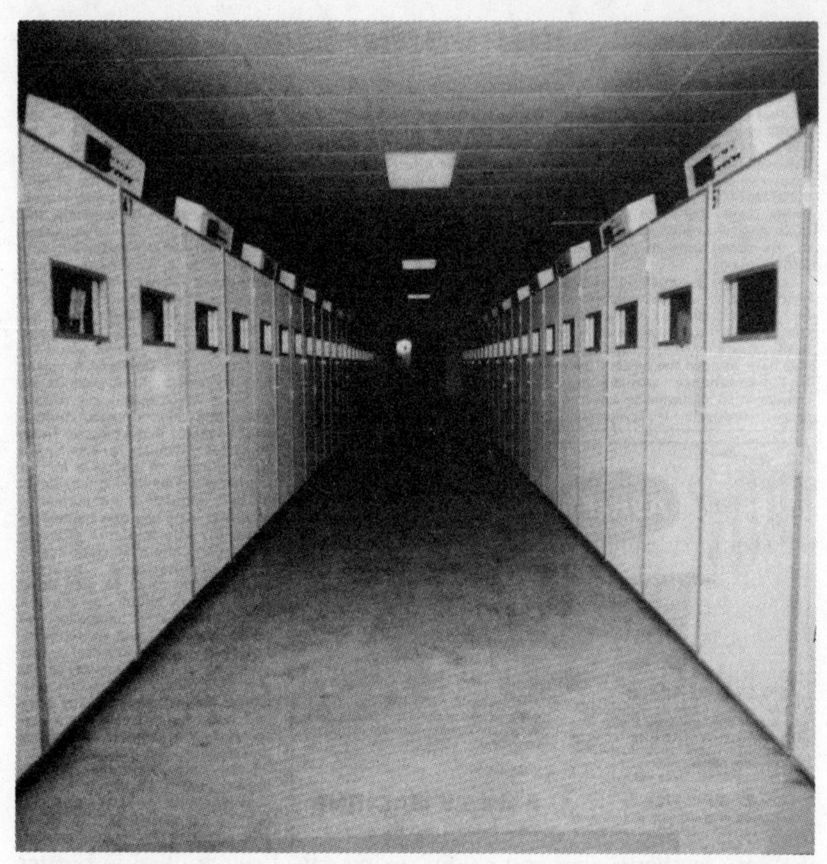

A modern sterilised incubator room with its mammoth machines which hatch chicks and turkeys by the millions throughout the world. Anyone entering a hatchery has to shower and have a complete change of clothes. A far cry from the few fluffy chicks under a hen or the early hatcheries of the 1920s through to the 1950s.

Earlier in the article, Stanhope argues that autosexing breeds did not make a great impact on the commercial poultry industry. The main reason, he says, is that they were never competitive with other commercial laying stock. Further, chick-sexing "machines" reduced the cost of sexing in the 1960s, and autosexing breeds became less relevant. This lack-of-competitiveness-in-performance argument is the same one that some Japanese poultrymen use when explaining why many chick buyers prefer layer replacement stock which has to be vent sexed.

As we have seen, worldwide, most vent sexing is for layer and broiler parent breeding stock (primary breeders) only. Also, there is considerable turkey sexing done by specialist chick sexers.

As Stanhope points out, the world's poultry breeding is in the hands of a very small number of large companies.

In Australia, and to a greater degree, Japan, there are a few independent breeders and hatcheries, but both countries depend on overseas breeders for their parent stock. Japan has a greater proportion of vent sexers working there than most other highly developed poultry-industry nations. Several poultrymen in Japan and America have indicated that there is a hint of a move back to using replacement layer stock which needs to be sexed by specialist chick sexers. This does not apply to the broiler industry, except for primary breeders.

If there was a swing back to using replacement layer pullets which were required to be vent sexed by specialist cloacal sexers a large and reliable supply of specialist sexers would be needed.

Consider chick sexing from the hatcheryman's position. If all pullet replacement chicks had to be sexed by the specialist chick sexer, as in the past, it would require at least three times the number of cloacal chick sexers the industry now employs. It is also generally accepted that since the mid-1940s there have been at least two occasions when there was a world shortage of specialist chick sexers.

I do not see a saving in the cost of sexing as the reason for using genetic sexing as opposed to vent sexing, as an issue, but rather who pays the cost of sexing: the breeder/hatcheryman, or the egg producer; and whether the costs are hidden or shown.

Most producers of layer replacement chicks would acknowledge that it is not the cost of employing the specialist chick sexers, but rather, I would suggest, the availability of fast, accurate chick sexers when and where they are required. Many present vent sexers are almost as fast as feather-sex operators. Colour sexing has the possibilities of being performed almost automatically if current trials are successful.

Chick sexers need to look at their occupation from a world perspective and be prepared to work at different localities at short notice if they are to be fully employed for most of the year. This is already happening, particularly with Japanese and Korean chick sexers, and to a lesser degree with English and Mexican chick sexers.

A world organisation of commercial chick sexers and classes is a future possibility. It need not interfere with the present independence of chick sexers from each country, and the various chick-sexing schools. This would add further to the professionalism and skill and ensure that there are always sufficient commercial chick sexers to meet the needs of the industry anywhere in the world.

The Japanese have shown what can be done with friendly cooperation between their own sexers, and yet they compete against one another and in teams at their annual chick-sexing competitions each year. The demand regulates the supply of chick sexers, but occasionally, for various reasons, there is suddenly a shortage. The breeders have found their solution to this sudden shortage but whether this solution remains viable is to be seen. The industry of course does not need any militant chick sexers.

There are some hatcheries in Europe which engage their specialist chick sexers to do their feather sexing, rather than employing supplementary staff on hatching days, but most have their feather sexing done by their own people.

In Australia, when feather sexing was first introduced, many hatcheries did use their chick sexers to do feather sexing as well, but with the rapid demise of vent sexers hatchery staff took this over.

When I asked the head of Hobo Chick Sexing, Takashi Hobo, what he saw as the future prospects for the chick sexers, he said he found it difficult to forecast.

He did think that sexing of commercial layer chicks would decline, because of colour and feather sexing. As he pointed out, the market share of brown chicks (colour sexing) is increasing.

He did say, however, that the cloaca sexing of broiler PS (primary parent stock) and GPS (grand primary parent stock) was increasing, because of the demand for feather-sexable commercial broilers. This increase in broiler PS is worldwide.

In most countries, almost all turkeys are sexed—a big plus for sexers.

But as Takashi Hobo and others have stressed, cloaca chick sexing will always be needed as both colour and feather sexing features last for only one generation.

There is no doubt that the aim of the geneticists working for the large breeding companies will continue to concentrate on breeding stock which can be colour or feather sexed. The German industry is even experimenting with using video equipment to do their colour sexing automatically.

Writing as a historian, rather than as a former specialist chick sexer, I have a historian's bias of looking at the past in order to see what may happen in the future. Historians try to avoid attempting to judge future trends by depending on what is the position at the moment. Anyone with a long involvement with the poultry industry would know the previous history of autosexing and feather-sexed strains and their lack of performance when measured against breeds where fewer things have to be considered when working towards breeding goals. For every gain in one area something has to be given up in another area.

Today's geneticists have a great deal more resources than poultry breeders of the past, but in the final analysis the geneticist breeding rules have not changed. Eventually many of their results will be the same as those of the less sophisticated poultry breeders of the past.

An executive of one of the world's largest poultry breeding companies, when asked to comment on the "future prospects" of the specialist chick sexer (as did Takashi Hobo) found it a difficult question to answer.

Stressing that these were personal views and that they may not reflect those of the company he said: "I believe that as long as primary breeding of chickens continues, then there will be limited opportunities for chicken sexers within those major organisations." And, "I believe that exceptionally accurate chick sexers will attract premium payments."

The executive director of the Zen-Nippon Chick Sexing Association, Hitoshi Miyata, was far more optimistic when asked the same question. As he said in this book's foreword, "It is more than 70 years or so since the vent-chick-sexing technique was developed in Japan. During this period, there was a time when dependence was placed on the so called sex-linkage applied autosexing, such as feather sexing and colour sexing, owing to a temporary shortage of vent sexers throughout the world. However, vent-sexed chickens have shown much better performance in egg productivity, cost effectiveness, and so on. We are optimistic about the future of commercial vent chick sexers throughout the world."

Whatever direction the pullet-replacement industry adopts in their future breeding programs, no-one would argue that there remains a need for many specialist chick sexers, far into the future.

Whether the future will go in the direction that Hitoshi Miyata and others believe, or continue the way Bill Stanhope's article suggests, specialist chick-sexing will remain a worthwhile occupation well into the next century.

Epilogue

This book is about men and women who made their livelihood from separating pullets from cockerels. It could just as easily have been about any other occupation and the methods used over time to solve a particular problem in a particular industry.

A new method comes along. It is used for a while, then bigger gains can be seen by again using past methods for new problems: using old techniques, but being better at them; the efficiencies of the new method being adapted as the standard for the former technique.

If this book has fallen short of some of its aims, the faults are mine alone. Whenever I asked for information, anywhere in the world, the men and women freely gave it and their time, photos, documents and stories.

While I, no doubt, have learnt something extra about chick sexing, I was also reminded that man's abilities are limited only by his thinking.

R.D.M.

Addresses

In alphabetical order

Amchick
220 South Line St.,
P.O. Box 905
Lonsdale, PA 19446
Tel: 215/855 5156
Fax: 215/362 0981

Chick Sexing Specialists (G.B.)
Marandellas, Pheasant Lane,
Maidstone,
Kent ME15 9QR UK
Tel: 0622 743561
Fax: 0622 69 1350

Association of British Chick Sexers
Secretary:
54 Mercia Avenue
Charlton, Nr Andover,
Hamshire SP10 4EJ
Tel: 0264 337160

Hobo Chick Sexing
b.v.b.a. pb 27 Wortegemseweg 51
B 8790 Waregem
Belgium
Tel: 056 60 52 41
Fax: 85 856

Korea Chick Sexer Services Association
RM 402 87 2 GA, Seongsoo
Dong Seongdong-Gu
Seoul.
Korea
Tel: 82 02 499 9951 -2
Fax: 82 2 533 5932

Mrs Hah's Sexing Service
4th Fl. Choryang Bldg.
172–3 Choryang 3 Dong. Dong
Ku, Pusan
South Korea
Tel: 051 462 2606
Fax: 051 464 4995

Zen-Nippon Chick Sexing Association
No 2 1-Chome,
Kanda-Surugadai
Chiyoda-Ku,
Tokyo
Tel: 03 3291 9826
Fax: 03 3291 9827

Index

This index is arranged alphabetically, word for word. **Bold** entries are the ones with the most information. *Italic* entries are illustrations.